Repr‹
Endo
and I
Handbook for Clinicians

Dan I. Lebovic, M.D., M.A.
Assistant Professor, Reproductive
Endocrinology and Infertility
Department of Obstetrics and Gynecology
University of Michigan
Ann Arbor, MI

John David Gordon, M.D.
Co-Director
Dominion Fertility
Arlington, VA

Associate Clinical Professor
Department of Obstetrics and Gynecology
The George Washington University
Washington, DC

Robert N. Taylor, M.D., Ph.D.
Professor and Vice Chair for Research
Department of Gynecology and Obstetrics
Emory University
Atlanta, GA

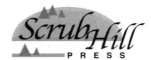

ISBN 0-9645467-0-1 (pocket edition)
ISBN 0-9645467-9-5 (desk edition)

Library of Congress Cataloging-in-Publication Data

Lebovic, Dan I.
  Reproductive endocrinology and infertility : handbook for clinicians / Dan I. Lebovic,
John D. Gordon, Robert N. Taylor.
       p. ; cm.
  Includes bibliographical references and index.
  ISBN 0-9645467-0-1
  1. Endocrine gynecology--Handbooks, manuals, etc. 2. Infertility, Female--Endocrine
aspects--Handbooks, manuals, etc. 3.   Human reproduction--Endocrine aspects--
Handbooks, manuals, etc.
  [DNLM: 1. Endocrine System Diseases--Handbooks. 2. Genital Diseases, Female--
Handbooks. 3. Infertility--Handbooks. 4. Reproduction--Handbooks. WP 39 L449r
2005] I. Gordon, John D. (John David) II. Taylor, Robert N., 1953- III. Title.
  RG159.L43 2005
  618.1--dc22

                                                                    2005004415

The opinions expressed in this book represent a broad range of opinions of the authors.
These opinions are not meant to represent a "standard of care" or a "protocol" but rather
a guide to common clinical conditions. Use of these guidelines is obviously influenced by
local factors, varying clinical circumstances, and honest differences of opinion.

The indications and dosages of all drugs in this book have been recommended in the medical literature and conform to all the practices of the general medical community. The medications described do not necessarily have specific approval by the Food and Drug
Administration for use in the diseases and dosages for which they are recommended. The
package insert for each drug should be consulted for use and dosage as approved by the
FDA. Because standards for usage change, it is advisable to keep abreast of revised recommendations, particularly those concerning new drugs.

Publisher: Scrub Hill Press, Inc.
Editorial Production: Silverchair Science + Communications
Cover Design: Silverchair Science + Communications and Christopher Carbone

Editorial offices:
Scrub Hill Press, Inc.
46 S. Glebe Road #301
Arlington, VA 22204
e-mail: johndavidgordon@erols.com
www.scrubhillpress.com
*Member of the American Medical
Publishers Association*

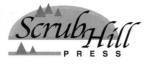

Inspiration for this book promoting "life" comes from the lives of four special people. From my maternal grandparents, I learned the value and honor of a life well-lived. From my paternal grandparents, who perished in the Holocaust, I strive to honor their memory by dedicating my life to the proliferation of life.

D.I.L.

Two percent of the profits from the sale of this book will be donated to the Daniel Pearl Foundation (http://www.danielpearl.org).

Contents

CONTENTS

Contributing Authors and Editors

Rajani Aatre-Keshavamurthy, M.Sc., M.S.
Genetic Counselor, Obstetrics and Gynecology
University of Michigan
Ann Arbor, MI
Chapter 32, Genetic Testing

Arnold P. Advincula, M.D.
Director of Minimally Invasive Surgery
Clinical Assistant Professor, Obstetrics and Gynecology
University of Michigan
Ann Arbor, MI
Chapter 15, Chronic Pelvic Pain

Pavna Kartha Brahma, M.D.
Resident, Obstetrics and Gynecology
University of Michigan
Ann Arbor, MI
Chapter 8, Abnormal Uterine Bleeding

Colleen L. Casey, M.D.
Fellow, Reproductive Endocrinology and Infertility
University of Vermont
Burlington, VT
Chapter 28, Hypothyroidism

Vanessa K. Dalton, M.D., M.P.H.
Lecturer, Obstetrics and Gynecology
University of Michigan
Ann Arbor, MI
Chapter 30, Management of Early Pregnancy Failure

Aimee D. Eyvazzadeh, M.D.
Fellow, Reproductive Endocrinology and Infertility
University of Michigan
Ann Arbor, MI
Chapter 20, Male Subfertility

CONTRIBUTING AUTHORS AND EDITORS

Senait Fisseha, M.D., J.D.
Fellow, Reproductive Endocrinology and Infertility
University of Michigan
Ann Arbor, MI
Chapter 35, Postmenopausal Osteoporosis

L. April Gago, M.D.
Clinical Assistant Professor, Reproductive Endocrinology and Infertility
University of Michigan
Ann Arbor, MI
Chapter 6, Turner Syndrome

Shahryar K. Kavoussi, M.D., M.P.H.
Fellow, Reproductive Endocrinology and Infertility
University of Michigan
Ann Arbor, MI
Chapter 25, Gamete Preservation

Kristie Keeton, M.D., M.P.H.
Robert Wood Johnson Clinical Scholar
University of Michigan
Ann Arbor, MI
Chapter 2, Puberty
Chapter 27, Hyperprolactinemia and Galactorrhea

Ania Kowalik, M.D.
Assistant Professor, Reproductive Endocrinology and Infertility
University of North Carolina
Chapel Hill, NC
*Chapter 37, Transvaginal Ultrasound in Reproductive
Endocrinology and Infertility*

William R. Meyer, M.D.
Associate Professor, Reproductive Endocrinology and Infertility
University of North Carolina
Chapel Hill, NC
Chapter 11, Exercise-Induced Amenorrhea

Tina Mitchell, M.D.
Practitioner, Obstetrics and Gynecology

CONTRIBUTING AUTHORS AND EDITORS

Women's Health Group of Southeast Georgia
Brunswick, GA
Chapter 9, Oral Contraceptives

Michael D. Mueller, M.D.
Associate Professor, Obstetrics and Gynecology
Director, Endometriosis Center
Frauenklinik Inselspital, University of Berne
Berne, Switzerland
Chapter 12, Ectopic Pregnancy

Liberato V. Mukul, M.D.
Assistant Professor, Obstetrics and Gynecology
University of Colorado Health Sciences Campus
Denver, CO
Chapter 39, Laparoscopy

Ringland S. Murray, M.D.
Clinical Instructor and Fellow, Reproductive Endocrinology
and Infertility
University of North Carolina
Chapel Hill, NC
Chapter 21, Diminished Ovarian Reserve

Maureen Phipps, M.D., M.P.H.
Assistant Professor, Obstetrics and Gynecology and
Community Health
Brown Medical School
Providence, RI
Chapter 40, Journal Club Guide

Elisabeth H. Quint, M.D.
Clinical Associate Professor, Obstetrics and Gynecology
University of Michigan
Ann Arbor, MI
Chapter 3, Pediatric and Adolescent Gynecology

Khurram Rehman, M.D.
Clinical Assistant Professor, Reproductive Endocrinology and Infertility
University of Texas Southwestern

CONTRIBUTING AUTHORS AND EDITORS

Dallas, TX
Chapter 34, Postmenopausal Hormone Therapy

John A. Schnorr, M.D.
Assistant Professor, Reproductive Endocrinology and Infertility
Medical University of South Carolina
Southeastern Fertility Center
Charleston, SC
Chapter 22, Assisted Reproductive Technologies

Danny J. Schust, M.D.
Associate Professor, Obstetrics and Gynecology, Reproductive Biology
Boston Medical Center
Boston, MA
Chapter 26, Luteal Phase Deficiency
Chapter 29, Recurrent Pregnancy Loss

Collin Smikle, M.D.
Reproductive Endocrinology and Infertility
Reproductive Science Center of the San Francisco Bay Area
San Ramon, CA
Chapter 23, Ovarian Hyperstimulation Syndrome

Yolanda R. Smith, M.D., M.S.
Associate Professor, Reproductive Endocrinology and Infertility
University of Michigan
Ann Arbor, MI
Chapter 3, Pediatric and Adolescent Gynecology

Arleen H. Song, M.D., M.P.H.
Clinical Instructor, Obstetrics and Gynecology
University of Michigan
Ann Arbor, MI
Chapter 17, Fibroids

Tony Tsai, M.D.
Director of Reproductive Endocrinology and Fertility
Laparoscopic and Laser Surgery, Obstetrics and Gynecology
New York Hospital Queens
Assistant Professor, Obstetrics and Gynecology

CONTRIBUTING AUTHORS AND EDITORS

Weill Medical College of Cornell University
New York, NY
Chapter 38, Hysteroscopy

Mary Ellen Wechter, M.D.
Clinical Instructor, Minimally Invasive Surgery
University of North Carolina
Chapel Hill, NC
Chapter 18, Polycystic Ovary Syndrome

Jennifer A. Williams, M.D.
Clinical Assistant Professor, Obstetrics and Gynecology
University of Michigan
Ann Arbor, MI
Chapter 36, Hot Flashes

Foreword

The degrees of complexity and diversity in science are a constant challenge. Most of us are searching for some underlying unity to make this diversity manageable. This minithesaurus of reproductive endocrinology and infertility (REI) is a remarkable, sod-busting achievement because it assumes that REI has an order that can be deciphered. Attempts to synthesize that order involve an enormous labor of sifting, combining, constructing, expunging, and correcting texts to achieve a final product. The authors have put a novel perspective on a mountain of facts, eliminated the spam, and provided the reader with an easier path to drawing knowledge from information.

Reproductive Endocrinology and Infertility: Handbook for Clinicians by Dan Lebovic and colleagues may be viewed by some as a survival guide to the overly challenged student of the specialty. However, more careful reading makes it clear that the text provides a fact-oriented outline that enables the reader to grasp a sense of the breadth and depth of the specialty. Putting facts and ideas together, the editors have created an anchoring scaffold to build a relevant knowledge base and to stimulate the student to look beyond the facts for their significance. In the future, *Reproductive Endocrinology and Infertility: Handbook for Clinicians* may be easily collapsed into an online starting point for the convenience of searchable archives and links to other resources. I am certain that the editors will continue to refine and evolve these modifications as new and alternative means of communication emerge. These modifications are important because teaching manuals are ultimately designed to be on hand, whereas scientific knowledge is provisional and changing.

Paul McDonough, M.D.
Professor Emeritus
Medical College of Georgia
Augusta, GA

Preface

Although there are several excellent texts devoted to reproductive endocrinology and infertility (REI), the present handbook was born out of a desire to provide a ready resource for clinicians to access the most important facts and figures. To accomplish this goal, the authors searched through textbooks, original articles, and erudite colleagues' brains for answers to specific queries. The *Reproductive Endocrinology and Infertility: Handbook for Clinicians* strives to be a literary Occam's razor: "Among competing hypotheses, favor the simplest one," or, in this case, an amalgam of REI information distilled into a handbook.

Scientific knowledge is constantly evolving, and REI is not immune to this phenomenon; this *Handbook* is simply a snapshot in time. The editors and authors have relied on evidence-based resources rather than tradition or dogma, and references are provided along with many original or adapted figures. Opinions from experienced clinicians were obtained when rigorous trials were not available. The value of this *Handbook* will depend on how often the pages are turned during training or practice. With time, the images and tables may become ingrained for easier recall. Despite strong efforts from the many contributors, this *Handbook* should not be considered a stand-alone resource, but a stepping stone to the words of Lee C. Bollinger: "You have to be willing to embarrass yourself in order to learn." Learning is not a spectator sport.

Apart from the generous contributors who offered their time to make this a better piece of work, I owe much to my teachers and colleagues and would like to acknowledge them by chronological order:

- Under the shade of the Campanile, through the arches of Sather Gate, and along Strawberry Canyon at **UC Berkeley:** Dr. Russ Baldocchi, Dr. Howard Bern, Dr. Julian Boyd, Dr. Marion Diamond, Dr. Satyabrata Nandi, Dr. Karl Nicoll, and Dr. Sharon Russell.
- Amidst Foggy Bottom at **George Washington University Medical School:** Dr. Frank Allen, Dr. Isaac Ben-Or, Dr. David Levy, and Dr. Frank Slaby.
- As a surgical intern in "Live Free or Die" **Dartmouth-Hitchcock Medical Center:** Dr. Thomas Collachio and Dr. Robert Crichlow, Dr. Wendy Dean, Dr. Horace Enriques, and Dr. Paul Manganiello.
- Beside the Blue Ridge Mountains at the **University of Virginia:** Dr. Willie Andersen, Dr. John Bourgeois, Dr. Guy Harbert, Dr. James Kitchin, Dr. Lisa Kolp, Dr. Elizabeth Mandell, Dr. Howard Montgomery, Dr. Laurel Rice, Dr. Peyton Taylor, and, Dr. Paul Underwood.
- In the fog of **UC San Francisco:** Dr. Joe Conaghan, Dr. Seth Feigenbaum, Dr. Simon Henderson, Dr. Robert Jaffe, Dr. John Kim, and Dr. Sae Sohn.

PREFACE

- Presently, beside the Big House at the **University of Michigan:** Dr. Rudi Ansbacher, Dr. Greg Christman, Dr. Steven Domino, Dr. Tim Johnson, Dr. Dana Ohl, Dr. John Randolph, Jr., Dr. Tim Schuster, and Dr. Gary Smith.

Many thanks to Kate Sallwasser at Silverchair Science + Communications for her impeccable attention to detail and style. And I thank my coeditors, Dr. John Gordon for his editing talents and allowing this project to reach prime time, and my mentor from fellowship days, Dr. Rob Taylor, who continues to inspire, entertain, and comfort me beyond any imaginable call of duty.

Finally, I would like to acknowledge the loving support of my brother Stan and my parents, Alex and Ida Lebovic.

Dan Israel Lebovic, M.D., M.A.

1. Sexual Differentiation: From Gonad to Phallus

EMBRYOLOGY

- Bipotential: gonads and external genitalia (urogenital sinus; two labioscrotal swellings; genital tubercle)
- Unipotential: internal genitalia (wolffian and müllerian ducts)

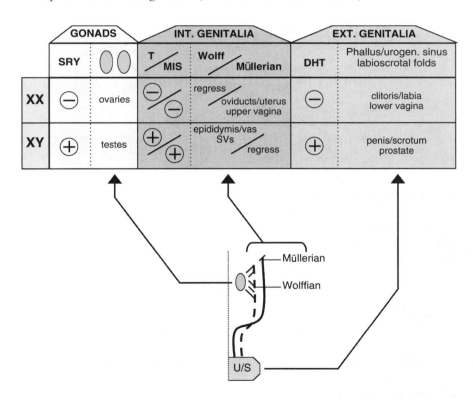

SEXUAL DIFFERENTIATION

Gonads
- Formation of a testis occurs in the presence of the Y chromosome (46,XY).
- Formation of an ovary occurs in the absence of the Y chromosome and the presence of a 2nd X chromosome (46,XX).
- Gonads begin development during wk 5–6 of gestation.

Testicular Determinants
- Sex-determining region of Y (*SRY*) is the gene involved in testis determination (short arm [p] of Y chromosome) (Page et al., 1985; Tilford et al., 2001).

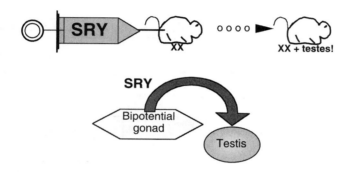

Ovarian Determinants
- Unless *SRY* is expressed, ovarian development ensues (assuming XX is present).
- **2nd X chromosome** required for ovarian maintenance.
- **Autosomal genes** (see diagram on three facets of sexual differentiation).

Internal Genitalia
- Wolffian ducts (dependent on testosterone [T] from testes) → epididymis/vas deferens/seminal vesicles (internal genitalia)
- MIS = müllerian inhibiting substance, produced by Sertoli cells (may act as an antitumor agent)
- Müllerian ducts (in absence of MIS) → fallopian tubes/uterus/upper vagina (internal genitalia)
- Müllerian and wolffian development begins simultaneously; they are local phenomena (i.e., they occur *ipsi*laterally depending on presence of T/MIS).

External Genitalia
- Female external genitalia develop in absence of DHT (dihydrotestosterone).
- DHT is produced in sufficient amounts from gestational wks 7–8 until birth.
- Human chorionic gonadotropin (hCG) stimulates Leydig cells → ↑ T

SEXUAL DIFFERENTIATION

- Feminization of external genitalia completed by approximately 14 wks.
- Masculinization of external genitalia completed by approximately 16 wks.
- T, insulin-like 3 ligand, and its receptor (Lgr8) mediate descent of testes.

THREE FACETS OF SEXUAL DIFFERENTIATION
1. Gonadal differentiation
2. Genital differentiation
3. Behavioral differentiation
   - Sexual or gender identity:
     - Sense of oneself as male or female
     - Established by age 2 1/2
     - Derived through internalization of social cues based on the external genitalia
       ⇨ Patients with 5α-Reductase (5αR) deficiency or 17β-hydroxysteroid dehydrogenase (17βHSD) deficiency may change from female to male gender identity at puberty, however; therefore, there is a *hormonal role* in sexualization of brain.
   - Sexuality:
     - Libido driven by T
     - Intimacy driven by estradiol

SEXUAL DIFFERENTIATION

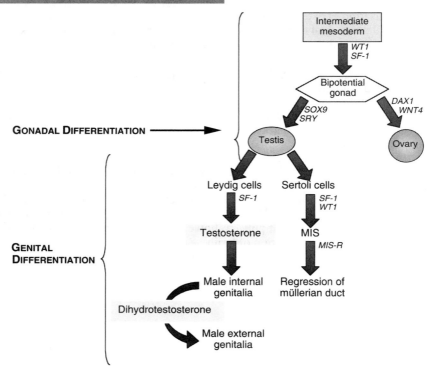

Factors involved in the determination of male sex. HOX, homeobox transcription factor; MIS, müllerian inhibiting substance gene; MIS-R, MIS-receptor; SF-1, steroidogenic factor 1; SOX9, SR homeobox gene (on autosomes); SRY, sex-determining region of the Y chromosome, in Y chromosome, "testis-determining factor"; WT1, Wilms' tumor 1. (Source: Adapted from Federman DD. Three facets of sexual differentiation. *N Engl J Med* 350[4]:323, 2004.)

SEXUAL DIFFERENTIATION TIMELINE

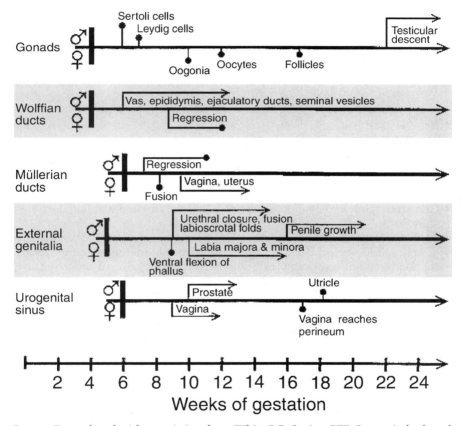

Source: Reproduced with permission from White PC, Speiser PW. Congenital adrenal hyperplasia due to 21-hydroxylase deficiency. *Endocr Rev* 21:245, 2000.

SEXUAL DIFFERENTIATION

SEXUAL DIFFERENTIATION GONE AWRY
46,XX: Masculinized Female
• Abnormal sexual differentiation in 46,XX:

	Site of Defect
Congenital adrenal hyperplasia	21-Hydroxylase (*CYP21*) deficiency
	11β-Hydroxylase (*CYP11β1*) deficiency
	3β-Hydroxysteroid dehydrogenase
	(*3βHSDII*) deficiency
Maternal androgen excess	Virilizing adrenal or ovarian tumor
46,XX gonadal dysgenesis	
46,XX true hermaphroditism	

Source: Adapted from Migeon CJ, Wisniewski AB. Human sex differentiation and its abnormalities. *Best Pract Res Clin Obstet Gynaecol* 17(1):1, 2003.

Congenital Adrenal Hyperplasia
• Gonads develop into ovaries; müllerian ducts present; and wolffian ducts regress
• *21-hydroxylase (CYP21)* deficiency: 90% of congenital adrenal hyperplasia [CAH]; salt-losing form of CAH from diminished aldosterone secretion; most common cause of sexual ambiguity and most common cause of endocrine neonatal death; autosomal recessive, chromosome 6p
• *11β-hydroxylase (CYP11β1)* deficiency: 5% of CAH cases; hypertensive form of CAH from excess corticosterone and 11-deoxycorticosterone secretion
• *3β-hydroxysteroid dehydrogenase (3βHSDII)* deficiency: least frequent form of CAH; salt-losing form of CAH
• Mechanism of abnormal sexual differentiation: ↓ Cortisol → ↑ adrenocorticotropic hormone (ACTH) → ↑ adrenal androgens → virilization of external genitalia (fusion of labioscrotal folds, clitoral enlargement), normal ovaries and müllerian ducts
• Only the external genitalia are affected, because internal genitalia differentiation is completed by the 10th wk, whereas the adrenal cortex does not begin functioning until the 12th wk.

SEXUAL DIFFERENTIATION

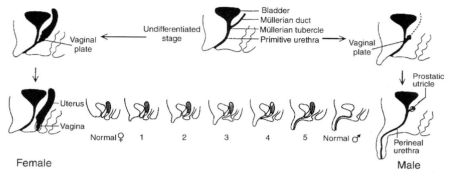

Female

Male

Normal and abnormal differentiation of the urogenital sinus and external genitalia (cross-sectional view). Diagrams of normal female and male anatomy flank a series of schematics of different degrees of virilization of females, graded using the scale developed by Prader (Prader, 1954). Note: The uterus persists in virilized females despite the external genitalia having a completely masculine appearance (Prader grade 5). (Source: Reproduced with permission from White PC, Speiser PW. Congenital adrenal hyperplasia due to 21-hydroxylase deficiency. *Endocr Rev* 21[3]: 245, 2000.)

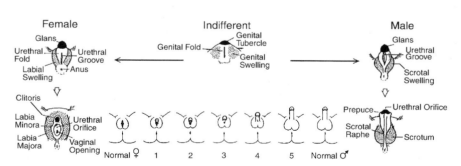

Normal and abnormal differentiation of the external genitalia (external view). (Source: Reproduced with permission from White PC, Speiser PW. Congenital adrenal hyperplasia due to 21-hydroxylase deficiency. *Endocr Rev* 21[3]:245, 2000.)

SEXUAL DIFFERENTIATION

- Untreated CAH:
  - Pubic hair by age 2–4, then axillary hair → body hair/beard
  - Premature epiphyseal closure
  - Male habitus
  - Acne; deep voice; primary amenorrhea and infertility

Maternal Androgen Excess

- Maternal ingestion of androgenic substances
  - Placenta is unable to aromatize synthetic androgens into estrogens.
- Androgen-producing neoplasia
  - Placenta is able to aromatize T into estrogens, therefore protecting the female fetus from masculinization.
  - Luteomas secrete DHT, and the placenta is unable to aromatize this, so there is masculinization of female fetus.
  - Treatment: surgical correction of abnormal external genitalia

46,XX: True Hermaphroditism

- Possess both testicular tubules and ovarian follicles (either separately or together as an **ovotestis**)
- 46,XX is the most common karyotype, although 46,XY and mosaic 45,XO/46,XY chromosome complements also are associated with true hermaphroditism.
- Etiology: difficult to explain
- Internal genitalia depending on gonad of that side
- External genitalia masculinize to varying degrees *in utero*, depending on the amount of T secreted by the testicular portions of the gonads.

46,XX: Gonadal Dysgenesis

- Present as female but fail to achieve female puberty
- Elevated gonadotropins and streak gonads similar to 45,XO
- Differs from 45,XO given absence of multiple congenital malformations

SEXUAL DIFFERENTIATION

46,XY: Undermasculinized Male

- Abnormal sexual differentiation in 46,XY:

	Site of Defect
Complete/partial gonadal dysgenesis	SRY, SF-1, SOX9, DMRTI/DMRT2, DAX-1, WnT4
Androgen insensitivity syndrome: Complete Partial	Androgen receptor (AR)
5α-Reductase deficiency	5α-reductase-2
Leydig cell hypoplasia (Sertoli cell only syndrome)	Genes for LHRH, GnRH receptor, LH, LH receptor
Abnormalities of Leydig cell function	StAR, CYP11A, 3βHSDII, CYP17, 17βHSDIII
Isolated persistence of müllerian ducts	MIS or MIS receptors I and II
46,XY true hermaphroditism	SRY
Maternal ingestion of estrogens and progestins	

GnRH, gonadotropin-releasing hormone; LH, luteinizing hormone; MIS, müllerian inhibiting substance.
Source: Adapted from Migeon CJ, Wisniewski AB. Human sex differentiation and its abnormalities. *Best Pract Res Clin Obstet Gynaecol* 17(1):1, 2003.

Gonadal Dysgenesis: Complete and Partial Deficiency

- Mutation of several transcription factors (see table above) can block the differentiation of a bipotential gonad into a testis and can result in either complete gonadal dysgenesis (Swyer syndrome, *SRY* deletion) or in partial gonadal dysgenesis.
  - Note: Must make sure there is a müllerian system present (i.e., cervix and uterus)! Otherwise, Swyer syndrome patients could instead be XY with an inactivating mutation in the luteinizing hormone (LH) receptor (also known as Leydig cell hypoplasia). If the patient is actually the latter, the gonads need to be removed but will most likely benefit from the help of Urology, as these cases can be difficult.
- Ramifications of diminished Leydig cell and Sertoli cell development:
  - Complete: no T, therefore, female external genitalia and persistence of müllerian ducts due to absence of Sertoli cell MIS
  - Partial: partial masculinization of external genitalia and partial development of wolffian ducts on account of diminished testicular androgens and MIS

Androgen Insensitivity Syndrome
Complete Androgen Insensitivity Syndrome
- X-linked recessive mutation of the AR gene located on chromosome Xq near the centromere

9

SEXUAL DIFFERENTIATION

- Incidence: 1 in 60,000
- Bilateral testes located in the abdomen or inguinal area; female external genitalia with blind-ending vagina; because there are normal amounts of MIS, there is no müllerian duct development, as well as no wolffian duct development from lack of T responsiveness; absence of pubic or axillary hair
- **Gonadectomy after pubertal feminization** (>18 yrs old) to allow for female secondary sexual characteristics

Partial Androgen Insensitivity Syndrome (Reifenstein's Syndrome)

- Ambiguous external genitalia with phallic development; normal T and DHT levels and elevated LH concentrations
- Partial virilization at puberty with female-typical breasts
- **Orchiectomy for partial androgen insensitivity syndrome (PAIS) should be done before puberty** but after breast development to prevent virilization
- Note: 17-Ketosteroid reductase deficiency can closely mimic the clinical picture of androgen insensitivity syndrome (AIS), although AIS patients have normal serum androgens.

5α-Reductase Deficiency

- $5\alpha R$ (*5α-reductase-2*) deficiency = *huevos a los doce* ("eggs at twelve"; in this case, the "eggs" are actually testes)
- Autosomal recessive, chromosome 2p
- ↓ Conversion of T into DHT (more potent androgen) leading to undermasculinization of the external genitalia during fetal development, whereas the wolffian ducts develop normally (T dependent)
- Puberty → ↑ 5αR-2 that leads to sufficient DHT and pubertal virilization (growth of the phallus, ↑ muscle mass, and deepening of the voice)
- Pseudovagina
- Erections + ejaculations from perineal urethra with normal sperm in adulthood

Leydig Cell Hypoplasia

- Sertoli cell–only syndrome
- Mutation in genes for gonadotropin-releasing hormone (GnRH), GnRH receptor, LH, LH receptor

Abnormalities of Leydig Cell Function

- Mutation in enzymes needed for the biosynthesis of T in Leydig cells (see table)
  - ↓ **Steroidogenic acute regulatory protein (StAR) or CYP11A** → no gonadal or adrenal steroids = *lipoid adrenal hyperplasia*
    - ⇨ Female external genitalia
    - ⇨ ↓ Adrenal steroids → adrenal crises at birth

SEXUAL DIFFERENTIATION

- ↓ 3βHSDII → inability to metabolize Δ5 steroids (pregnenolone, 17-hydroxypregnenolone, dehydroepiandrosterone) into Δ4 steroids (progesterone, 17-hydroxyprogesterone [17-OHP], androstenedione)
  ⇨ Usually, other genes can compensate for the 3βHSDII enzyme outside of the gonads and adrenals, so female fetuses are slightly masculinized and male fetuses are markedly undermasculinized at birth.
  ⇨ Salt-wasting due to ↓ cortisol and aldosterone
  ⇨ Also covered in the section on CAH.
- ↓ CYP17 → deficient 19-carbon steroids (androgens), 18-carbon steroids (estrogens), and cortisol
  ⇨ Adrenal crisis at birth
  ⇨ Female external genitalia in a 46,XY subject
  ⇨ Note: Isolated 17,20 desmolase deficiency only compromises androgen and estrogen secretion, so that 46,XY individuals present with female-appearing genitalia but no adrenal abnormality (preserved aldosterone and cortisol formation)
- ↓ 17βHSDIII → inability to convert androstenedione into T
  ⇨ Lack of androgenic effects during fetal development
  ⇨ Usually present with partial enzyme abnormality and resulting ambiguous genitalia at birth
  ⇨ Marked pubertal masculinization if testes not removed, because several 17βHSD genes are more active at puberty than during fetal life.

Isolated Persistence of Müllerian Ducts: Hernia Uteri Inguinale
- Detected at the time of hernia repair (remnants of a uterus and fallopian tubes are found in the hernia sac)
- May be due to a mutation of *MIS* or MIS receptors
- Normal testes function and masculinized external genitalia

46,XY: True Hermaphroditism
- Possess well-defined seminiferous tubules and ovarian follicles (resulting in **ovotestis** formation)
- Wolffian duct development and degree of masculinization depend on the extent of testicular Leydig cell function.
- Müllerian duct development also depends on the level of Sertoli cell MIS production.

SEXUAL DIFFERENTIATION

Abnormal Sex Chromosome Complement

- See also Chapter 6, Turner Syndrome, and Chapter 32, Genetic Testing.
- Abnormal sexual differentiation (external genitalia) associated with unusual sex chromosome complement:

Female
- 45,X (Turner syndrome) and variants
- 47,XXX ("super female")
- 46,XY$_{p-}$ or 46,Xi(Y$_9$)
- 45,X/46,XY

Ambiguous
- 46,XX/46,XY
- Triploidy 69,XXY/69,XYY

Male
- 47,XXY (Klinefelter's syndrome)
- 47,XYY
- 46,XX males

Source: Adapted from Migeon CJ, Wisniewski AB. Human sex differentiation and its abnormalities. *Best Pract Res Clin Obstet Gynaecol* 17(1):1, 2003.

45,X: Turner Syndrome

- Absence of oocytes (streak gonads) is secondary to increased oocyte atresia, not failure of germ cell formation; normal müllerian duct system (lack of MIS) and small female external genitalia
- Incidence: 1 in 5000 live births
- Etiology: paternal or maternal meiotic nondysjunction; curiously, 80% of liveborn 45,X individuals have lost a *paternal* sex chromosome.
- Approximately 1/2 of these patients have a 45,X karyotype, with the remaining individuals having a variant of this karyotype (i.e., 46,XX with variable deletions of the long or short arm of an X chromosome).
- Failure of secondary sexual development
- $\downarrow$ Estrogen and androgen; $\uparrow$ follicle-stimulating hormone (FSH) and LH
- $\uparrow$ Relative risk for diabetes, thyroid disease, and essential hypertension
- Turner stigmata: growth failure, epicanthal folks, high arched palate, low nuchal hair line, webbed neck, shield-like chest, coarctation of aorta, ventriculoseptal defect, renal anomalies, pigmented nevi, lymphedema, hypoplastic nails, ptosis of the upper eyelid, cubitus valgus, inverted and widely spaced nipples, autoimmune diseases, hypertension, etc. (see Chapter 6, Turner Syndrome)

SEXUAL DIFFERENTIATION

46,XY$_{p-}$ or 46,Xi(Y$_q$)

- *SRY* gene is located at the tip of the short arm (p) of the Y chromosome; with its deletion, there is complete gonadal dysgenesis with female external genitalia, müllerian duct development, and no wolffian duct

47,XXY: Seminiferous Tubule Dysgenesis (Klinefelter's Syndrome)

- 47,XXY or 46,XY/47,XXY or 46XnY
- Androgen deficiency
- Fertilization possible using testicular aspirated sperm and intracytoplasmic sperm injection (Ron-El et al., 2000)

Other Anomalies of the Female Genitalia

Imperforate Hymen

- Results in hydrocolpos/hydrometrocolpos
- Treatment: cruciform surgical incision (Note: do not drain with needle only)

Transverse Vaginal Septa

- Incidence: 1 in 80,000 women
- Usually at junction of upper $\frac{1}{3}$ and lower $\frac{2}{3}$ of vagina
- Hydrocolpos/hydrometrocolpos
- Treatment: resection of septa with mucosal reanastomosis

Longitudinal Vaginal Septa

- Frequency: 0.2–0.5/1000 live births
- Treatment: surgical transection

Vaginal Atresia

- Failure of urogenital sinus to form distal vagina
- Treatment: surgery if there is a cervix, uterus, and fallopian tubes; otherwise, hysterectomy necessary

Müllerian Agenesis or Hypoplasia

- No uterine corpus/cervix, upper vagina
- Treatment: surgical or nonsurgical with vaginal dilators

Incomplete Müllerian Fusion

- Unicornuate, bicornuate, didelphic, septate uteri
- The high number of ectopic pregnancies in both rudimentary horn and tube warrants the removal (laparoscopy) of the rudimentary horn and its tube when diagnosed (Heinonen, 1997); unilateral renal agenesis is associated with such anomalies.

Diethylstilbestrol-Associated Anomalies

- Most common = squamous metaplasia and vaginal adenosis
- Rare = clear cell adenocarcinoma of vagina and cervix

SEXUAL DIFFERENTIATION

- T-shaped endometrial cavity; uterine constrictions; bulbous dilation of lower cervical segment

DIFFERENTIAL

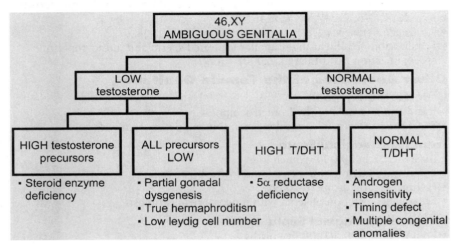

DHT, dihydrotestosterone; T, testosterone. (Source: Adapted from Migeon CJ, Wisniewski AB. Human sex differentiation and its abnormalities. *Best Pract Res Clin Obstet Gynaecol* 17[1]:1, 2003.)

- Laboratory tests
  - **Karyotype** (deletion syndromes; 46,XY; 46,XX/46,XY; 46,XX)
  - Hormone markers of testes:
    ⇨ 3–4 mos of age, T ≥20 ng/dL; MIS ≥10 ng/mL
    ⇨ Later childhood, hCG stimulation test → T ≥20 ng/dL
  - T precursors:
    ⇨ **Androstenedione, 17-OHP, 17-hydroxypregnenolone**
      ❖ CAH can be identified via a.m. **17-OHP:**
        <2 ng/mL → not NCAH (nonclassic adrenal hyperplasia)
        2–4 ng/mL → ACTH testing
        >4 ng/mL → NCAH
  - Abnormally **high T/DHT ratio** in peripheral blood before and/or after hCG administration to rule out 5αR deficiency
  - **SRY gene** detection via fluorescence *in situ* hybridization (FISH) is a reliable way to determine the genetic sex of a child.

- Further genital evaluation:
  - hCG IM × 5 days: looking for androgen enzyme deficiency by evaluating enzyme precursor/product values
  - Short course of T ointment applied to genital tubercle: check for competency of androgen receptors
  - Send genital skin biopsy for androgen receptor studies.
- Blood/fibroblasts for DNA extraction and analysis using gene probes

MANAGEMENT STRATEGIES

- **46,XX:** usually due to CAH
  - Optimize growth and fertility.
    - ⇨ Hydrocortisone (Solu-Cortef) t.i.d. twice the normal secretion rate due to gastric metabolism
    - ⇨ Fludrocortisone (Florinef) (9α-fluroro-cortsol acetate), 0.05–0.15 mg PO q.d.
    - ⇨ Suppress excess androgens.
    - ⇨ Maintain 17-OHP between 500 and 1000 ng/dL and androstenedione at 10–50 ng/dL.
    - ⇨ Monitor plasma rennin activity for control of salt-water retention.
    - ⇨ Dual-energy x-ray absorptiometry (DXA) scan every year
    - ⇨ Monitor growth rate with stadiometer and bone-age measurement.
    - ⇨ Adrenalectomy is a possibility.
    - ⇨ Phallus-reducing surgery should be avoided in infancy, and vaginoplasty should wait until adolescence or older.
- **46,XY**
  - **Female genitalia:** complete lack of masculinization (complete androgen insensitivity syndrome [CAIS], Swyer syndrome, complete T biosynthesis defect)
  - No cosmetic external genitalia surgery except for possible vaginal lengthening
  - Female sex rearing is advised.
  - Estrogen treatment for female sexual characteristics, bone preservation, and menses if uterus present
    - ⇨ Gonadectomy?

Note on gonadal tumors: Gonadal tumors are found in 30% of individuals with XY gonadal dysgenesis and are particularly frequent (55%) in H-Y antigen–positive patients. These are almost always gonadoblastomas or dysgerminomas. Neoplasia occurs in patients with CAIS but rarely in those with PAIS or $5\alpha R$ deficiency. In CAIS, the risk of malignant tumors is small before age 25; after age 25, the risk is approximately 2–5% (Verp and Simpson, 1987).

SEXUAL DIFFERENTIATION

Disorder	Gonads	T Produced?	Puberty?	Gonadectomy before Age 30?
Swyer syndrome	Dysgenesis	No	No	Yes
Luteinizing hormone receptor inactivation mutation	Testes	No	No	Yes
AI	Testes	Yes	Dependent on degree of AI	Yes[a]

AI, androgen insensitivity.

[a]For complete AI, allow for pubertal feminization first. For partial AI, allow for breast development first; gonadal tumors occur late in those with AI.

- **Ambiguous genitalia**
  ⇨ Female sex rearing (with estrogen treatment) is recommended if there is incomplete masculinization and stretched phallus <1.9 cm.
  ⇨ More masculinized infants may be reared as males with T treatment except those with 5αR or 17βHSD deficiency; individuals with 5αR deficiency can be fertile if reared as males.

SUMMARY

	SRY	MIS	T	Gonads	INT	EXT	
XX	—	—	—	♀	♀	♀	
XY	+	+	—	♂	♂	♂	
XO, Turner syndrome	—	—	—	undiff	♀	♀	
Swyer's	—	—	—	dysgen	♀	♀	Gonadectomy
XY-LH-R inact	+	+	—	♂	undiff	♀	Gonadectomy
AI	+	+	+	♂	mild ♂	♀	Gonadectomy after puberty
XY; 5αR def	+	+	+	♂	♂	♀	Huevos a los doce
Müllerian Agen	—	—	—	♀	undiff	♀	♀T levels; no gonadectomy

Agen, agenesis; AI, androgen insensitivity; DHT, dihydrotestosterone; dysgen, dysgenesis; EXT, external; INT, internal; LH-R inact, luteinizing hormone receptor inactivation; MIS, müllerian inhibiting substance; SRY, sex determining region of Y; 5αR def, 5α-reductase deficiency; T, testosterone; undiff, undifferentiated.

2. Puberty

DEFINITION
- Puberty is the process of biologic and physical development through which sexual reproduction first becomes possible.
- Progression:
  - thelarche → adrenarche → peak growth spurt → menarche → ovulation

FACTORS AFFECTING TIME OF ONSET
- Genetics (average interval between menarche in monozygotic twins is 2.2 mos compared with 8.2 mos in dizygotic twins) (McDonough, 1998)
- Race (African-American girls enter puberty 1.0–1.5 yrs before white girls) (Herman-Giddens et al., 1997)
- Nutritional state (earlier with moderate obesity; delayed with malnutrition)
- General health
- Geographic location (urban, closer to the equator, lower altitudes earlier than rural, farther from the equator, higher altitudes)
- Exposure to light (blind earlier than sighted)
- Psychological state
- Several pathologic states influence the timing of puberty either directly or indirectly, contributing to a gaussian distribution (Palmert and Boepple, 2001).

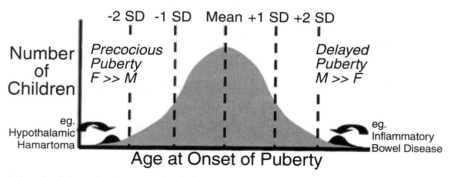

F, female; M, male; SD, standard deviation. (Source: Reproduced with permission from Palmert MR, Boepple PA. Variation in the timing of puberty: clinical spectrum and genetic investigation. *J Clin Endocrinol Metab* 86:2364, 2001.)

PUBERTY

PHYSICAL CHANGES DURING PUBERTY

- Thelarche to menarche requires approximately 2–3 yrs.
  - Accelerated growth
  - Breast budding (thelarche)
  - Pubic and axillary hair growth (pubarche and adrenarche)
  - Peak growth velocity
  - Menarche
  - Ovulation (half the cycles are ovulatory approximately 1–3 yrs after menarche) (McDonough, 1998)
- Adrenarche can precede thelarche.
  - Prevalent in girls of African descent (McDonough, 1998)
- Average age of appearance of pubertal events:

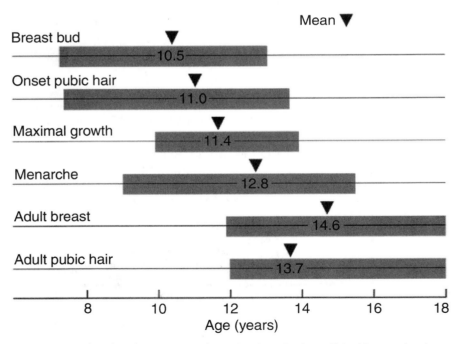

Source: Reproduced with permission from Gordon JD, Speroff L. Abnormal puberty and growth problems. In *Handbook for Clinical Gynecologic Endocrinology & Infertility* (6th ed). Philadelphia: Lippincott–Raven, 2002:199.

- Tanner staging (Marshall and Tanner, 1969)
  - Developed in 1969
  - Based on cohort of 192 British children of low socioeconomic status

Classification	Description
Breast growth	
B1	Prepubertal: elevation of papilla only.
B2	Breast budding.
B3	↑ Breast with glandular tissue, without separation of breast contours.
B4	2nd mound formed by areola.
B5	Single contour of breast and areola.
Pubic hair growth	
PH1	Prepubertal: no pubic hair.
PH2	Labial hair present.
PH3	Labial hair spreads over mons pubis.
PH3	Slight lateral spread.
PH4	Further lateral spread to form inverse triangle and reach medial thighs.

B, breast; PH pubic hair.

PUBERTY

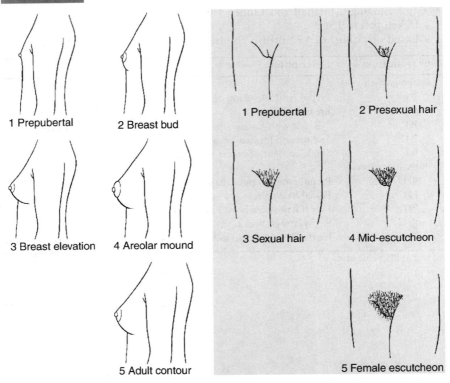

1 Prepubertal   2 Breast bud

3 Breast elevation   4 Areolar mound

5 Adult contour

1 Prepubertal   2 Presexual hair

3 Sexual hair   4 Mid-escutcheon

5 Female escutcheon

Source: Reproduced with permission from Gordon JD, Speroff L. Abnormal puberty and growth problems. In *Handbook for Clinical Gynecologic Endocrinology & Infertility* (6th ed). Philadelphia: Lippincott–Raven, 2002:205.

Pubertal Intervals	Mean ± Standard Deviation (Yrs)
B2 to peak height velocity	1.0 ± 0.8
B2 to menarche	2.3 ± 1.0
B2–PH5	3.1 ± 1.0
B2–B5 (average duration of puberty)	4.5 ± 2.0

B, breast; PH, pubic hair.

MECHANISMS UNDERLYING PUBERTY

- Early in puberty, the sensitivity of the gonadostat to the negative effects of low estradiol (E_2) decreases.
- Late in puberty, maturation of positive E_2 feedback → luteinizing hormone (LH) surge.
- Basal levels of follicle-stimulating hormone (FSH) and LH ↑ throughout puberty due to ↑ gonadotropin-releasing hormone (GnRH) pulse **amplitude** rather than frequency.
- Gonadotropin levels during prenatal and postnatal development (Delemarre-van de Waal, 2002):

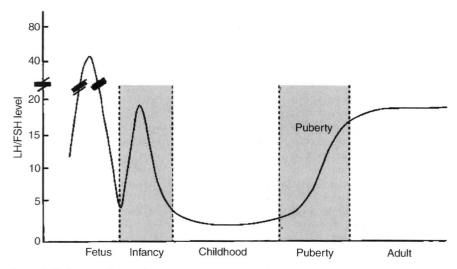

FSH, follicle-stimulating hormone; LH, luteinizing hormone. (Source: Reproduced with permission from Delemarre-van de Waal HA. Regulation of puberty. *Best Pract Res Clin Endocrinol Metab* 16:1, 2002.)

PUBERTY

ABERRATIONS OF PUBERTAL DEVELOPMENT
Delayed or Interrupted Puberty
- Difficult to define due to wide variation in normal development (most girls should enter puberty by 13 yrs; mean age of menarche is 16 yrs).

Eugonadal (Well-estrogenized [26%] [Reindollar et al., 1981])
- Müllerian agenesis or Mayer-Rokitansky-Kuster-Hauser syndrome (14%)
  - Second most common cause of primary amenorrhea after gonadal dysgenesis
  - Amenorrhea aside, pubertal development is normal (ovaries present).
  - 11–50% have skeletal abnormalities (scoliosis, phocomelia, lobster claw).
  - Up to 30% have unilateral renal agenesis or a single pelvic kidney.
  - Diagnosis: normal pubic hair (to differentiate from androgen insensitivity syndrome), ultrasound reveals absence of uterus and presence of ovaries
  - Treatment: counseling, creation of a neovagina (through dilators or surgery), possible assisted reproductive technology with use of a surrogate
  - Karyotype 46,XX
- Vaginal septum (3%)
- Imperforate hymen (0.5%)
- Androgen insensitivity syndrome (1%)
  - Etiology: receptor absence, receptor defect, postreceptor defect
  - Complete: testes, female external genitalia, blind vaginal pouch, no müllerian derivatives
  - Incomplete: above features as well as clitoral enlargement, labioscrotal fusion
  - Diagnosis: absent or significantly reduced pubic hair, male testosterone levels (to differentiate from müllerian agenesis), karyotype
  - Treatment: gonadectomy after breast development, estrogen replacement therapy (ERT)
  - Karyotype 46,XY
- Inappropriate positive feedback (7%): constitutional delay

Hypogonadal Hypoestrogenic (25%)
- Hypergonadotropic hypogonadism (FSH >30 mIU/mL) (13%)
  - Turner syndrome (45,X or mosaic)
    - ⇨ Lymphedema at birth, short stature, webbed neck, nevi and heart/kidney/skeletal/great vessel problems, streak ovaries secondary to oocyte depletion
    - ⇨ Check karyotype, complete physical exam, thyroid function tests (TFTs), glucose, liver function tests, and intravenous pyelogram (IVP) or renal ultrasound.
    - ⇨ Treatment: growth hormone (GH) for height, then estrogen (gradually increase to 2× postmenopausal dose); later, progestins; counseling

- Pure gonadal dysgenesis
  ⇨ 46,XX
    ❖ Idiopathic
    ❖ FSH and LH receptor mutations
    ❖ StAR, CYP17 (congenital adrenal hyperplasia [CAH]), and CYP19 mutations
  ⇨ 46,XY
    ❖ Swyer syndrome: point mutations in sex-related Y (SRY) or deletion of SRY
      No secondary sexual development, normal (or above average) height, normal but infantile female genitalia
    ❖ Wilms' tumor suppressor gene (WT1) mutations
      Hypogonadism, nephropathy, and Wilms' tumor
    ❖ Camptomelic dysplasia (SOX9 gene), SF-1, DAX1, Leydig cell hypoplasia
  ⇨ Treatment: estrogen, gonadectomy if XY (20–30% risk of developing a gonadal tumor)
  ⇨ Must differentiate **Swyer syndrome** (–SRY) from **LH-R mutation,** as the latter involves a more technically challenging surgery because of the lack of landmarks.
- **Hypogonadotropic hypogonadism** (LH and FSH <5 mIU/mL) (12%)
  - Physiologic or constitutional delay is most common, but it is important to exclude other causes.
  - Sustained malnutrition: gastrointestinal (GI) malabsorption, anorexia nervosa, excessive exercise
  - Endocrine disorders: hypothyroidism, Cushing's disease or syndrome, CAH, hyperprolactinemia
  - Hypothalamic-pituitary etiologies
    ⇨ Kallmann syndrome (anosmia, hypogonadism)
      ❖ Absence of GnRH neurons in hypothalamus
      ❖ Treatment: hormonal therapy (oral contraceptives)
      ❖ Fertility treatment: gonadotropins or pulsatile GnRH
    ⇨ Pituitary insufficiency
    ⇨ Pituitary tumors
      ❖ Craniopharyngioma
        Signs: headache, visual changes, growth failure, delayed puberty
        Treatment: surgical, radiation treatment

PUBERTY

Precocious Puberty

- Distribution of diagnoses in 80 girls referred for precocious puberty:

Diagnosis	%
Premature adrenarche	46
Premature thelarche	11
True precocious puberty	11
Early breast development	11
Pubic hair of infancy	6
Premature menses	6
No puberty	6

Source: Adapted from Kaplowitz P. Clinical characteristics of 104 children referred for evaluation of precocious puberty. *J Clin Endocrinol Metab* 89(8):3644, 2004.

- Most patients with Tanner stage 2 breast or pubic hair can be evaluated with only a history, physical exam, and review of the growth chart, without the need for hormonal studies and an estimate of bone age, provided that growth is normal (Kaplowitz, 2004).

Definitions

- Traditional: thelarche before 8 yrs, pubarche before 9 yrs
- New (Kaplowitz and Oberfield, 1999):
  - Pubarche or thelarche before 7 yrs (white girls) or 6 yrs (African-American girls)
  - After ages 7 (white) or 6 (African-American) in conjunction with:
    ⇨ Rapid progression of puberty
    ⇨ Central nervous system (CNS) findings: headache, neurologic symptoms, seizures
    ⇨ Pubertal progression that affects the emotional health of the family or girl

Central or True Precocious Puberty

- Premature stimulation by GnRH (GnRH dependent)
- Idiopathic is the most common.
- CNS tumors, infection, congenital abnormality, trauma, juvenile primary hypothyroidism, Russell-Silver syndrome

Peripheral Precocious Puberty

- GnRH independent
- Peripheral precocious puberty may result in GnRH-dependent precocious puberty if left untreated.

Isosexual Precocious Puberty

- Ovarian cysts

24

- McCune-Albright syndrome
  - ⇨ Gene mutation of the G protein α-subunit (leads to hormone receptor activation in absence of the hormone); toxic multinodular goiter, pituitary gigantism, Cushing's syndrome, polyostotic fibrous dysplasia, café au lait spots
  - ⇨ Treat with testolactone (aromatase inhibitor)
- Neoplasms (adrenal or gonadal); 11% of girls with precocious puberty have an ovarian tumor.
- Exogenous hormones (drugs, food)

Heterosexual Precocious Puberty

- Prepubertal production of androgens with pubarche, adrenarche, and skeletal maturation
- CAH:
  - 21-Hydroxylase deficiency (**virilizing, salt-wasting, nonclassic**)
  - 3β-Hydroxysteroid dehydrogenase (classic, **nonclassic**)
- Exogenous androgen ingestion
- Androgen secreting tumor (i.e., adrenal masculinizing tumor)

Pseudoprecocious Puberty

- Premature thelarche
  - Early isolated breast development
  - Normal bone age
  - Close follow-up to rule out true precocious puberty
- Premature adrenarche
  - Early isolated appearance of pubic or axillary hair (polycystic ovary syndrome [PCOS] precursor?)
  - Commonly seen in African-American girls
  - May be associated with excess androgen secretion secondary to deficiencies in other enzymes

Evaluation

- Check bone age (increase in growth or bone age is more dramatic in girls with central precocious puberty or ovarian disease)
- High basal and GnRH-stimulated serum LH concentration = gonadotropin-dependent precocious puberty

Treatment

- Incomplete precocity:
  - Premature thelarche or adrenarche → reexamine regularly
- GnRH- and gonadotropin-independent precocious puberty:
  - Tumors of adrenal or ovary → surgery
  - McCune-Albright syndrome → testolactone (aromatase inhibitor)

PUBERTY

- Central precocious puberty:
  - GnRH-agonist–induced pituitary-gonadal suppression ± GH when growth is slowed too much:
    - ⇨ Regression of secondary sexual characteristics
    - ⇨ Cessation of menstrual bleeding
  - Slowing of bone growth

3. Pediatric and Adolescent Gynecology

PEDIATRIC GYNECOLOGY
Physical Examination Specifics
- Weight and height → assess appropriate growth
- Breast examination → Tanner staging (see Chapter 2, Puberty, for diagram)
- External genitalia

Examination	Notes
Positioning	Frog-legged, knee-chest position (if girl takes a deep breath may actually see the cervix), mother on examination table with child, or child on mother's lap.
Pubic hair	Tanner staging (see Chapter 2, Puberty, for diagram).
Clitoris	Normal is ~3 mm × 3 mm.
Signs of estrogenization	Mucosal tissues in premenarchal child are thin and red.
Perineum	Look for hygiene.
Type of hymen	Crescent or posterior rim, annular, fimbriated or redundant, imperforate, microperforate, cribriform, septate.
Size of hymen opening	Upper limit of normal is 1 mm for each year of age, although controversy exists on method of measurement; standard → perform in prone knee-chest position with gentle traction on labia.
Vagina	Examine under anesthesia if more visualization of the vagina is needed; this allows for vaginoscopy, cultures, and biopsies as indicated.

- Rectoabdominal palpation:
  - Well tolerated if one needs to rule out a foreign body or a pelvic mass
  - Usually, only a small cervix should be palpable; ovaries should not be palpable.
  - With removal of the finger from the rectum, milk the vagina to see if there is a discharge.

Vulvovaginal Problems
Vulvovaginitis
Reasons for Susceptibility to Vulvovaginitis
- Anatomic (↑ bacterial colonization of the vagina):
  - Lack of protective fat pads and pubic hair
  - Thin vulvar skin

PEDIATRIC AND ADOLESCENT GYNECOLOGY

- Vaginal mucosa: atrophic, neutral pH
- Proximity of the vagina to the anus
- Hygiene:
  - Poor hand-washing
  - Inadequate cleansing of the vulva after voiding or bowel movements
  - Irritants against the vulva (i.e., soaps, bubble baths, sand, dirt)
- Foreign body
- Traumatization by tight clothing, irritating materials
- Sexual abuse

Nonspecific Infection
- ~50% of infections; culture shows normal urogenital flora.

Specific Infection
- Respiratory and enteric pathogens are the most common.

Caveats
- Enteric pathogens (*Shigella* and *Yersinia*) can result in bloody discharges.
- *Candida*: very uncommon prepubertal except after antibiotics, in insulin-dependent diabetes mellitus (IDDM), and in immunocompromised states
- Sexually transmitted diseases (STDs), herpes simplex virus, human papillomavirus (HPV), and *Trichomonas*:
  - Can be transmitted at birth; consider abuse
  - Must culture (not DNA probe) for gonorrhea and chlamydia
- Bacterial vaginosis: usually not associated with discharge but can be associated with abuse or be present in asymptomatic children

Laboratory Tests
- If no discharge and only mild mucus/erythema → try good hygiene instructions
- If persistent discharge → wet prep, Gram's stain, and obtain cultures
- If perianal pruritus → test for pin worms with tape test

Treatment
Specific Vaginitis
- Geared toward the causative organism

Nonspecific Vaginitis
- Initial: discuss hygiene (white cotton underwear, front-to-back wiping, urinating with legs apart), sitz baths, avoid soaps and bubble baths
- Persistent discharge for 2–3 wks: prescribe broad-spectrum antibiotic (i.e., amoxicillin, amoxicillin/clavulanate, cephalexin, or trimethoprim/sulfamethoxazole) × 10 days; may also try estrogen cream twice daily for 2 wks, then daily for 2 wks to thicken the mucosa
- Persistent/recurrent discharge: consider other causes—pelvic abscess, ectopic ureters, small foreign body; consider an examination under anesthesia (EUA)

PEDIATRIC AND ADOLESCENT GYNECOLOGY

Lichen Sclerosis
- Symptoms: itching, irritation, soreness, dysuria, vaginal discharge, and bleeding
- Examination: white, atrophic, parchment-like skin; fissures; chronic ulceration or inflammation; the perianal area is often involved
- Treatment:
  - Mild cases: eliminate local irritants, improve hygiene, and use protective ointments (i.e., A & D)
  - More severe cases: high-dose corticosteroids (i.e., clobetasol topical) for 4 wks with taper to milder topical steroids (although no randomized controlled trial [RCT] as yet)

Condyloma Acuminata
- If <24 mos old, may have been transmitted at birth; consider sexual abuse
- Evaluation: abuse history, culture for other STDs, and occasionally EUA to determine extent of disease and to treat
- Treatment:
  - Younger children: surgical with silver sulfadiazine (Silvadene) cream and oral analgesics for postoperative care
  - Older children: may use outpatient trichloroacetic acid (TCA)

Labial Adhesions
- Consists of agglutination of the labia minora; if labia are completely adhered, there can be urinary retention or mucocolpos
- Diagnosis by inspection
- Treat if large area is agglutinated:
  - Usually estrogen cream and gentle separation of the labia while the cream is applied
  - Apply twice daily × 3 wks → daily × 3 wks (some need longer treatment)
  - Once open, need good hygiene measures and daily application of a daily lubricant such as A & D ointment; if does not resolve, may need EUA and gentle separation

Vaginal Bleeding
- Look for signs of puberty (i.e., breast development, growth spurt).
- Vaginal bleeding with precocious puberty: see Chapter 2, Puberty
- Vaginal bleeding not associated with precocious puberty:
  - *Neonatal hormone withdrawal:* most common in first 2 wks of life as a result of withdrawal from maternal estrogen
  - *Vaginitis:* Group A beta-hemolytic streptococcus (usually presents after an upper respiratory illness [URI]) and *Shigella* (only associated with diarrhea 25% of the time)
  - *Lichen sclerosus* (bleeding secondary to trauma)

- *Condyloma acuminata* (bleeding secondary to trauma)
- *Trauma:* accidental trauma (i.e., bicycles, slides, bathtub edge) may result in straddle injuries; consider sexual abuse
- *Foreign body:* often associated with foul-smelling discharge; may try gentle outpatient vaginal irritation with a small Foley catheter in the vagina if the patient is cooperative; otherwise, an EUA is necessary
- *Tumors:* sarcoma botryoides
- *Urethral prolapse:* Peak incidence in children is 1:3000 between ages 5 and 8 yrs; it is more common in African-American girls. Symptoms include dysuria, bleeding, and pain. Treatment includes sitz baths, topical estrogen or antibiotics, and oral antibiotics. If there is necrotic tissue, then surgery may be indicated. Resolution occurs in 1–4 wks.
- *Precocious menarche:* cyclical vaginal bleeding without signs of puberty. May be a response to transient production of estrogen by the ovary. Sometimes associated with hypothyroidism. Usually self-limiting in approximately 2–10 mos. Follow closely to confirm diagnosis.

PEDIATRIC AND ADOLESCENT GYNECOLOGY

ADOLESCENT GYNECOLOGY
Abnormal Uterine Bleeding

Cause	Notes
Dysfunctional uterine bleeding	Most common cause in adolescents. Caused by anovulation secondary to an immature H-P-O axis. Maturation of the H-P-O axis takes 2–5 yrs (Apter et al., 1978).
Coagulation disorders	20–40% of adolescents with severe menorrhagia have coagulation disorders (most common: platelet disorders).
Pregnancy	Always rule out with β-human chorionic gonadotropin test.
Reproductive tract pathology	Rare.
Endocrine disorders	Most common: thyroid disease. PCOS may be difficult to diagnose in adolescents secondary to the relative hyperinsulinemia normally seen at this time and acne from adrenal androgens also common in adolescents. There is no randomized controlled study on the use of metformin in adolescents with PCOS.
Hypothalamic dysregulation	Eating disorders. Excessive exercise. Chronic illness. Psychological stress.

H-P-O, hypothalamic-pituitary-ovarian; PCOS, polycystic ovary syndrome.

Evaluation
- **Complete blood count (CBC)** with platelets; coagulation profile if acute hemorrhage or hemoglobin (Hb) <10%, including a prothrombin time (PT)/partial thromboplastin time (PTT) and bleeding time; additional coagulation evaluation may be considered.
- **von Willebrand's** testing is less accurate if the patient is taking estrogen.
- **Thyroid-stimulating hormone (TSH), prolactin, androgens**—if endocrine testing is indicated.
- **STD screening** if sexually active.
- **Pelvic ultrasound** if high suspicion for anatomic abnormality and pelvic examination is not possible or inadequate.

Treatment
- If irregular bleeding neither heavy nor prolonged, may give reassurance and observe.

31

- If more severe and anemia (Hb, 10–12 mg/dL): oral contraceptives (OCs) or cyclic progestins
- If acute severe menorrhagia (acute blood loss or Hb <10 mg/dL): IV conjugated estrogen (Premarin) or OC taper
- Iron supplementation
- Surgical dilatation and curettage (D&C) is last resort if medical therapy unsuccessful.

Dysmenorrhea

- Most common gynecologic complaint among adolescents (Klein and Litt, 1981)

Primary Dysmenorrhea

- Painful menses in the absence of anatomic pathology; believed to be caused by prostaglandins; most common type of dysmenorrhea in adolescents

Treatment

- First-line treatment is nonsteroidal antiinflammatory drugs (NSAIDs [i.e., propionic acids, such as ibuprofen and naproxen, and fenamates such as mefenamic acid and meclofenamate]); may have gastrointestinal (GI) or central nervous system (CNS) side effects.
- If severe dysmenorrhea, should start NSAIDs the day before menses or right at menses and continue for 1–3 days around the clock.
- OCs if unresponsive to NSAIDs.
- If no success with either, consider causes of secondary dysmenorrhea.

PEDIATRIC AND ADOLESCENT GYNECOLOGY

Secondary Dysmenorrhea

- Painful menses in the presence of anatomic pathology

Cause	Notes
Endometriosis	See Chapter 16, Endometriosis. In adolescents, gonadotropin-releasing hormone agonists are not used without laparoscopic confirmation of the diagnosis and are generally not used until bone density is maximum (~16 yrs old). Endometriotic lesions are generally red or clear (early lesions). Advanced endometriosis is rare.
Ovarian cysts	Pelvic ultrasound. Most are functional and resolve spontaneously or with oral contraceptives. Often, these are actually paratubal cysts.
Sexually transmitted infections	Screen all sexually active teens.
Pelvic adhesions	History very helpful. Laparoscopy to diagnose and treat.
Congenital obstructive müllerian anomaly: duplicated uterus (didelphic or septate) with an oblique vaginal septum obstructing one of the cervices → cyclic menses with worsening, severe cyclic dysmenorrhea	In adolescents with severe pelvic pain, a pelvic ultrasound can rule out a müllerian anomaly and collection of blood behind a septum; if an ultrasound is abnormal, magnetic resonance imaging provides the best information concerning anatomy. This anomaly requires surgical correction. Do not drain with a needle, as this may introduce bacteria into the obstructed menstrual blood and result in severe infection or abscess formation. Almost always associated with absence of the kidney on the side with the obstruction.

4. Müllerian Agenesis

SYNONYMS
- Müllerian agenesis (MA)
- Mayer-Rokitansky-Küster-Hauser syndrome
- Vaginal agenesis

DEFINITION
- Lack of fallopian tubes, uterus, and upper vagina

EMBRYOLOGY
- Sertoli cells (SCs) in fetal testis → müllerian inhibiting substance (MIS) → regression of ipsimüllerian structures *in utero*

ANATOMY (Griffin et al., 1976)
- Normal external female genitalia
- Normal ovarian function; thus, normal female secondary sexual characteristics
- Absence of fallopian tubes, uterus, internal vagina → some variations in degree of müllerian structure regression
- 1/3 of MA patients have renal anomalies (renal agenesis, malrotations, ectopic kidneys).
- Possible spinal and skeletal anomalies
- Diagnosis usually due to presentation with primary amenorrhea; need to differentiate from those with imperforate hymen, transverse vaginal septum, or complete androgen insensitivity syndrome

MÜLLERIAN INHIBITING SUBSTANCE
- From SCs and granulosa cells of postnatal ovaries
- Likely acts via mesenchyme
- Glycoprotein cleaved into two different protein products:
  - Embryonic testis → larger MIS protein
  - Postnatally → smaller MIS protein (function unknown)
- Target cells may contain the enzyme to cleave the MIS precursor molecule.
- MIS receptor found in SCs, fetal and postnatal granulosa cells, and the mesenchyme around müllerian ducts
- Effects exerted at 8–10 wks of fetal life
- *Male:* smaller MIS protein elevated for several years after birth, then very low levels during puberty

- *Females:* circulating levels of MIS (large or small form) below limits of assay sensitivity until onset of puberty (but still below fetal levels); possible role in ovarian gametogenesis

ETIOLOGY

- *MIS gene mutations* may lead to inappropriate time of MIS production (i.e., too early), but this cannot explain the lack of virilization, as MIS causes aromatase suppression that would lead to elevated testosterone levels in a female fetus.
- *MIS-receptor gene mutations* may lead to constitutively active MIS receptor.

MANAGEMENT

- Nonsurgical or surgical treatment usually delayed until perisexual activity time of life.
- Nonsurgical management (usually preferred):
  - Must continue to use dilators in absence of routine sexual intercourse to ensure continued patency.
    - ⇨ *Frank's vaginal dilation technique* (Frank, 1938): increasing sizes of vaginal dilators (from 0.5-in. diameter and 4- to 5-in. length up to 1-in. diameter and 4- to 5-in. length):
      - ❖ Pressure to vaginal dimple t.i.d. × 20 mins
        Total time: 6–8 wks
        Normal sexual function: 76%
    - ⇨ *Ingram's modified Frank's technique:* bicycle seat stool for constant perineal pressure; total daily time of 2 hrs
    - ⇨ *Jaffe's modified Frank's technique:* increasing sizes of syringe containers
    - ⇨ Estradiol (E_2) cream for vaginal epithelial transformation
- Surgical management:
  - *Abbe-McIndoe technique* with split-thickness skin graft
  - *Modifications to split-thickness skin graft:* human amnion, peritoneum, segments of colon, gracilis, rectus abdominus, myocutaneous flaps, Interceed
  - *Vecchietti operation/acrylic olive traction device:* continuous pressure to the vaginal dimple (with a plastic "olive") with strings attached laparoscopically to the suprapubic region; this traction device is tightened daily (1 cm/day)

5. Septate Uterus

PREVALENCE
- ~1% in women with normal fertility and subfertility
- 3.3% in women with recurrent pregnancy loss (RPL)

BACKGROUND
- Congenital uterine anomalies resulting from müllerian fusion defects are the most common types of malformations of the reproductive system (Rock and Jones, 1977).
- Septate uterus is the most common and is associated with the poorest reproductive outcome:
  - 25% incidence of 1st trimester (TM) loss; 6% incidence of 2nd TM loss
  - Spontaneous abortion (SAB) >60% (Green and Harris, 1976)
- Correlation of septate uterus in three patient populations:

	Fertile	Recurrent Pregnancy Loss	Subfertile
Septate	1.5%	2.0%	0.6%

Note: No statistically significant difference.
Source: Adapted from Raga F, Bauset C, et al. Reproductive impact of congenital Mullerian anomalies. *Hum Reprod* 12(10):2277, 1997.

- Mechanism of pregnancy loss: implantation into a poorly vascularized, fibrous septum (Fedele et al., 1996b)
- Bicornuate uterus is not generally associated with RPL (Proctor and Haney, 2003).

EMBRYOLOGY
- Müllerian ducts develop by in-folding of the coelomic epithelium overlying the *urogenital ridge,* and, in the absence of müllerian inhibiting factor (from Sertoli cells), duct growth proceeds caudally and medially, reaching the *urogenital sinus* to form the müllerian tubercle. Fusion and resorption begin at the isthmus and proceed simultaneously in both the cranial and caudal directions (Muller et al., 1967).
- Failure of fusion → bicornuate uterus; failure of resorption → septate uterus
- Abnormal müllerian differentiation is associated with urologic/renal malformations (up to 30%) (Li et al., 2000); however, because septum resorption usually occurs after urologic development is completed, there is no need to obtain a renal ultrasound in women with septate uteri.

HISTOLOGY

- Contrary to the conventional view that the septum consists of fibrous tissue, there may actually be more muscle fibers in the septum than previously believed (Dabirashrafi et al., 1995).

DIAGNOSIS

Hysteroscopy + Laparoscopy

- Gold standard for differentiating between a bicornuate and a septate uterus

Ultrasound

- Septate uterus appears as two cavities without sagittal notching and with a fundal myometrium; intercornual distance usually <4 cm.
  - If the fundal midpoint/indentation is >5 mm above a line joining both ostia → septate uterus (**see part c of diagram**) (Homer et al., 2000).

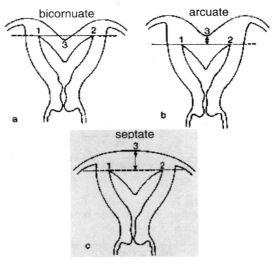

Source: Reproduced with permission from Homer HA, Li TC, Cooke ID. The septate uterus: a review of management and reproductive outcome. *Fertil Steril* 73(1):1, 2000.

SEPTATE UTERUS

Hysterosalpingogram
- Hysterosalpingogram (HSG) cannot reliably differentiate between a septate and a bicornuate/arcuate uterus (55% accuracy).
  - If the angle of divergence of the two uterine cavities seen on HSG is ≤75 degrees, the defect is most likely a septate uterus.
  - If the angle of divergence is >75 degrees and <105 degrees, a diagnosis cannot be made.

Magnetic Resonance Imaging
- Accurate, noninvasive means of classification and obtaining information on septal morphometry (proportion of myometrial vs. fibrous tissue) (Carrington et al., 1990)
- If the septum extends to ≥30% of the cavity length, it should be resected (Dr. Greg Christman, *personal communication,* 2002).

MECHANISM OF ADVERSE OUTCOMES
- Septate uterus is associated with
  - 1st- and 2nd-TM loss (usually between 8–16 wks; two-thirds in the 1st TM)
  - Premature delivery
  - Abnormal presentation
  - Intrauterine growth restriction
  - Infertility
- Reproductive performance of septate uterus:

	Spontaneous Abortion	Preterm Delivery	Live Birth
Septate	25.5%	14.5%	62.0%

Source: Adapted from Raga F, Bauset C, et al. Reproductive impact of congenital Mullerian anomalies. *Hum Reprod* 12(10):2277, 1997.

INDICATIONS FOR SURGERY
- If septate uterus is found in association with adverse reproductive outcome (greater than one loss) or in women >35 yrs old.

	Miscarriages	Preterm Delivery
Untreated septa (pooled data)	79%	9%

PREOPERATIVE PREPARATION
- Surgery during early proliferative phase
- Gonadotropin-releasing hormone (GnRH) agonist not essential unless there is a wide septum or septum involving the lower third of the cavity and/or cervical canal

38

OPERATIVE TECHNIQUE: RESECTOSCOPE METROPLASTY

- 0- or 12-degree lens preferred.
- Dissection complete when
  - Hysteroscope can be moved freely from one cornu to the other without obstruction.
  - Both ostia viewed simultaneously.
  - Bleeding indicates that incision has reached the myometrium.
- Residual septum <1 cm does not seem to impair outcome (Fedele, 1996a).
- Ultrasound helpful: stop incision when distance = 1 cm between dissection and serosal surface (Querleu et al., 1990).
- Either ultrasound or laparoscopy is necessary to guide surgeon; turn laparoscope light off and observe hysteroscopic transillumination.
- With complete septate uterus, it is recommended that the cervical portion of the septum be spared and the dissection start at the internal os to avoid cervical incompetence. Place a No. 8 Foley catheter into one cavity (prevents leakage of distending medium), inject indigo carmine into this cavity, and enter the other cavity with the resectoscope to incise the septum at the level of the isthmus (see diagram) (Romer and Lober, 1997).

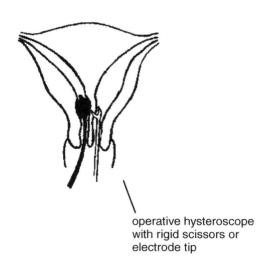

operative hysteroscope
with rigid scissors or
electrode tip

SEPTATE UTERUS

- Resection of the cervical portion may be indicated, as the incidence of cervical incompetence after removal of the cervical septum is rare (1 of 43 cases [Homer, 2000]; 0 of 10 cases [Nisolle and Donnez, 1996]).
- Excision is rarely indicated because the septum typically retracts with incision.

POSTOPERATIVE MANAGEMENT (Dr. Michael DiMattina, *personal communication*, 2004)

Hormonal Treatment
- One prospective, randomized study suggests no benefit.
- Estradiol valerate (Delestrogen), 5 mg IM immediately postoperation

No. 14-16 Foley Catheter
- Use 4–8 cc of sterile water for balloon.
- Maintain for 5–7 days.
- Doxycycline, 100 mg PO b.i.d., for duration of catheter use
- Nonsteroidal antiinflammatory drug to ↓ pain/adhesions (?)

Antibiotics
- Unnecessary unless Foley catheter left in place

Intrauterine Device
- No role (may increase formation of synechiae)

Follow-Up Examination
- Ultrasound satisfactory
- No reason to delay conception for more than two cycles

TRADITIONAL METROPLASTIES

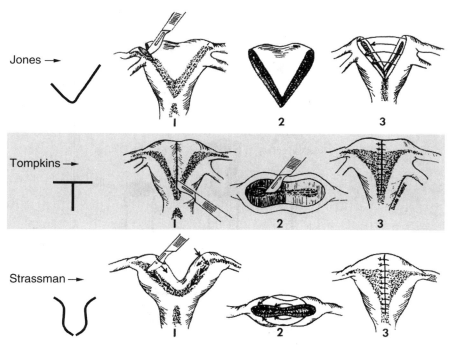

Source: Adapted from Rock JA, Zacur HA. The clinical management of repeated early pregnancy wastage. *Fertil Steril* 39(2):123, 1983.

- Jones, wedge metroplasty; Tompkins, fundal bivalve metroplasty (no excision of septum); Strassman, unification of (bicornuate or didelphic) uterine horns

SEPTATE UTERUS

AMERICAN SOCIETY FOR REPRODUCTIVE MEDICINE
CLASSIFICATION OF UTERINE MALFORMATIONS

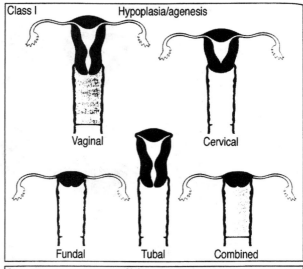

Class I   Hypoplasia/agenesis

Vaginal   Cervical

Fundal   Tubal   Combined

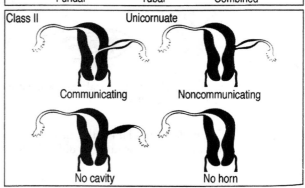

Class II   Unicornuate

Communicating   Noncommunicating

No cavity   No horn

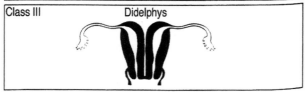

Class III   Didelphys

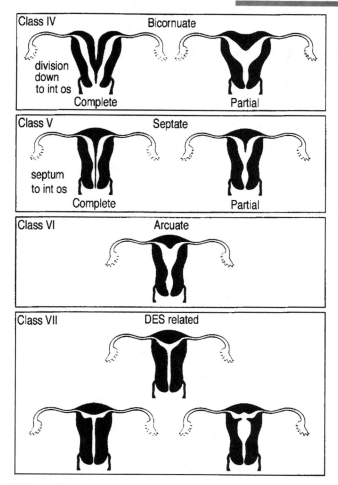

DES, diethylstilbestrol. (Source: Reproduced with permission from Gordon JD, Speroff L. Abnormal puberty and growth problems. In *Handbook for Clinical Gynecologic Endocrinology & Infertility* [6th ed]. Philadelphia: Lippincott–Raven, 2002:443.)

6. Turner Syndrome

DEFINITION AND INCIDENCE (Ranke and Saenger, 2001)
- Turner syndrome (TS; also known as *Ulrich-Turner syndrome*): combination of characteristic physical features (short stature and gonadal dysgenesis) and complete or partial absence of 2nd X chromosome
- 1 in 2500 live births
- 1% of 45,X fetuses survive to term.
- 10% of spontaneous losses have 45,X karyotype (most common aneuploid in 1st trimester [TM] loss).
- *Not* associated with advanced maternal or paternal age
- http://www.turner-syndrome-us.org

DIAGNOSIS (Ranke and Saenger, 2001)
- *Ultrasound findings suggestive:* ↑ nuchal translucency, cystic hygroma, coarctation of aorta ± left-sided cardiac defects, brachycephaly, renal anomalies, polyhydramnios, oligohydramnios, growth retardation
- *Karyotype (chorionic villus sampling [CVS]/amniocentesis):* necessary for diagnosis (confirm postnatally, if clinical suspicion is high and peripheral blood karyotype normal, then 2nd tissue should be checked)
- *Potential mosaic karyotypes:* 45,X/46,XX; 45,X/46,XY (mixed gonadal dysgenesis); 45,X/46,XX; 45,X/46,Xxiq (phenotype, including stature, impossible to predict with mosaics, although there is clearly a ↓ fertility rate with ↑ risk of spontaneous loss and premature ovarian failure)

Indications for a Karyotype
- If *virilization* or *fragment of sex chromosome of unknown origin (X or Y) is present*, probe for Y chromosome (risk of gonadoblastoma → 7–10% [Gravholt et al., 2000]; if present, recommend gonadectomy).
- Any female patient with unexplained growth failure or pubertal delay
- Newborn/infant:
  - Edema of the hands/feet, nuchal folds, left-sided cardiac anomalies, coarctation of aorta, hypoplastic left heart, low hairline, low-set ears, small mandible
- Childhood:
  - Growth velocity <10th percentile for age
  - Markedly ↑ follicle-stimulating hormone (FSH)
  - Cubitus valgus, nail hypoplasia, hyperconvex uplifted nails, multiple pigmented nevi, characteristic facies, short 4th metacarpal, high arched palate

- Adolescence:
  - No breast development by 13 yrs old, pubertal arrest, or primary or secondary amenorrhea with ↑ FSH
  - Unexplained short stature

PEDIATRIC MANAGEMENT (Ranke and Saenger, 2001)
Cardiac Disease
- Congenital heart defects occur in ~30%.
- Left-sided obstructive defects predominate, especially bicuspid aortic valves (30–50%).
- Coarctation of aorta (30%)
  - All TS patients should have an echocardiogram (ECHO) in childhood and repeat ECHO in adolescence (12–15 yrs old) if no cardiovascular malformation diagnosed earlier.
  - Annual blood pressure (BP) monitoring (upper and lower extremity BPs)

Renal Disease
- Up to 30% have congenital anomalies of the urinary system (most common are rotational abnormalities and double collecting systems).
- ↑ Risk of hypertension (HTN), urinary tract infection (UTI), hydronephrosis
  - Screening renal ultrasound and additional evaluation as indicated
  - Urine culture every 3–5 yrs

Thyroid
- 10–30% develop primary hypothyroidism, generally associated with antithyroid antibodies:
  - Thyroid-stimulating hormone (TSH), free thyroxine (FT_4) checked at diagnosis and every 1–2 yrs

Hearing
- Conductive and sensorineural hearing loss is common in girls with TS (50–90%).
- Otitis media is common and may progress to mastoiditis and/or cholesteatoma formation; typically between 1 and 6 yrs of age; peak incidence is at 3 yrs of age.
  - Aggressive treatment of otitis media is appropriate.
  - Short girls with extensive otitis media should be evaluated for TS.

Speech
- Speech problems are common in TS.
  - Referral to ear, nose, and throat (ENT) clinic and speech therapist is recommended.

45

TURNER SYNDROME

Vision
- Strabismus, amblyopia, and ptosis are common in TS.
  - Ophthalmology evaluation

Orthopedic
- ↑ Risk of congenital hip dislocation and may be associated with degenerative arthritis of the hips in older women
- 10% develop scoliosis, most commonly in adolescence.
  - Evaluate for orthopedic problems with annual examination.

Weight
- Predisposition for obesity

Lymphedema
- Most common in infancy but may occur at any age
  - Initiation of growth hormone (GH) or estradiol (E_2) may exacerbate; usually controlled with support stockings/diuretics; surgery not of proven benefit

Glucose Intolerance
- Possible ↑ risk of insulin resistance, but frank diabetes rare
  - Routine glucose tolerance test (GTT) not necessary

Plastic Surgery
- High risk of keloid formation
- Even small elective procedures should be used judiciously.

SHORT STATURE (Ranke and Saenger, 2001)
- 95% of TS; overall, ↓ final height ~20 cm below female average/ethnic group
- Comprised of mild intrauterine fetal growth retardation (IUGR), slow growth in infancy, delayed onset of childhood growth, growth failure during adolescence
- Impacts on socialization and academic achievement
- All girls with short stature (<3% or –2 standard deviations [SD] on growth curves) should have karyotyping if any other features of TS are present. (If –2.5 SD, even in absence of other features, karyotyping should be done.)
- Recombinant human GH and/or steroid treatment (risks/benefits) should be discussed with the patient and family at an early age, with a goal of achieving normal height before estrogenization. Long-term effects of supraphysiologic insulin-like growth factor-I (IGF-I) are unknown.

TURNER SYNDROME

PUBERTY MANAGEMENT (Ranke and Saenger, 2001)

- 90% of TS patients have gonadal failure; however, 30% undergo spontaneous pubertal development and 2–5% have spontaneous menses and potential for pregnancy without medical intervention (Hovatta, 1999).
- Check an FSH, if normal, then ultrasound ovaries to assess status.
- If gonadal failure is diagnosed and estrogen treatment is required for pubertal development, the dosing and timing should attempt to mimic normal puberty.
  - Goal of achieving idealized height first (±GH), followed by estrogen therapy slowly initiated for appropriate pubertal development (results in closure of epiphyses).
  - Percutaneous E_2 gel leads to the development of secondary sexual characteristics and uterine growth in a gradual progress mimicking natural puberty (Piippo et al., 2004).

ADULT MANAGEMENT (Ranke and Saenger, 2001)

- Transition from pediatric care to adult at approximately 18 yrs of age; care should include a gynecologist with expertise in fertility
- Annual history and physical examination (H&P) with attention to particular areas of concern:
  - Congenital heart disease (CHD)
  - Thyroid
  - Ophthalmologic abnormalities
  - Skeletal problems
  - Routine gynecologic care
  - Cardiac evaluation
  - Dental abnormalities
  - Hearing loss
  - Breast examination
  - HTN
  - Osteoporosis
- Lifestyle education regarding diet and exercise for prevention of diabetes, osteoporosis, and HTN
- ECHO every 5 yrs for evaluation of aortic root; more frequent if previous diagnosis
- If known renal anomalies, frequent screening for UTI
- Bone mineral density at 45 yrs and every 3–5 yrs as needed
- Low-dose oral contraceptives started at the age of 12 yrs if the child has previously been treated with recombinant human GH and at the age of 14 if she has not
- Otologic assessment every 3–5 yrs if loss noted; if normal, then every 10 yrs
- Laboratory tests every 2 yrs: hemoglobin (Hb), blood urea nitrogen (BUN)/creatinine (Cr), fasting glucose, lipid profile, liver enzymes, TSH, FT_4

TURNER SYNDROME

PREPREGNANCY MANAGEMENT (Ranke and Saenger, 2001)
- Preconceptual ECHO for evaluation of aortic root, as this can pose a risk for aortic dissection during pregnancy
- Evaluate renal function, thyroid, and glucose tolerance.
- Genetic counseling on risks of miscarriage and chromosomal anomalies in offspring
  - Out of 160 pregnancies (Tarani et al., 1998):
    - ⇨ 29%: Spontaneous loss
    - ⇨ 20%: Malformed babies (TS, trisomy 21, and so forth)
    - ⇨ 7%: Perinatal death
- Women with nonfunctional ovaries: adequate hormones 3–4 mos before embryo transfer from donated oocytes/embryos to ↑ size and improve blood flow to uterus; ↑ dose of E_2 until endometrium ≥7 mm
- Vaginal delivery possible, but cesarean section frequent due to narrow pelvis

COGNITIVE AND ACADEMIC PERFORMANCE (Ranke and Saenger, 2001)
- No ↑ prevalence of mental retardation except in those with small ring X chromosome that fails to undergo inactivation
- Impaired nonverbal, visual-spatial processing; defects in social cognition (failure to appreciate subtle social cues)
- Many TS patients achieve high professional status.

7. Menstrual Cycle

CHARACTERISTICS OF THE NORMAL MENSTRUAL CYCLE

- Purpose: renewal of uterine lining to optimize embryonic implantation
- Mechanism: closely coordinated interactions between the hypothalamus, pituitary gland, and ovaries producing cyclic changes in target tissues of the reproductive tract → endometrium, cervix, and vagina
- Fast facts:
  - Mean age of **menarche** = 12.8 yrs old; mean age of **menopause** = 51 yrs old
  - Cycle day 1 = first day of vaginal bleeding; mean duration of flow = 4 ± 2 days
  - Cycle length:
    ⇨ Least variable between ages 20 and 40 yrs (gradual decrease in length)
    ⇨ 90% have menstrual cycles between **24 and 35 days**; 15% have 28-day cycles.
  - Irregular cycles: **just after menarche** (2 yrs); **just before menopause** (3 yrs); changes in diet, exercise, emotions; postpartum; postabortion
  - Menstrual cycle phases:
    ⇨ Follicular phase: variable length (7–21 days); key determinant of cycle length
    ⇨ Ovulation
    ⇨ Luteal phase: more constant (≥12 days)
- Ovulation: The female gamete is released from the ovarian follicle at monthly intervals.
- Mitotic division of the germ cells ceases by the 7th mo of fetal life, although this has recently been challenged by data indicating the presence of germline stem cells allowing follicular renewal in the postnatal rodent ovary (Johnson et al., 2004a).
- Gonadotropin-releasing hormone (GnRH) pulsatility:

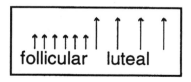

- Follicle-stimulating hormone (FSH) half-life ($t_{1/2}$) = 3 hrs; luteinizing hormone (LH) $t_{1/2}$ = 20 mins

MENSTRUAL CYCLE

FOLLICULAR PHASE

- Folliculogenesis occurs in waves and is actually initiated in the last few days of the preceding cycle and may be a few cycles antecedent (Gougeon, 1986).
- Small ↑ in FSH initiates follicular **recruitment,** growth, and development ↑ of a cohort of 3–30 follicles.
- **Dominant follicle is selected** from cohort, while remaining ones undergo **atresia.**
- Site of ovulation is random in consecutive cycles (Baird, 1987).
- LH: slow rise
- ↓ FSH in response to estradiol (E_2) negative feedback and from inhibin secretion from developing follicle
- The concentration of inhibin B in individual follicular fluid is highest in follicular fluid samples from the early follicular phase. Inhibin B appears to be the predominant form of inhibin in the preovulatory follicle. The source of inhibin is granulosa cells (GCs) (Groome et al., 1996).
- E_2: ↑ due to ↑ production from GCs in dominant follicle in response to FSH stimulation
- FSH stimulates GCs → ↑ FSH receptors and LH receptors (in presence of E_2), progesterone (P_4), 17-hydroxyprogesterone (17-OHP), androgens
- In the late stages of follicle development, once antral ovarian follicle diameter increases beyond roughly 10 mm, GCs become receptive to LH stimulation, and LH becomes capable of exerting its actions on both theca cells and GCs (Filicori and Cognigni, 2001).
- E_2 may not be required for follicular growth and development:

Granulosa Cells	ER-Alpha	ER-Beta
Preantral	—	+++
Antral	+	+++

ER, estradiol receptor; –, absent; +, present; +++, high levels.
Source: Adapted from Rosenfeld CS, Wagner JS, et al. Intraovarian actions of oestrogen. *Reproduction* 122(2):215, 2001.

- If not E_2, then what is responsible for follicular growth and development?
  - Activin, inhibin, insulin-like growth factors (IGF-I, II), IGF-binding proteins

OVULATION   (Yoshimura and Wallach, 1987)

Timings

- E_2 positive feedback: E_2 (≥ 200 pg/mL) sustained for >50 hrs constitutes the ovarian signal for initiating the midcycle gonadotropin surge, and a small increment of P_4 secreted by the preovulatory follicle is required to establish the normal dimension of the surge. Thus, P_4, although essential for creating a normal gonadotropic surge, operates by synergizing the obligatory action of E_2 (Nakai et al., 1978; Liu and Yen, 1983).
- LH surge has three phases (Hoff et al., 1983):
  1. Rapidly ascending limb of 14 hrs
  2. Plateau of 14 hrs
  3. Descending phase of 20 hrs
- Site of ovulation from cycle to cycle is random (Ecochard and Gougeon, 2000).
- *Mittelschmerz:* dull, unilateral pain at time of ovulation lasting few minutes to hours; cause may be follicular expansion before ovulation or leakage of follicular fluid and associated blood into abdominal cavity at time of ovulation.

Ovulation

- *Stigma:* a small protrusion on follicular wall representing site of rupture; present well in advance of ovulation
- Follicle becomes extensively vascularized before ovulation.
- GCs → plasminogen activator (in response to FSH) → proteolytic breakdown of follicular wall
- LH → ↑ prostaglandin $F_{2\alpha}$ ($PGF_{2\alpha}$), prostaglandin E_2 (PGE_2), proteolytic enzymes → contractions of smooth muscle of follicular wall (therefore, avoid periovulatory prostaglandin synthetase inhibitors in patient seeking pregnancy) (Pall et al., 2001)
- Serum LH rises to a median of 32 hrs and peaks at 16.5 hrs before ovulation.

MENSTRUAL CYCLE

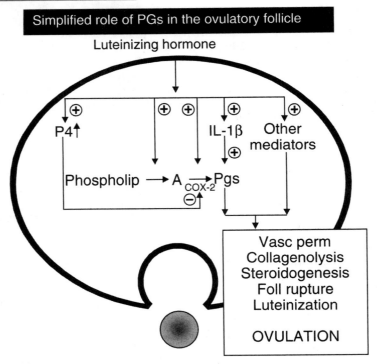

Simplified role of PGs in the ovulatory follicle

Luteinizing hormone

P4↑

IL-1β   Other mediators

Phospholip → A —COX-2→ Pgs

Vasc perm
Collagenolysis
Steroidogenesis
Foll rupture
Luteinization

OVULATION

A, arachidonic acid; COX-2, cyclooxygenase-2; Foll, follicle; IL-1β, interleukin-1β; P4, progesterone; PGs, prostaglandins; Phospholip, phospholipids; Vasc perm, vascular permeability.

• Basal body temperature (BBT) nadir is an inaccurate method for predicting ovulation time because ovulation is between 6 days before and 4 days after the nadir (Guermandi et al., 2001).

LUTEAL PHASE

- Begins with expulsion of the oocyte
- Corpus luteum (CL; "yellow body"): luteinized GCs, theca interna/externa
- CL $\rightarrow P_4$ to prepare endometrium for conceptus; P_4 begins to rise 12 hrs before the LH surge.
- P_4 peak secretion is ~1 wk after LH surge (parallel $\uparrow$ in estrone [E_1], E_2, 17-OHP).
- Degeneration $\rightarrow$ corpus albicans formation
- LH and human chorionic gonadotropin (hCG) stimulate P_4 secretion in a pulsatile fashion (paralleling LH).
- Ovulatory women: P_4 >3 ng/mL at midluteal phase (Israel et al., 1972)

MENSTRUAL CYCLE

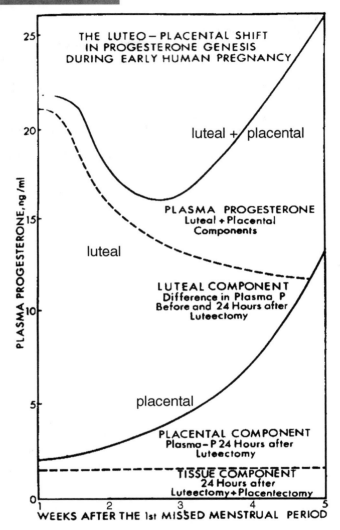

P, progesterone. (Source: Reproduced with permission from Csapo AI, Pulkkinen M. Indispensability of the human corpus luteum in the maintenance of early pregnancy. Luteectomy evidence. *Obstet Gynecol Surv* 33:69, 1978.)

MENSTRUAL CYCLE

- Luteoplacental shift in P_4 begins at 6 wks' estimated gestational age (EGA) and is far advanced by the 9th wk of gestation (Csapo and Pulkkinen, 1978). The ovarian source of P_4 is dispensable >9 wks. If a luteectomy is performed before this time, P_4 replacement can be administered as follows:

Estimated Gestational Age	Progesterone Replacement (until Wk 12)
<9 wks	Crinone 8% q.h.s. per vagina
	Prometrium (wet tablet per vagina) or progesterone vaginal suppository:
	Non–down-regulated cycles: 100 mg q12 hrs
	Gonadotropin-releasing hormone–agonist cycles: 200 mg q12 hrs
	Agonadal: 200 mg q6 hrs
≥9 wks	None

CYCLIC CHANGES IN TARGET ORGANS
Ovary
Early Development

Oocytes (No.)	Time
6 million	Wk 20 of fetal life.
2 million	Birth.
400,000	Menarche.
400	Normal reproductive life span involves ~400 oocytes ovulated.

Adult Ovary

- Each primordial follicle contains a small primary oocyte arrested in **prophase of meiosis I** (diplotene stage).
- Primordial follicle (50 μm) → primary follicle
  - Independent of gonadotropin control
  - *Zona pellucida:* translucent "shell" of glycoproteins surrounding the oocyte; 150 μm diameter
  - Within 36 hrs of the onset of the LH surge, the oocyte completes the first meiotic division (reducing to 22,X chromosomes), and the first polar body is extruded.
  - Second meiotic division occurs if oocyte is fertilized by a spermatozoon.
  - If fertilization occurs, hCG is secreted by the developing blastocyst even before implantation (Fishel et al., 1984).

55

MENSTRUAL CYCLE

Endometrium

- Of the three layers of the endometrium, only the basal layer is *not* shed at menstruation.
- Follicular phase: Basal layer regenerates the superficial layer of compact epithelial cells and intermediate layer of spongiosa; endometrial glands proliferate in response to E_2.
- First histologic sign that ovulation has occurred is the appearance of **subnuclear intracytoplasmic glycogen vacuoles.**
- Luteal phase: glands become coiled and secretory, $\uparrow$ vascularity and edema of stroma in response to P_4; late luteal phase: stroma becomes edematous, glandular and endothelial necrosis occurs, and bleeding ensues.
- Noncoagulability of menstruum due to peak in fibrinolytic activity of endometrium (Todd, 1973).

Cervix and Cervical Mucus

- $E_2 \rightarrow \uparrow$ vascularity and edema of cervix leads to $\uparrow$ cervical mucus (10–30× in quantity), which becomes clear, and its elasticity (*spinnbarkeit*) increases; "palm-leaf" arborization ("ferning") becomes marked just before ovulation (secondary to NaCl).
- $P_4 \rightarrow$ mucus thickens, becomes opaque, and loses its elasticity and ability to fern.

Vagina

- Early follicular phase: thin/pale
- Late follicular phase: thickens/dusky ($\uparrow E_2$)
- Luteal phase: $\uparrow$ percentage of cornified cells; increased numbers of precornified intermediate epithelial cells and polymorphonuclear cells ($\uparrow P_4$)

OVARIAN STEROIDOGENESIS

Androgens   (Erickson et al., 1985)

- Androstenedione (A_4) and testosterone = 19-C steroids
- Serve as substrates for GCs and aromatization
- Major ovarian androgen = A_4; can be converted to testosterone in peripheral tissues

Estrogens   (McNatty et al., 1979)

- Aromatization in GCs of A-ring and androgens diffusing from theca cells
- Contain 18-C atoms
- Definition: stimulate proliferation of the endometrium

Progesterone

- Follicular phase $\rightarrow$ 2–3 mg/day

- Midluteal phase → 25–30 mg/day
- Pregnancy at term → 250–300 mg/day
- LH stimulation is required (therefore, those without pituitary function need luteal phase support for fertility).

CENTRAL AND FEEDBACK CONTROL OF OVULATION (Filicori et al., 1986)

- Hypothalamic signals: pulsatile (every 1–4 hr) gonadotropin secretion due to pulsatile GnRH secretion

MENSTRUAL MIGRAINES

- Treatment: 0.1-mg E_2 patch/day before menses

PROTOCOL FOR HALTING VAGINAL BLEEDING IN HEMATOLOGY/ONCOLOGY/BONE MARROW TRANSPLANT PATIENT

- Acute induction (no admission warning):
  - If not bleeding at admission:
    - ⇨ Ortho-Novum 1/35 → q.d. × 6 wks without break
    - ⇨ Nafarelin (Synarel), 200 μg to dimish LH and FSH release→ alternate nostril b.i.d. × 6 wks
    - ⇨ Note: Tell patient she may have menses-like flow after Synarel.
  - If bleeding at admission:
    - ⇨ 1st wk:
      - ❖ Ortho-Novum 1/35:
        Light bleeding → 2 pills q.d.
        Heavy bleeding → 3 pills q.d.
    - ⇨ 2nd wk:
      - ❖ Taper Ortho-Novum 1/35 by one pill (if bleeding stops before end of 1st wk, may go to a more rapid taper)
      - ❖ Synarel 200 μg → alternate nostril b.i.d.
    - ⇨ 3rd wk:
      - ❖ Taper Ortho-Novum 1/35 to one pill and give continuously until wk 6.
      - ❖ Continue Synarel until wk 6.
- Elective consolidation or bone marrow transplant (normal blood counts with 3- to 4-wk admission warning)
  - Leuprolide (Lupron) or nafarelin acetate (Synarel) 3–4 wks before hospitalization; doses:
    - ⇨ Lupron, 3.75 mg IM q4 wks; repeat dose 1–2 days after admission
    - ⇨ Synarel, 200 μg b.i.d.; continue until discharge

MENSTRUAL CYCLE

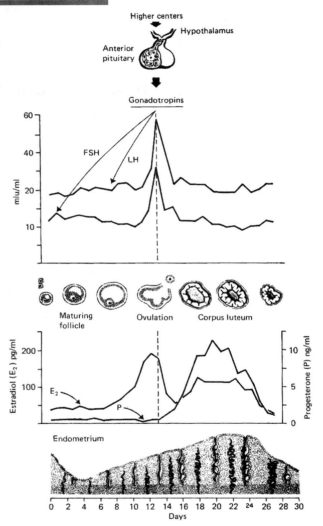

FSH, follicle-stimulating hormone; LH, luteinizing hormone. (Source: Reproduced with permission from Couchman GM, Hammond CB. Physiology of reproduction. In Scott JR, DiSaia PD, Hammond CB, Spellacy WN, eds. *Danforth's Obstetrics and Gynecology* [7th ed]. Philadelphia: JB Lippincott Co, 1990:48.)

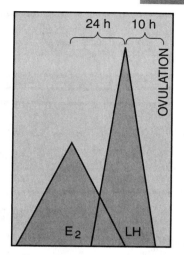

Source: Adapted from Speroff L, Glass RH, et al. Reproduction and the thyroid. In *Clinical Gynecologic Endocrinology & Infertility* (6th ed). Philadelphia: Lippincott–Raven, 1999:209.

⇨ The rise in **serum** LH occurs approximately 36 hrs before ovulation.

⇨ The LH surge appears in **urine** 12 hrs after it appears in serum.

⇨ Therefore, **a positive urine LH-kit occurs approximately 24 hrs before ovulation.**

⇨ Ovulation occurs 34–46 hrs after hCG administration (mean of 36 hrs) (Andersen et al., 1995).

MENSTRUAL CYCLE

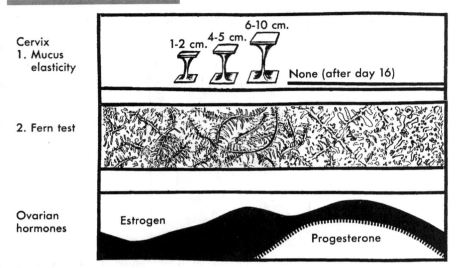

Cervix
1. Mucus
   elasticity

1-2 cm. 4-5 cm. 6-10 cm.

None (after day 16)

2. Fern test

Ovarian
hormones

Estrogen

Progesterone

Source: Adapted from Schneeberg NG, ed. *Essentials of Clinical Endocrinology* (1st ed).
St. Louis: Mosby, 1970:367.

8. Abnormal Uterine Bleeding

DEFINITION
- *Dysfunctional uterine bleeding* is simply abnormal uterine bleeding (AUB) unrelated to systemic medical illness, endocrinopathy, or structural uterine anomaly → *diagnosis of exclusion.*

TYPES OF ABNORMAL UTERINE BLEEDING

Term	Menses Pattern
Oligomenorrhea	>35-day cycle length
Polymenorrhea	<24-day cycle length
Menorrhagia	↑ Flow[a] or duration at regular intervals
Metrorrhagia	Regular flow at irregular intervals
Menometrorrhagia	↑ Flow or duration at irregular intervals

[a]Blood loss >80 mL.

ENDOMETRIAL SLOUGHING
- Intense spiral arteriole vasoconstriction (prostaglandin [PG] E_2 and $PGF_{2\alpha}$) precedes the onset of menses (Markee, 1940).
- Two theories for the trigger of menstruation:
  1. Apoptosis, tissue regression, and release of PGs and proteases
  2. Spiral arteriole constriction and necrosis
- More than 90% of menstrual blood loss occurs during the first 3 days (Haynes et al., 1977).
- Different hemostatic mechanisms in the endometrium compared to the rest of the body:
  - Initial suppression of platelet adhesion
  - With ↑ blood extravasation, damaged vessels are sealed by intravascular plugs of platelets and fibrin.
  - 20 hrs after the onset of menses, hemostasis is achieved by further intense spiral arteriole vasoconstriction.
  - 36 hrs after the start of menses, tissue regeneration is initiated.

ABNORMAL UTERINE BLEEDING

SYSTEMIC ETIOLOGIES FOR ABNORMAL UTERINE BLEEDING

Coagulation disorders
  von Willebrand's disease
  Thrombocytopenia
  Acute leukemia
  Advanced liver disease
Endocrinopathies
  Thyroid disease, hyperprolactinemia
  Polycystic ovary syndrome or elevated circulating androgens
  Cushing's syndrome
Anovulation or oligoovulation
  Idiopathic
  Stress, exercise, obesity, rapid weight changes
  Polycystic ovary syndrome or endocrinopathies as above
Drugs
  Contraception: oral/transdermal/vaginal contraceptive, intrauterine device, medroxy-
    progesterone acetate (Depo-Provera)
  Anticoagulants
  Antipsychotics
  Chemotherapy
  Drugs related to dopamine metabolism: tricyclic antidepressants, phenothiazines, anti-
    psychotic drugs
Trauma
  Sexual intercourse
  Sexual abuse
  Foreign bodies
  Pelvic trauma
Other
  Urinary system disorders: urethritis, cystitis, bladder cancer
  Inflammatory bowel disease, hemorrhoids

ABNORMAL UTERINE BLEEDING

GENITAL TRACT DISORDERS LEADING TO ABNORMAL UTERINE BLEEDING

	Uterus	Cervix	Vagina	Vulva
Infection	Endometritis	Cervicitis	Bacterial vaginosis, STDs, atrophic vaginitis	STD
Benign	Polyps, endometrial hyperplasia, adenomyosis, leiomyomas	Polyps, ectropion, endometriosis	Gartner's duct cysts, polyps, adenomyosis	Skin tags, condylomata, angiokeratoma
Cancer	Adenocarcinoma, sarcoma	Invasive or metastatic cancer	Vaginal cancer	Vulvar cancer

STD, sexually transmitted disease.

ABNORMAL UTERINE BLEEDING

CAUSES OF ABNORMAL UTERINE BLEEDING BY AGE GROUP (APGO, 2002)

- Neonates:
  - Estrogen withdrawal
- Premenarchal:
  - Foreign body
  - Adenomyosis
  - Trauma, abuse
  - Vulvovaginitis
  - Cancer (i.e., sarcoma botryoides)
  - Precocious puberty
- Early postmenarche:
  - Anovulation: hypothalamic immaturity (>90% of cases)
  - Stress: exercise induced
  - Pregnancy
  - Infection
  - Coagulation disorder
- Reproductive age:
  - Anovulation
  - Pregnancy
  - Endocrine disorder
  - Polyps/fibroids/adenomyosis
  - Medication related (oral contraceptives)
  - Infection
  - Sarcoma, ovarian
  - Coagulation disorder
- Perimenopausal:
  - Anovulation leading to unopposed estrogen and hyperplasia
  - Polyp/fibroid/adenomyosis
  - Cancer
- Postmenopausal:
  - Atrophy
  - Cancer/polyp
  - Estrogen therapy
  - Selective estrogen receptor modulators (SERMs)

ABNORMAL UTERINE BLEEDING

INITIAL EVALUATION

History

- Timing: frequency, temporal pattern, last menstrual period
- Nature of bleeding: duration, postcoital, quantity, temporal pattern
- Associated symptoms: pain, fever, vaginal discharge, changes in bowel/bladder function
- Pertinent medical history, history of bleeding disorders (family history as well), and medication history
- Changes in weight, excessive exercise, chronic illness, stress

Physical Examination

- General: signs of systemic illness, ecchymosis, thyromegaly, evidence of hyperandrogenism (hirsutism, acne, male pattern balding), acanthosis nigricans
- Pelvic: determine site of bleeding; assess contour, size, and tenderness of the uterus; any suspicious lesions or tumors

Laboratory Testing

- Urine pregnancy test to rule out pregnancy-related bleeding
  - Serum β-human chorionic gonadotropin (βhCG) if there has been a recent pregnancy (rule out trophoblastic disease)
- Pap smear
- Complete blood count (CBC) and platelets (PLTs)
- Thyroid-stimulating hormone (TSH) to exclude hypothyroidism
- If history of menorrhagia since onset of menses, mucocutaneous bleeding, or family history of coagulopathy (Kouides et al., 2000), check prothrombin time (PT)/partial thromboplastin time (PTT), factor VIII, and von Willebrand's factor antigen (especially in adolescents).
- Liver function tests (LFTs) in those with chronic liver or renal disease
- Determine ovulatory status (see also Chapter 26, Luteal Phase Deficiency)
  - Menstrual cycle charting: >10 days of variance from one cycle to the next suggests anovulatory cycles.
  - Normal menstrual cycle length: 24–35 days
  - Luteinizing hormone (LH) urine predictor kit: False positives include premature ovarian failure, menopause, and polycystic ovary syndrome (on occasion).

Endometrial Biopsy

- Perform in all women >35 yrs of age
- History of unopposed estrogen exposure
- Risk factors for endometrial hyperplasia:

ABNORMAL UTERINE BLEEDING

- Obesity, chronic anovulation, history of breast cancer, SERM (tamoxifen) use
- Family history of endometrial, ovarian, breast, or colon cancer (Farquhar et al., 1999)

Summary of Initial Evaluation

History and physical
Pregnancy tests: exclude pregnancy or trophoblastic disease
Pap smear
CBC/PLTs
TSH
LFTs (those with chronic liver or renal disease)
PT/PTT, factor VIII, von Willebrand's factor antigen (if suspicious history)
Ovulatory status
Menstrual charting
Luteal phase length (24–35 days)
LH urine predictor kits
Endometrial biopsy
Transvaginal ultrasound (possible sonohysterogram or hysteroscopy)

SECONDARY EVALUATION

- **Transvaginal ultrasound** (TVS) evaluates for structural lesions in the setting of abnormal pelvic examination or normal endometrial biopsy.
  - Can demonstrate a thickened endometrial lining; cannot reliably distinguish between submucous fibroids, polyps, adenomyosis, and neoplastic change
  - Utility of TVS in excluding endometrial abnormalities is more reliable in postmenopausal women.
  - In premenopausal women, TVS should be performed on cycle days 4–6; if returns with an endometrial stripe >5 mm → obtain sonohysterogram.
    - ⇨ In 200 premenopausal women with AUB, 16 of 80 women (20%!) with an endometrial stripe <5 mm had an endometrial polyp or submucosal fibroid seen on sonohysterogram (Breitkopf et al., 2004).
- **Sonohysterography** allows for careful evaluation of cavity by infusing sterile saline into the endometrial cavity and monitoring by TVS.
  - Can better detect smaller lesions such as polyps or small submucosal fibroids
  - Advantage: higher sensitivity in detecting polyps than TVS alone (94% vs. 75%, respectively) (Kamel et al., 2000)
  - Disadvantage: no tissue for histologic diagnosis
- **Hysteroscopy:** direct visualization of the endometrial cavity
  - Considered the gold standard for the diagnosis of AUB
  - Can biopsy or excise lesions identified

ABNORMAL UTERINE BLEEDING

TREATMENT
Acute Menorrhagia
- High-dose intravenous, intramuscular, or oral estrogen
- 30-cc Foley balloon catheter (tamponade) until medical or surgical therapy can be performed
- Resuscitate with blood transfusion as needed
- Surgical: if persistent heavy vaginal bleeding, may consider dilatation and curettage (D&C)

Chronic Menorrhagia
Medical Options

	↓ Blood Flow (%)	Comments
Oral contraceptives	50	Continuous or cyclic[a]
Levonorgestrel intrauterine device	80–90	May induce amenorrhea
Nonsteroidal antiinflammatory drugs	20–50	Effective in ovulatory women
Cyclic progestin	—	Particularly in anovulatory bleeding
Antifibrinolytics (tranexamic acid, 1 g q.i.d. cycle days minus 1–4)	50	Side effects: nausea, leg cramps, potential deep venous thrombosis risk
Gonadotropin-releasing hormone agonists and antagonists	—	Hypoestrogenemia side effects: hot flashes, osteopenia; limit use to 6 mos

[a]May need an oral contraceptive with a more estrogenic progestin, such as ethynodiol diacetate; if the endometrium is thick on oral contraceptives, then a higher dose of progestin (1 mg norethindrone) may be necessary.

Failed Medical Therapy or Known Surgical Indication
- Hysteroscopy/D&C
- Endometrial ablation
- Approximately 20% of patients require further surgery, with 10% needing hysterectomy.
- Hysterectomy: definitive surgery

A. Diagnostic Algorithm for Premenopausal Bleeding

ABNORMAL UTERINE BLEEDING

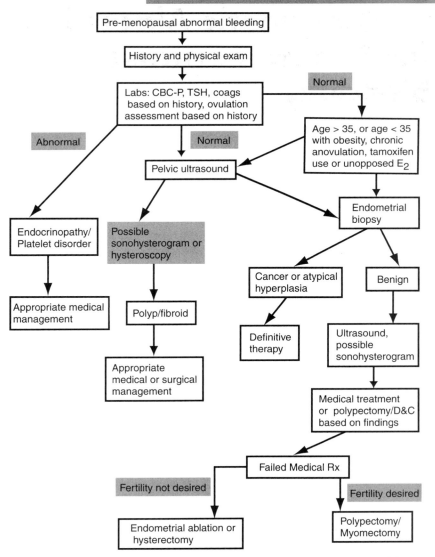

CBC-P, complete blood count/platelets; coags, coagulation disorders; D&C, dilatation and curettage; E_2, estradiol; Rx, treatment; TSH, thyroid-stimulating hormone.

B. Diagnostic Algorithm for Postmenopausal Bleeding

ABNORMAL UTERINE BLEEDING

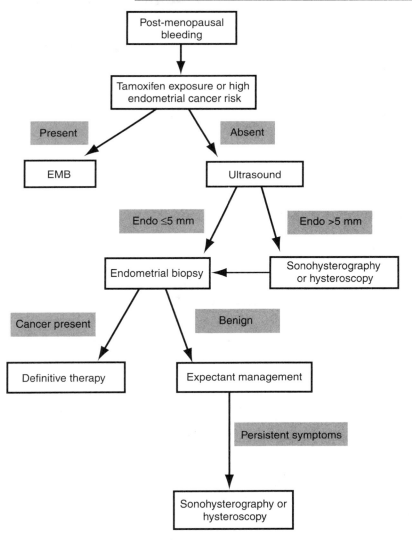

EMB, endometrial biopsy; Endo, endometrium.

71

9. Oral Contraceptives

STEROID COMPONENTS OF ORAL CONTRACEPTIVES
Estrogen Component
- Peak serum levels in 1.2–1.7 hrs
- Estradiol (E_2) is the most potent natural estrogen (E) and the major E secreted by the ovaries. An ethinyl group at the C-17 position makes E_2 orally active. All current oral contraceptives (OCs) use ethinyl estradiol (EE).
- Physiologic effects:
  - Potentiates the action of the progestogenic component by ↑ progesterone (P_4) receptors
  - Stabilizes the endometrium to minimize breakthrough bleeding (BTB) and irregular shedding

Progestin Component (Dorflinger, 1985)
- Peak serum levels in 2 hrs
Synthetic Progestins

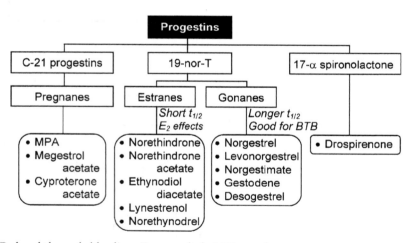

BTB, breakthrough bleeding; E_2, estradiol; MPA, medroxyprogesterone acetate; $t_{1/2}$, terminal half-life.

ORAL CONTRACEPTIVES

- Physiologic effects:
  - Contraception but not an absolute anovulatory effect (with current lower EE doses)
    ⇨ Ovulation still occurs in approximately 3% of cycles (Teichmann et al., 1995).
  - Turbidity of cervical mucus
  - Inhibit *spinnbarkeit*
  - Suppression of endometrial gland maturation → decidualized

Generation Terminology
- 1st generation: ≥50 μg E
- 2nd generation: <50 μg E and any progestin except norgestimate, desogestrel, or gestodene
- 3rd generation: <50 μg E and progestin of a levonorgestrel derivative (norgestimate, desogestrel, or gestodene)

Potency
- Potency varies depending on the target organ and endpoint being studied.
  - The biologic effect of the various progestational components in current low-dose OCs is approximately the same.

Multiphasic Formulations
- The aim is to alter steroid levels to ↓ metabolic effects and ↓ BTB/amenorrhea.

Mechanism of Action
- E and progestin are given every day for 3 of 4 wks.
- Contraception efficacy derived from the negative feedback actions of progestins
- Bleeding is controlled by the E component.
- P_4 inhibits luteinizing hormone (LH).
- E inhibits follicle-stimulating hormone (FSH) and LH.
- E minimizes irregular shedding of endometrium and BTB.
- E is required to potentiate the action of progestin via ↑ progestin receptors (thus allowing ↓ progestin dose).

Efficacy
- Annual failure rate = 0.1% (with typical use, 3.0% in 1st yr)

ORAL CONTRACEPTIVES

PATIENT MANAGEMENT

Practice Guidelines for Oral Contraceptive (OC) Selection: Summary

1 = first choice, combination formulation containing 30–35 µg of ethinyl estradiol except where noted. See footnotes.
2 = second choice, combination formulation containing 30–35 µg of ethinyl estradiol except where noted. See footnotes.

Patient Characteristics	Progestin Androgenic Activity		
	Low	Medium	High
	Norgestimate Desogestrel Norethindrone 0.4–0.5 mg monophasic	Levonorgestrel triphasic Norethindrone 1 mg monophasic or triphasic Norethindrone acetate 1 mg Ethynodiol diacetate 1 mg	Norgestrel 0.3 mg Norethindrone acetate 1.5–2.5 mg Levonorgestrel 0.15 mg

General formulation selections for women initiating OC use

New start	1	2
Adolescent	1	2
Perimenopause	1	2
Postpartum (lactating)	If no supplemental feedings and no menses, conception unlikely for 2–3 mos; if OC desired, progestin-only pill recommended 6 wks after delivery. Replace with combination pill when supplemental feeding introduced.	
Postpartum (nonlactating) (start at 2 wks)	1	2

Formulation selections in minimizing or managing unwanted OC side effects

Breakthrough bleeding	1[a]	1[a]
Weight gain	1	2
Acne/hirsutism	1	2
Headaches/common migraine	1[b, c]	2
Nausea	1[b, d]	2
Breast tenderness	1[b, d]	2
Mood change	1[b]	2

Formulation selections in minimizing or managing OC adverse effects

Adverse lipid/lipoprotein effects (except hypertri-glyceridemia)	1	2
Adverse carbohydrate effects	No current formulations have a clinically significant effect on glucose metabolism.	
Adverse thrombotic effects	Thrombotic effects are primarily related to the dose of the estrogen component; use OC containing <50 µg estrogen or other method.	

[a]The lowest incidence of breakthrough bleeding appears to be with formulations containing either levonorgestrel, norgestimate, or desogestrel. If breakthrough bleeding persists after switching from one such formulation to another—and if poor compliance, infection, and other potential problems have been ruled out—placement of the patient on a preparation containing 50 µg estrogen may be considered.
[b]A formulation containing a progestin with low androgenic activity remains the agent of choice, but evidence for a clear advantage in this parameter is lacking; if the problem persists, switching to a pill containing a different type of progestin may be beneficial in some individuals.
[c]If headache occurs exclusively during the pill-free interval, use daily, continuous, combined OCs to avoid cyclicity.
[d]This effect is largely estrogenic and infrequent with low-estrogen-dose OCs. If the problem persists, a 20- µg ethinyl estradiol formulation may be tried.

74

ORAL CONTRACEPTIVES

Practice Guidelines for Oral Contraceptive (OC) Selection: Summary

1 = first choice, combination formulation containing 30–35 μg of ethinyl estradiol except where noted. See footnotes.
2 = second choice, combination formulation containing 30–35 μg of ethinyl estradiol except where noted. See footnotes.

Patient Characteristics	Progestin Androgenic Activity		
	Low	Medium	High
	Norgestimate Desogestrel Norethindrone 0.4–0.5 mg monophasic	Levonorgestrel triphasic Norethindrone 1 mg monophasic or triphasic Norethindrone acetate 1 mg Ethynodiol diacetate 1 mg	Norgestrel 0.3 mg Norethindrone acetate 1.5–2.5 mg Levonorgestrel 0.15 mg

Formulation selections for women with medical conditions

	Low	Medium	High
Acne/hirsutism	1	2	
Obesity	1	2	
History of vascular disease (e.g., thromboembolism, coronary artery disease)	Contraindication		
Hypertension (uncontrolled)	Contraindication		
Hypertension (controlled or history of pregnancy-induced)	1	2	
Hypercholesterolemia	1	2	
Hypertriglyceridemia	OCs contraindicated above 350–600 mg/dL, depending on panel member's view and presence/absence of other factors (e.g., low HDL); with mild elevations, a norgestimate-containing OC may be preferred.		
Smoker >35 yrs of age	Contraindication		
Smoker 30–35 yrs of age	1[a]	1 (<50 μg estrogen)	
Heavy smoker <30 yrs of age	1[a]	1 (<50 μg estrogen)	
Family history of coronary heart disease	1	2	
Classic migraine	Contraindication		
Common migraine	1[b]	2	
Depression	1[b]	2	
Family history of breast cancer	1[b, c]	2	
Personal history of breast cancer	Contraindication		
Benign breast disease	1[b, d]	2	
Diabetes/gestational diabetes	1[b]	2	
Antiepileptic drug use	Formulation containing 50 μg estrogen may be preferable.		
Family history of ovarian cancer	1	2	
Sickle cell	1	2	
Prosthetic heart valve	1	2	
Anticoagulant use	1	2	
Mitral valve prolapse	1	2	

[a]There is no epidemiologic evidence indicating that there is a difference in risk of venous thrombosis in 20-μg ethinyl estradiol and 30–35-μg ethinyl estradiol OCs in smokers as well as nonsmokers.

continued

75

ORAL CONTRACEPTIVES

[b]A formulation containing a progestin with low androgenic activity remains the agent of choice, but evidence for a clear advantage in this parameter is lacking; if the problem persists, switching to a pill containing a different type of progestin may be beneficial in some individuals.
[c]A formulation containing a progestin with low androgenic activity remains the agent of choice, but there is no evidence that any particular OC formulation is preferable in women with a family history of breast cancer.
[d]OCs generally protect against the development of benign breast disease; a formulation containing a progestin with low androgenic activity remains the agent of first choice.

Practice Guidelines for Oral Contraceptive (OC) Selection: Summary

1 = first choice, combination formulation containing 30–35 µg of ethinyl estradiol except where noted. See footnotes.
2 = second choice, combination formulation containing 30–35 µg of ethinyl estradiol except where noted. See footnotes.

Patient Characteristics	Progestin Androgenic Activity		
	Low	Medium	High
	Norgestimate Desogestrel Norethindrone 0.4–0.5 mg monophasic	Levonorgestrel triphasic Norethindrone 1 mg monophasic or triphasic Norethindrone acetate 1 mg Ethynodiol diacetate 1 mg	Norgestrel 0.3 mg Norethindrone acetate 1.5–2.5 mg Levonorgestrel 0.15 mg

Formulation selections in women for whom OCs are being considered in some measure for therapeutic purposes

	Low	Medium	High
Ovulatory dysfunctional uterine bleeding	1	2	
Persistent anovulation	1	2	
Premature ovarian failure	1	2	
Dysmenorrhea	1[a, b]	1[a, b]	
Functional ovarian cysts	1 (monophasic only)		2 (monophasic only)
Mittelschmerz	1[a]	2	
Endometriosis (pain)		1 (monophasic continuous)	2 (monophasic continuous)
Bleeding with blood dyscrasias		1 (continuous)	2 (continuous)

[a]A formulation containing a progestin with low androgenic activity remains the agent of choice, but evidence for a clear advantage in this parameter is lacking; if the problem persists, switching to a pill containing a different type of progestin may be beneficial in some individuals.
[b]A formulation containing a progestin with low androgenic activity remains the agent of first choice and may be used in combination with a prostaglandin synthetase inhibitor. If dysmenorrhea persists, options include the use of an agent with higher androgenic activity plus a prostaglandin synthetase inhibitor or diagnostic tests to rule out endometriosis.
Source: Adapted from Mishell DR, Darney PD, et al. Practice guidelines for OC selection: update. Dialogues Contracept 5(4):7, 1997.

ORAL CONTRACEPTIVES

CURRENTLY AVAILABLE ORAL CONTRACEPTIVES

Product	Manufacturer	Estrogen (µg)	Progestin (mg)
Combined oral contraceptives: monophasic extended cycle			
Seasonale	Duramed	30 EE	0.15 LNG
Combined oral contraceptives: monophasic products			
Alesse	Wyeth	20 EE	0.1 LNG
Aviane	Barr	20 EE	0.1 LNG
Lessina	Barr	20 EE	0.1 LNG
Levlite	Berlex	20 EE	0.1 LNG
Loestrin	Pfizer	20 EE	1 NEA
Loestrin Fe 1/20	Pfizer	20 EE	1 NEA
Junel 1/20	Barr	20 EE	1 NEA
Junel Fe 1/20	Barr	20 EE	1 NEA
Microgestin 1/20	Watson	20 EE	1 NEA
Microgestin Fe 1/20	Watson	20 EE	1 NEA
Levlen 28	Berlex	30 EE	0.15 LNG
Levora 21	Watson	30 EE	0.15 LNG
Nordette	Monarch	30 EE	0.15 LNG
Portia	Barr	30 EE	0.15 LNG
Desogen	Organon	30 EE	0.15 DSG
Ortho-Cept	Ortho-McNeil	30 EE	0.15 DSG
Apri	Barr	30 EE	0.15 DSG
Cryselle	Barr	30 EE	0.3 NOR
Lo/Ovral	Wyeth	30 EE	0.3 NOR
Low-Ogestrel	Watson	30 EE	0.3 NOR
Loestrin 1.5/30	Pfizer	30 EE	1.5 NEA
Loestrin Fe 1.5/30	Pfizer	30 EE	1.5 NEA
Junel 1.5/30	Barr	30 EE	1.5 NEA
Junel Fe 1.5/30	Barr	30 EE	1.5 NEA
Microgestin Fe 1.5/30	Watson	30 EE	1.5 NEA
Yasmin	Berlex	30 EE	3 DRO
MonoNessa	Watson	35 EE	0.25 NGM
Ortho-Cyclen	Ortho-McNeil	35 EE	0.25 NGM
Spirintec	Barr	35 EE	0.25 NGM
Ovcon 35	Warner Chilcott	35 EE	0.4 NE
Brevicon	Watson	35 EE	0.5 NE
Modicon	Ortho-McNeil	35 EE	0.5 NE
Necon 0.5/35	Watson	35 EE	0.5 NE

77

ORAL CONTRACEPTIVES

Product	Manufacturer	Estrogen (μg)	Progestin (mg)
Nelova 10/11	Warner Chilcott	35 EE	0.5, 1 NE
Necon 1/35	Watson	35 EE	1 NE
Norinyl 1+35	Watson	35 EE	1 NE
Nortrel 1/35	Barr	35 EE	1 NE
Ortho-Novum 1/35	Ortho-McNeil	35 EE	1 NE
Genora 1/35	Physicians Total Care	35 EE	1 NE
Nelova 1/35	Warner Chilcott	35 EE	1 NE
Demulen 1/35	Pfizer	35 EE	1 ED
Zovia 1/35E (21/28)[a]	Watson	35 EE	1 ED
Ovral	Wyeth	50 EE	0.5 NOR
Ogestrel 0.5/50	Watson	50 EE	0.5 NOR
Demulen 1/50	Pfizer	50 EE	1 ED
Zovia 1/50E	Watson	50 EE	1 ED
Ovcon 50	Warner Chilcott	50 EE	1 NE
Genora 1/50	Physicians Total Care	50 MES	1 NE
Necon 1/50	Watson	50 MES	1 NE
Nelova 1/50M	Warner Chilcott	50 MES	1 NE
Norinyl 1+50	Watson	50 MES	1 NE
Ortho-Novum 1/50	Ortho-McNeil	50 MES	1 NE

Combined oral contraceptives: biphasic products with 2-day hormone-free interval

Kariva	Barr	10, 20 EE	0.15 DSG
Mircette	Organon	10, 20 EE	0.15 DSG

Combined oral contraceptives: biphasic products

Necon 10/11	Watson	35 EE	0.5, 1 NE
Ortho-Novum 10/11	Ortho-McNeil	35 EE	0.5, 1 NE
Jenest-28	Organon	35 EE	0.5, 1 NE

Combined oral contraceptives: triphasic products: constant estrogen with a phasic progestin dose

Cyclessa	Organon	25 EE	0.1, 0.125, 0.15 DSG
Velivet	Barr	25 EE	0.1, 0.125, 0.15 DSG
Ortho Tri-Cyclen Lo	Ortho McNeil	25 EE	0.18, 0.215, 0.25 NGM
Ortho Tri-Cyclen	Ortho McNeil	35 EE	0.18, 0.215, 0.25 NGM
Tri-Sprintec	Barr	35 EE	0.18, 0.215, 0.25 NGM
Ortho-Novum 7/7/7	Ortho McNeil	35 EE	0.5, 0.75, 1 NE

ORAL CONTRACEPTIVES

Product	Manufacturer	Estrogen (μg)	Progestin (mg)
Nortel 7/7/7	Barr	35 EE	0.5, 0.75, 1 NE
Necon 7/7/7	Watson	35 EE	0.5, 0.75, 1 NE
Tri-Norinyl	Watson	35 EE	0.5, 1, 0.5 NE

Triphasic products: phasic estrogen dose with a progestin dose

Trivora	Watson	30, 40, 30 EE	0.05, 0.075, 0.125 LNG
Triphasil	Wyeth	30, 40, 30 EE	0.05, 0.075, 0.125 LNG
Tri-Levlen	Berlex	30, 40, 30 EE	0.05, 0.075, 0.125 LNG
Enpresse	Barr	30, 40, 30 EE	0.05, 0.075, 0.125 LNG

Triphasic products: constant progestin with a phasic estrogen dose

Estrostep Fe	Pfizer	20, 30, 35 EE	1 NEA

Oral contraceptives: progestin only

Ovrette	Wyeth	—	0.075 NOR
Camila	Barr	—	0.35 NE
Errin	Barr	—	0.35 NE
Nor-QD	Watson	—	0.35 NE
Jolivette	Watson	—	0.35 NE
Nora-BE	Watson	—	0.35 NE
Ortho-Micronor	Ortho-McNeil	—	0.35 NE

COC, combined oral contraceptive; DRO, drospirenone; DSG, desogestrel; ED, ethynodiol diacetate; EE, ethinyl estradiol; LNG, levonorgestrel; MES, mestranol; NE, norethindrone; NEA, norethindrone acetate; NGM, norgestimate; NOR, norgestrel.

ORAL CONTRACEPTIVES

METABOLIC EFFECTS OF ORAL CONTRACEPTIVES

Myocardial Infarction

- 2nd-generation OCs ↑ risk of myocardial infarction by approximately twofold among users even after controlling for cardiovascular risk factors (Tanis et al., 2001).
- Major mortality risk in smokers >35 yrs of age

Ischemic Stroke

- Risk of ischemic stroke is not significantly different in women with simple migraine (no aura) compared to those with classic migraine (with aura) (Curtis et al., 2002).
- OCs should not be used for women with visual changes or focal neurologic deficits associated with migraines.

Hemorrhagic Stroke (Farley et al., 1999)

- <35 yrs old → no increased risk for OC users
- >35 yrs old → 2.2-fold higher risk for users (95% confidence interval [CI], 1.5–3.3)

Venous Thromboembolism

- Minimal risk of thrombosis associated with OCs (3/10,000 vs. 8/10,000 in pregnancy). If a patient develops a thrombotic complication while taking OCs, should check antithrombin (AT) III, protein C, protein S, activated protein C resistance, factor V Leiden, prothrombin G20210A mutation, and homocysteine.
- For those with a heterozygous or homozygous factor V Leiden mutation (5% prevalence), the risk of thrombosis on OCs is 28.5/10,000) (Vandenbroucke et al., 1994).
- Progestins alone are associated with a lower risk of venous thrombosis; however, the risk among women with a history of thrombosis is unknown.
- **In the absence of a clear family history of venous thrombosis, there is little justification to screen for prothrombotic mutations.**

Hypertension

- No ↑ incidence of clinically significant hypertension (HTN) has been reported to date.
- Hormonal contraception can safely be provided based on careful review of medical history and blood pressure (BP) measurement; for most women, no further evaluation is necessary (Stewart et al., 2001).

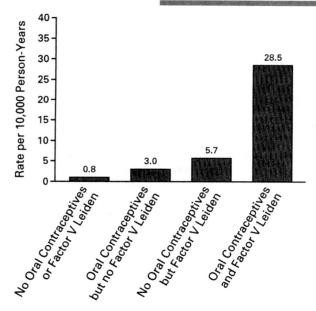

Source: Reproduced with permission from Vandenbroucke JP, Rosing J, Bloemenkamp KW, Middeldorp S, et al. Oral contraceptives and the risk of venous thrombosis. *N Engl J Med* 344:1527, 2001.

Carbohydrate Metabolism

- Insulin resistance and glucose changes with low-dose monophasic and multiphasic OCs are so minimal that it is now believed that they are of no clinical significance.
- OCs do not increase risk of diabetes mellitus (DM).

Other Effects

- Minimally ↑ risk of gallbladder disease (secondary to change in composition of bile due to ↑ cholesterol from E), although low-dose OCs yet to be tested.
- OCs contraindicated in acute or chronic cholestatic liver disease.
- Nausea and breast discomfort are most intense within first few months and usually disappear (lower incidence with low-dose pills).
- No causal association between OCs and weight gain (Gupta, 2000).
- ↑ Erythrocyte sedimentation rate (ESR)/total Fe-binding capacity; ↓ prothrombin time (PT)

ORAL CONTRACEPTIVES

- Telangiectasia; melasma
- Thick cervical mucus (leukorrhea)
- Rarely → depression/↓ libido
- Progestin-associated side effects: mood swings, depression, fatigue, ↓ libido, weight gain

ORAL CONTRACEPTIVES AND CANCER (Mishell, 1982)

Breast Cancer (Schlesselman, 1995)

- After 2 yrs of use, there is a 40% reduction in fibrocystic disease.
- Conflicting data, but epidemiologic studies have generally not demonstrated an association between OC use and breast cancer.
- A case-control study on a total of 4575 women aged 35–64 yrs found current or former OC use was not associated with a significant ↑ risk of breast cancer: odds ratio (OR), 1.0 (0.8–1.3) (Marchbanks et al., 2002).

Cervical Cancer

- Risk for dysplasia and carcinoma *in situ* ↑ with use of OCs for >1 yr; invasive cancer may be ↑ after 5 yrs of use, reaching a twofold ↑ after 10 yrs; ↑ risk for both adenocarcinoma and squamous cell carcinoma (Smith et al., 2003; Green et al., 2003).
- It is uncertain if the ↑ risk persists after discontinuation of OCs.
- Risk in human papillomavirus (HPV)-positive OC users may be related to the 16α-hydroxyestrone metabolite of E_2, which can act as a cofactor with oncogenic HPV to promote cell proliferation (Newfield et al., 1998).
- There are many confounding variables, and the conclusions regarding cervical cancer are not definite.

Endometrial Cancer

- ↓ Cancer risk (adenocarcinoma, adenosquamous carcinoma, and adenoacanthoma) by 56%, 67%, and 72% with use of combined OCs for 4, 8, and 12 yrs (Schlesselman and Collins, 1999).
- Protection persists for up to 20 yrs after discontinuation (Schlesselman and Collins, 1999).
- Lower dose (30–35 µg) OCs provide comparable protection (Weiderpass et al., 1999).

Ovarian Cancer (Ness et al., 2000; Royar et al., 2001)

- ↓ Cancer risk (serous, endometrioid, mucinous, and clear cell) by 41%, 54%, and 61% with use of OCs for 4, 8, and 12 years (Schlesselman and Collins, 1999).
- Protection persists for up to 20 yrs after discontinuation (Schlesselman and Collins, 1999).

- There may not be a protective effect for those with *BRCA1* or *BRCA2* mutation (Modan et al., 2001), although a case-control study found a 50% ↓ in risk in past OC users with *BRCA* mutations compared with OC nonusers with the same mutations (Narod et al., 1998).

Colorectal Cancer

- OCs may protect women from developing colorectal cancer:
  - Relative risk (RR) of colon cancer in OC users: 0.82 (95% confidence interval [CI], 0.74–0.92) (Fernandez et al., 2001)

Tumors of the Liver

- Hepatocellular adenoma risk (1/1 million OC users) is related to duration and dose of the pill; no such tumor found to date with low-dose formulations.
- World Health Organization (WHO) found no association between OCs and hepatocellular carcinoma.

Summary of Oral Contraceptives and Cancer

Form of Cancer	Risk with Oral Contraceptives (OCs)
Breast	OCs ↑ risk of breast cancer (24%) for women <30 yrs, but the added risk declines to no increase 10 or more yrs after stopping OCs. Current or past use in women 35–64 yrs does not alter risk of breast cancer compared with never-users.
Cervical	OCs ↑ risk of cervical cancer (10%) and may be associated with an additional six cases (primarily for those with papillomavirus infection) in 100,000 pill users aged 25–50 yrs.
Endometrial	OCs ↓ endometrial cancer (60%) and prevent 25 cases in 100,000 pill users, aged 25–50 yrs.
Ovarian	OCs ↓ ovarian cancer (40%) and prevent 14 cases in 100,000 pill users, aged 25–50 yrs.

Source: Based on data from the National Cancer Institute.

ORAL CONTRACEPTIVES

ENDOCRINE EFFECTS

Adrenal Gland
- ↑ Free and active cortisol (F) levels but still within normal limits
- Normal pit-adrenal reaction to stress in women taking OCs

Thyroid Gland
- No change in free thyroxine

ORAL CONTRACEPTIVES AND REPRODUCTION

Inadvertent Use while Pregnant
- Initial reports linking OCs to congenital malformations have not been substantiated.
- Risk of a significant congenital anomaly is no greater than the general rate of 2–3%.

Subsequent Fertility
- Delay in achieving pregnancy: 90% conceive by 15 mos compared with 90% by 12 mos if discontinuing condoms or other method.
- 50% conceive by 3 mos; after 2 yrs, maximum of 15% (nulliparous) and 7% (multiparous) fail to conceive.
- Spontaneous loss: no ↑ (actually less, 0.3% vs. 1.0% for non-OC users)
- Pregnancy outcome: ↑ dizygotic twinning (1.6% vs. 1.0%) in women who conceive soon after cessation of OCs.

Oral Contraceptives and Breast-Feeding
- ↓ Quantity and quality of lactation (no matter the starting month), although no impairment of infant growth
- ↓ Lactation at 3.7 mos vs. 4.6 mos for controls
- It has been argued that the threshold for ovulation suppression is ≥5 feedings for ≥65 mins/day of suckling duration.
- Amenorrheic women who exclusively breast feed at regular intervals, including nighttime, during the first 6 mos have the contraceptive protection equivalent to that provided by OCs; with menstruation or after 6 mos, the risk of ovulation increases.
- The progestin-only pill has no negative impact on breast milk, and some studies show ↑ milk production.

Initiation of Oral Contraceptives in Postpartum Period
- Rule of 3s for postpartum (pp) contraception:
  - Full breast-feeding → begin OCs *3 mos* pp
  - Partial or no breast-feeding → begin in *3rd wk* pp

ORAL CONTRACEPTIVES

Postpill Amenorrhea
- No evidence that OCs cause secondary amenorrhea
- Women who have not resumed menstrual function within 6 mos should be evaluated as any other patient with secondary amenorrhea.

ORAL CONTRACEPTIVES AND INFECTION
Bacterial Sexually Transmitted Diseases
- ≥12 mos' use necessary to achieve protection in OC users against pelvic inflammatory disease (PID); mechanism unknown:
  - Cervical mucus thickening?
  - Decreased menstruum?

Viral Sexually Transmitted Diseases
- No proven association between OCs and human immunodeficiency virus (HIV)/HPV/hepatitis B virus (HBV)

PATIENT MANAGEMENT

Absolute contraindications
  Thrombophlebitis.
  Markedly impaired liver function.
  Breast cancer (see table below).
  Undiagnosed vaginal bleeding.
  Pregnancy.
  Smokers >35 yrs old.
  Vascular disease associated with lupus (use progesterone-only pill or intrauterine device).
  Current or past deep vein thrombosis or pulmonary embolus.

Relative contraindications
  Migraines: ↑ risk stroke vs. improvement.
  Hypertension in those >35 yrs old (see table below).
  Diabetes mellitus: the effective contraception outweighs the small risk in diabetic women <35 yrs old.
  Elective surgery: probably less important with today's low-dose pill.
  Antiepileptic drugs may ↓ effectiveness of OCs.
  Sickle cell disease or sickle C: protection warrants use of low-dose pill.
  Gallbladder disease.

ORAL CONTRACEPTIVES

American College of Obstetricians and Gynecologists Guidelines	Comment
Smoker >35 yrs old	Risk unacceptable
Hypertension	
BP controlled	Risk acceptable
BP uncontrolled	Risk unacceptable
History of stroke, ischemic heart disease, or venous thromboembolism	Risk unacceptable
Diabetes	Risk acceptable if no other CV risk factors and no end-organ damage
Hypercholesterolemia	Risk acceptable if low-density lipoprotein <160 mg/dL and no other risk factors
Multiple CV risk factors	Not addressed
Migraine headache	
<35 yrs old	Risk acceptable
>35 yrs old	Risk outweighs benefit
With aura	Risk unacceptable
Breast cancer	
Current disease	Risk unacceptable
Past disease, no active disease for 5 yrs	Risk unacceptable
Family history of breast or ovarian cancer	Risk acceptable

BP, blood pressure; CV, cardiovascular.
Note: Progestin-only pill or intrauterine devices are preferable for those with a prior stroke, diabetes with vascular disease, diabetes and >35 yrs old, or hypertensive with vascular disease.

Surveillance
• Every year for pelvic examination, Pap smear, blood pressure evaluation

Proper Pill Taking
• Effective contraception is present during the first cycle of pill use, provided the pills are started ≤5th day of cycle; Sunday starts usually avoid weekend bleeding.
• Postponing a period can be achieved by omitting the 7-day hormone-free interval.
• Missed pills:
  ▪ 1 Missed pill → take 1 pill as soon as possible, then resume.
  ▪ 2 Missed pills (in first 2 wks) → take 2 pills × 2 days with backup × 7 days.
  ▪ 3 Missed pills (in 3rd wk or more than 2 anytime) → backup × 7 days

CLINICAL PROBLEMS
Breakthrough Bleeding

- Most frequently occurs in first few months of use (10–30% in 1st mo, 1–10% in 3rd mo).
- Occurs due to tissue breakdown as the endometrium adjusts its architecture.
- If BTB just before end of pill cycle → stop pills, wait 7 days, and start new cycle.
- Control of BTB: estradiol valerate, 5 mg IM × 1 dose.
- There is no evidence that any specific formulation is significantly superior to any other in terms of the rate of BTB; in general, pills with high doses of E and P_4 have the lowest rates of BTB.

Amenorrhea

- There is no harmful, permanent consequence of developing amenorrhea while taking OCs.
- Incidence: 1st yr = 1%; several years = 5%
- A simple test for pregnancy is to assess the basal body temperature (BBT) during the end of the pill-free week:
  - <98°F (36.8°C): pregnancy

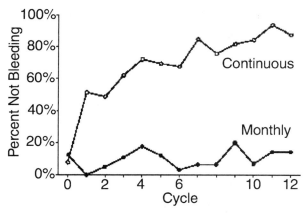

Rates of amenorrhea for continuous vs. monthly oral contraceptives. (Source: Reproduced with permission from Miller L, Hughes JP. Continuous combination oral contraceptive pills to eliminate withdrawal bleeding: a randomized trial. *Obstet Gynecol* 101[4]:653, 2003.)

ORAL CONTRACEPTIVES

Weight Gain
- No association between OCs and weight gain

Acne
- Improvement shown (even with 20-μg-EE OCs) (Thorneycroft et al., 1999)
  - $E_2 \rightarrow \downarrow$ gonadotropins + $\uparrow$ sex hormone–binding globulin (SHBG) to bind T
  - Progestins $\rightarrow \downarrow$ gonadotropins + $\uparrow$ T metabolism + $\downarrow$ 5α-reductase
  - Yasmin (ethinyl estradiol, 30 μg; drospirenone, 3 mg) may be OC of choice for treament of hirsutism/acne.

Ovarian Cysts
- Functional ovarian cysts occur less frequently in women taking higher-dose OCs.

Drugs Possibly Decreasing Oral Contraceptive Efficacy
- Rifampin/phenobarbital/phenytoin (Dilantin)/primidone/carbamazepine (Tegretol)

Alternative Route of Administration
- One pill per vagina every day if patient has significant nausea/vomiting with the oral route (Coutinho et al., 1993); equivalent efficacy against conception

SUMMARY OF ORAL CONTRACEPTIVE BENEFITS

Control of Menstrual Cycle Symptoms
- $\downarrow$ Dysmenorrhea
- $\downarrow$ Menorrhagia
- $\downarrow$ *Mittelschmerz*
- $\downarrow$ Anemia
- Possible $\downarrow$ in premenstrual syndrome (PMS)

Beneficial Effects on the Breasts
- $\downarrow$ Benign breast disease

Cancer Prevention
- $\downarrow$ Endometrial cancer
- $\downarrow$ Ovarian cancer

Reduction in Gynecologic Conditions
- $\downarrow$ Ectopic pregnancies
- $\downarrow$ Endometriosis
- Possibly $\downarrow$ fibroids
- Possibly $\downarrow$ ovarian cysts with higher-dose E_2

Other Benefits
- Treatment of androgen excess disorders
- $\uparrow$ Bone density

ORAL CONTRACEPTIVES

- Possibly ↓ rheumatoid arthritis

PROGESTIN-ONLY PILL
- Ovrette: Neogest: 0.075 mg norgestrel
- Micronor, NOR-QD: 0.35 mg norethindrone

Mechanism of Action
- Endometrium involutes and becomes hostile to implantation; cervical mucus becomes thick and impermeable (within 2–4 hrs).
- ~40% ovulate normally.
- Because of the low dose, the minipill must be taken q.d. at the same time of day.
- Immediate return to fertility on discontinuation
- Useful alternative for those:
  - Who are breast-feeding
  - Who have uncontrolled HTN
  - Who have persistent nausea while taking combination OCs
  - Who are smokers >35 yrs old
  - Who have a history of thromboembolic disease
  - Who have migraines

Efficacy
- In *motivated women,* the failure rate = that of combination pills.

Pill Taking
- Start on day 1 of menses with 7-day backup.
- If ≥2 missed pills and there is no menstrual bleeding in 4–6 wks → pregnancy test
- If >3 hrs late in taking pill → use backup × 48 hrs

Problems
- Bleeding:
  - 40% → normal ovulatory cycles
  - 40% → short, irregular cycles
  - 20% → irregular bleeding/spotting/amenorrhea

Clinical Decisions
- Progestin-only pills are a good choice for
  - Lactating women
  - Those >40 yrs old
  - Those for whom E is contraindicated
  - Those who complain of gastrointestinal (GI) upset/breast tenderness/headaches with OCs

ORAL CONTRACEPTIVES

POSTCOITAL EMERGENCY CONTRACEPTION
- Single act of intercourse 1–2 days before ovulation is associated with the following pregnancy rate:
  - Fertile couples = 8% (Wilcox et al., 1995)
  - Women 19–26 yrs old = 50% (Dunson et al., 2002)

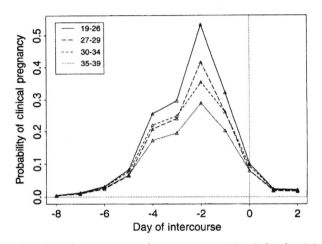

Source: Reproduced with permission from Dunson DB, Colombo M, Baird DD. Changes with age in the level and duration of fertility in the menstrual cycle. *Hum Reprod* 17:1399, 2002.

Yuzpe Method
- Within 72 hrs of coitus:
  - Preven (100 µg EE + 0.5 mg levonorgestrel) or Plan B (0.75 mg levonorgestrel) given twice, 12 hrs apart
  - Alternate: 8 tabs (4 given 12 hrs apart) of Lo/Ovral; Nordette; Levlen; Triphasil; Tri-Levlen
  - Antiemetic

ORAL CONTRACEPTIVES

- Success rate by timing:

Timing (Hrs)	Pregnancy Rate (%)
<72	0.8
72–120	1.8

Source: Adapted from Rodrigues I, Grou F, et al. Effectiveness of emergency contraceptive pills between 72 and 120 hours after unprotected sexual intercourse. *Am J Obstet Gynecol* 184(4):531, 2001.

Product	Manufacturer	Estrogen (μg)	Progestin (mg)	Pills per Dose[a]
Emergency contraception: progestin-only products				
Plan B	Women's Capital	—	0.75 mg LNG	1
Ovrette	Wyeth	—	0.075 mg NOR	20
Emergency contraception: combined estrogen-progestin products				
Preven	Gynétics	50 EE	0.25 LNG	2
Ogestrel	Watson	50 EE	0.5 NOR	2
Ovral	Wyeth	50 EE	0.5 NOR	2
Low-Ogestrel	Watson	30 EE	0.3 NOR	4
Lo/Ovral	Wyeth	30 EE	0.3 NOR	4
Levlen	Berlex	30 EE	0.15 LNG	4
Levora	Watson	30 EE	0.15 LNG	4
Nordette	Monarch	30 EE	0.15 LNG	4
Trivora	Watson	30 EE	0.125 LNG	4
Triphasil	Wyeth	30 EE	0.125 LNG	4
Tri-Levlen	Berlex	30 EE	0.125 LNG	4
Alesse	Wyeth	20 EE	0.1 LNG	5
Aviane	Barr	20 EE	0.1 LNG	5
Lessina	Barr	20 EE	0.1 LNG	5
Levlite	Berlex	20 EE	0.1 LNG	5

[a]Treatment consists of two separate doses taken 12 hrs apart.

- Advised for condom breakage/sexual assault/dislodged diaphragms or cervical caps
- Alternate method → mifepristone (RU486), 600 mg PO
- Mechanism of action:
  - Interference with implantation

ORAL CONTRACEPTIVES

- 2% failure rate
- The next menses after treatment usually occurs within 1 wk before or after the expected date.

Intrauterine Device Method

- Copper intrauterine device (IUD) (progestin IUD not studied as yet) may be placed within 5 days of unprotected intercourse.
- Mechanism of action:
  - Toxic to sperm
  - Inflammatory response initiated
- <1% failure rate
- Contraindications: multiple partners, active pelvic infection, victim of sexual assault

ORAL CONTRACEPTIVES FOR OLDER WOMEN (>40 YRS OLD)

- Use low-dose OCs or minipill
- Note: The E dose in even the low-dose OCs is at least four times greater than that necessary for postmenopausal treatment.
- Summary of benefits of OCs in perimenopausal women:
  - Effective contraception
  - Treatment of irregular menses/dysfunctional uterine bleeding (DUB), menorrhagia, and/or dysmenorrhea
  - ↓ Vasomotor symptoms
  - High bone density/fewer fractures (Michaelsson et al., 1999)
  - Prevention of ovarian and endometrial cancers
  - Treatment of acne

WHEN TO CHANGE TO HORMONE REPLACEMENT THERAPY FOR POSTMENOPAUSAL WOMEN

- Menopause diagnosis while on OCs: day 8 of pill-free interval (Creinin, 1996) → menopausal if:
  - FSH:LH >1, or
  - E_2 <20 pg/mL, or
  - FSH >30 mIU/mL
- Can also empirically switch to hormone replacement therapy (HRT) when patient enters mid-50s

ORAL CONTRACEPTIVES

ANOVULATION AND BLEEDING

- In an anovulatory women (serum P_4 <3 ng/dL measured 1 wk before menses) with proliferative or hyperplastic endometrium (without atypia), treat with 10 mg medroxyprogesterone (Provera) q.d., first 10 days of each month; if progestin treatment is ineffective, more aggressive treatment is warranted.
- Monthly progestin treatment should be continued until withdrawal bleeding ceases or menopausal symptoms are experienced.
- The use of a low-dose OC is recommended for contraception/prophylaxis against irregular, heavy anovulatory bleeding and the risk of endometrial hyperplasia.

NEWER METHODS OF CONTRACEPTION

Continuous Oral Contraception: Seasonale

- Levonorgestrel, 150 µg, and EE, 30 µg
- 84 days (active tablet) → 7 days (inert tablet)
- Use for dysmenorrhea, menorrhagia, menstrual migraines, premenstrual symptoms, anemia, ovarian cysts, endometriosis, or polycystic ovary syndrome (PCOS).
- Interrupt with a 5-day hiatus if there is BTB >4 days.

Monthly Injectable: Lunelle (0.5-cc aqueous solution; currently removed from the market)

- Estradiol cypionate, 5 mg; medroxyprogesterone, 25 mg
- IM injection every 23–33 days
- Physiologic level of E_2
- Initial irregular bleeding due to initial ↑ E_2 and subsequent E_2 plummet
- 5-yr pregnancy rate: 0.2%
- Ovulation 2 mos after last month of administration

Levonorgestrel Intrauterine Device: Mirena

- 20 µg/day levonorgestrel
- Use for menorrhagia, HRT with E_2
- ~90% Decreased menstrual blood loss by 1 yr
- 5-yr pregnancy rate: 0.71/100 women; ectopic rate: 0.02/100 women years

Vaginal Ring: NuvaRing

- Progestin: etonogestrel, 120 µg/day (serum: ~1500 pg/mL), and EE, 15 µg/day (serum: ~20 pg/mL)

ORAL CONTRACEPTIVES

- Worn for 3 of 4 wks and, although off-label (extended-cycle use is under study), if the ring is left for longer than 3 wks, the user is likely still protected from pregnancy for up to 35 days from the same ring.

Patch: Ortho Evra

- Progestin: norelgestromin, 20 µg/day, and EE, 20 µg/day
- Once-a-week administration for 3 of 4 wks
- 4- × 5-cm patch

10. Amenorrhea

DEFINITION
- Absence or suppression of menstruation; broadly classified as *primary* (a patient who has never menstruated) or *secondary* (a patient who previously had normal menstrual function).

PHYSIOLOGIC AMENORRHEA
- Prepubertal (menarche range, 9–17 yrs old)
- During lactation and pregnancy
  - When amenorrhea is present in a woman of child-bearing age, must first rule out pregnancy
- Postmenopausal

GENERAL CLASSIFICATION OF PATIENTS
- Physical examination is necessary only if primary amenorrhea with breast development

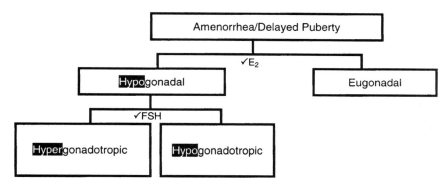

E_2, estradiol; FSH, follicle-stimulating hormone.

AMENORRHEA

HYPERGONADOTROPIC HYPOGONADISM

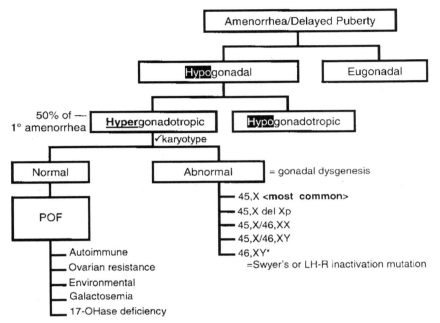

60% of multiple endocrine neoplasia (MEN) type I have associated premature ovarian failure (POF); 4% of MEN type II have associated POF; 15% of autoimmune polyglandular syndrome type I have associated POF; and 5% of autoimmune polyglandular syndrome type II have associated POF. LH-R, luteinizing hormone receptor; 17-OHase, 17-hydroxylase. *Abnormal for phenotype.

HYPOGONADOTROPIC HYPOGONADISM

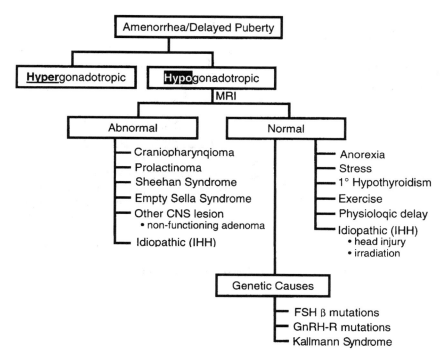

CNS, central nervous system; FSH, follicle-stimulating hormone; GnRH-R, gonadotropin-releasing hormone receptor; IHH, idiopathic hypogonadotropic hypogonadism; MRI, magnetic resonance imaging.

AMENORRHEA

EUGONADAL

```
                 Amenorrhea/Delayed Puberty
        ┌──────────────────────┴──────────────────────┐
   Hypogonadal                              Eugonadal
                              ┌──────────────────┴──────────────────┐
            ✓EmBx─  Chronic                          Outflow Tract
                    Anovulation                      Abnormality
                         ├─ PCOS                           ├─ Imperforate hymen
                         ├─ Stromal Hyperthecosis          ├─ Transverse vag. septum
                         └─ Insulin Resistance             ├─ Müllerian Agenesis
                                                           ├─ Androgen insensitivity
                                                           │    syndrome (Measure T)
                                                           └─ Intrauterine synechiae
```

EmBx, endometrial biopsy; PCOS, polycystic ovary syndrome; T, testosterone.

INITIAL EVALUATION

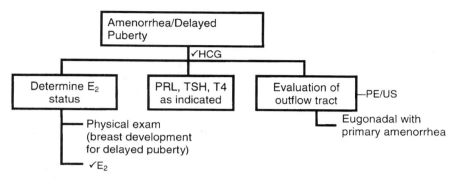

E_2, estradiol; HCG, human chorionic gonadotropin; PE/US, pelvic examination/ultrasound; PRL, prolactin; T4, thyroxine; TSH, thyroid-stimulating hormone.

DIAGNOSTIC ALGORITHM FOR AMENORRHEA

- Majority of cases accounted for by polycystic ovary syndrome (PCOS), hypothalamic amenorrhea, hyperprolactinemia, and ovarian failure.
  - β-Human chorionic gonadotropin (β-hCG), prolactin (PRL), thyroid-stimulating hormone (TSH), follicle-stimulating hormone (FSH), estradiol (E_2)
    ⇨ If there is gonadal failure, check karyotype.
    ⇨ If PRL is elevated, check somatomedin C (rule out growth hormone microadenoma) and magnetic resonance imaging (MRI).
  - Genital examination:
    ⇨ Blind or absent vagina with breast development usually indicates müllerian agenesis, transverse vaginal septum, or androgen insensitivity syndrome.

AMENORRHEA

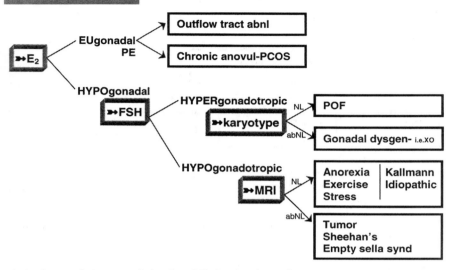

abnl, abnormal; E_2, estradiol; FSH, follicle-stimulating hormone; MRI, magnetic resonance imaging; NL, normal; PCOS, polycystic ovary syndrome; PE, pelvic examination; POF, primary ovarian failure; synd, syndrome.

DISTRIBUTION OF CAUSES OF PRIMARY AMENORRHEA

Category	Frequency (%)
Breast development	30
Müllerian agenesis	10
Androgen insensitivity	9
Constitutional delay	8
Vaginal septum	2
Imperforate hymen	1
No breast development: high FSH	40
Abnormal	20
46,XX	15
46,XY	5
No breast development: low FSH	30
Constitutional delay	10
Prolactinomas	5
Kallmann syndrome	2
Other central nervous system disorder	3
Stress, weight loss, anorexia	3
Polycystic ovary syndrome	3
Congenital adrenal hyperplasia	3
Other	1

FSH, follicle-stimulating hormone.
Source: Adapted from Reindollar RH, Novak M, et al. Adult-onset amenorrhea: a study of 262 patients. *Am J Obstet Gynecol* 155(3):531, 1986; and Bachmann GA, Kemmann E. Prevalence of oligomenorrhea and amenorrhea in a college population. *Am J Obstet Gynecol* 144(1):98, 1982.

PRIMARY AMENORRHEA
Definition
- Absence of menses by 15 yrs old in the presence of normal secondary sexual development (breasts)
- Within 5 yrs after breast development if that occurs before age 10
- Failure to initiate breast development by age 13

AMENORRHEA

Gonadal Abnormalities

- 60% of primary amenorrhea patients cannot synthesize ovarian steroids.

Gonadal Dysgenesis (Turner Syndrome)

- Most common error in fetal gonadal differentiation, karyotype 45,XO

Pure Gonadal Dysgenesis

- *Pure gonadal dysgenesis* is a term used to describe sexually immature girls with normal karyotype but elevated FSH levels.

XY Gonadal Dysgenesis (Swyer Syndrome)

- Phenotypically, patients are female, with normal female internal/external genitalia and streak ovaries. Always verify presence of cervix/uterus in the event of rare inactivating mutation of luteinizing hormone (LH) receptor, which would require urology assistance to find gonad.

Mixed Gonadal Dysgenesis

- Rare anomaly of asymmetric gonadal development, with a germ-cell tumor or testis on one side and a streak or no gonad on the other side.
- Such persons usually are mosaics with XO/XY karyotypes. They have anomalous external genitalia and exhibit virilization at or after puberty.

Ovarian Insensitivity Syndrome (Savage Syndrome)

- Functional ovarian failure. Perhaps an ovarian cell membrane gonadotropin-receptor defect. The ovary is unable to respond to the gonadotropin stimulus.

CYP17 (17α-Hydroxylase) Deficiency

- Primary amenorrhea, no secondary sexual characteristics, female phenotype, hypertension, hypokalemia. $\downarrow$ Cortisol production $\rightarrow$ $\uparrow$ adrenocorticotropic hormone (ACTH) $\rightarrow$ $\uparrow$ mineralocorticoids (therefore, Na^+-retention, K^+-loss, hypertension).

Extragonadal Anomalies

- 40% of primary amenorrhea cases

Congenital Absence of the Uterus and Vagina

- Müllerian agenesis (Mayer-Rokitansky-Küster-Hauser syndrome) is the most common defect (Griffin et al., 1976) (see Chapter 4, Müllerian Agenesis).

Male Pseudohermaphroditism (Androgen Insensitivity) (Morris and Mahesh, 1953)

- Inadequate or inappropriate feminization of the urogenital sinus and external genitalia may be caused by enzymatic deficiencies in gonadal or adrenal steroidogenesis. The most common cause of this condition is the *androgen insensitivity syndrome*.

Note: Normal-appearing female without a uterus:
  Androgen insensitivity: XY (5α-reductase [5αR] deficiency); (–) pubic and axillary hair; normal male-range testosterone
  Müllerian agenesis: XX; (+) pubic and axillary hair; female-range testosterone

Female Pseudohermaphroditism

- Extraovarian sources of androgen may virilize the external genitalia in genetically normal females with normal internal genitalia. Congenital adrenal hyperplasia is the most common cause. Excess adrenal androgen secretion is usually associated with defective cortisol synthesis due to P450c21 (21-hydroxylase) or P450-11β (11β-OHase) deficiency.

Abnormal Hypothalamic-Pituitary Function

- Central nervous system (CNS) and pituitary lesions. Kallmann syndrome (olfactogenital dysplasia); pituitary dysfunction, manifested by isolated gonadotropin deficiency; and destruction of the anterior pituitary by neoplasms (craniopharyngioma) or metastases all resulting in hypogonadotropic hypogonadism.

AMENORRHEA

DISTRIBUTION OF CAUSES OF SECONDARY AMENORRHEA

Category	Frequency (%)
Low or normal FSH	66
Weight loss/anorexia	
Nonspecific hypothalamic	
Chronic anovulation, including polycystic ovary syndrome	
Hypothyroidism	
Cushing's syndrome	
Pituitary tumor, empty sella, Sheehan syndrome	
Gonadal failure: high FSH	12
46,XX	
Abnormal karyotype	
High prolactin	13
Anatomic	7
Asherman syndrome	
Hyperandrogenic states	2
Ovarian tumor	
Nonclassic adrenal hyperplasia	
Undiagnosed	

FSH, follicle-stimulating hormone.
Source: Adapted from Reindollar RH, Byrd JR, et al. Delayed sexual development: a study of 252 patients. *Am J Obstet Gynecol* 140(4):371, 1981.

SECONDARY AMENORRHEA
Definition
- Absence of menses for 3 mos
- Oligomenorrhea <9 cycles/yr
- Most commonly → PCOS, hypothalamic amenorrhea, hyperprolactinemia, and ovarian failure

Secondary Amenorrhea with Normal Ovarian Function
Intrauterine Synechiae (Asherman Syndrome)
- Ovarian function is normal. Amenorrhea is caused by intrauterine adhesions that obliterate the uterine cavity. Adhesions usually secondary to an induced abortion or postpartum curettage complicated by endometritis and intrauterine scarification. More common after pregnancy due to ↓ estrogen. Those with normal-appearing endometrium above the level of obstruction on transvaginal

ultrasound are likely to have successful hysteroscopic treatment and resumption of menses (Schlaff and Hurst, 1995).

- Four out of seven patients undergoing uterine artery embolization were subsequently found to have intrauterine adhesions (Honda et al., 2003).
- See end of chapter for American Society of Reproductive Medicine (ASRM) classification of intrauterine adhesions.

Endometrial Destruction Due to Infection

- *Tuberculosis* (TB) may occasionally cause sufficient endometrial scarification to cause amenorrhea.
- *Uterine schistosomiasis* is another rare cause of secondary amenorrhea.
- Irradiation

Secondary Amenorrhea with Decreased Ovarian Function

High Gonadotropin Levels (Premature Ovarian Failure)

- 10% of cases of secondary amenorrhea.
- An autoimmune mechanism has been suggested for the etiology.
- Surgical or radiation castration also causes high gonadotropin levels.

Low or Normal Gonadotropin Levels

- Patients with hypothalamic-pituitary dysfunction. Diagnosis of hypothalamic amenorrhea is usually made by exclusion. Hypothalamic amenorrhea $\rightarrow \uparrow$ cortisol. 83% of women with hypothalamic amenorrhea have trabecular bone density below the mean for controls.

Psychogenic Amenorrhea

- Stress can produce amenorrhea, perhaps due to corticotropin-releasing hormone (CRH) decreasing LH levels.

Weight Loss–Related Amenorrhea (Warren and Vande Wiele, 1973)

- Probably hypothalamic in origin. The *ratio* between *body fat and lean mass* plays a critical role in the onset and maintenance of menses. Gonadotropin levels are low-normal. Patients exhibit failure of pulsatile LH output. 30% of anorectics remain amenorrheic despite weight gain.
- 17% body fat is needed to initiate menses; 22% to maintain cycles (Frisch and McArthur, 1974).

Exercise-Induced Amenorrhea (Loucks et al., 1989)

- A persistent depression of circulating levels of E_2, progesterone (P_4), LH, and FSH is characteristic of exercise-induced amenorrhea.
- Surprisingly, $\downarrow$ bone loss, rather than $\uparrow$ in bone density, can result from vigorous exercise in amenorrheic athletes as compared to eumenorrheic athletes.

AMENORRHEA

- Menarche is delayed by exercise begun before menarche. May be sport specific (runners [50%] vs. swimmers [12%] [Sanborn and Jankowski, 1994]).

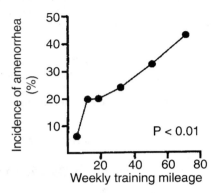

Correlation between training mileage and amenorrhea (Source: Reproduced with permission from Feicht CB, Johnson TS, Martin BJ, et al. Secondary amenorrhoea in athletes. *Lancet* 2[8100]:1145, 1978.)

Pseudocyesis
- The patient is overanxious to conceive and develops amenorrhea, morning sickness, abdominal enlargement, breast changes, and even perception of fetal movements. The pulsatile pattern of LH and PRL is markedly elevated, whereas FSH remains normal.

Central Nervous System Lesions
- Pituitary or parapituitary (i.e., craniopharyngioma) tumors are the CNS lesions most frequently associated with amenorrhea. Galactorrhea is frequently seen. Elevated PRL levels interfere with cyclicity at central and ovarian levels. Usually, there are other symptoms present.
- Sheehan syndrome: most commonly, a postpartum hemorrhage leading to pituitary apoplexy; mammary involution and failure of lactation are the earliest signs; loss of pubic and axillary hair common (see Chapter 13, Sheehan Syndrome).

Amenorrhea with Other Endocrinopathies
- Systemic endocrinopathies involving extragonadal glands. Abnormalities in thyroid function—either *hyperthyroidism* or *hypothyroidism* (Poretsky et al., 1986)—may produce amenorrhea; amenorrhea is more often seen in hyperthyroidism with exophthalmos. *Adrenal cortisol overproduction (Cushing's syndrome) or underproduction (Addison's syndrome)* may also interfere with

AMENORRHEA

normal menstrual function. *Juvenile diabetes mellitus* (DM) is associated with amenorrhea in 50% of cases.

Drug-Induced Amenorrhea

- Phenothiazine derivatives, reserpine, ganglionic blocking agents, and alkylating agents affect the hypothalamus and may cause amenorrhea.

Acute and Chronic Disease

- Amenorrhea is often associated with generalized, systemic illnesses such as lung disease, cardiac disease, renal disease, chronic uremia, severe infections, malabsorption syndromes involving poor nutrition, and neoplasms.

Secondary Amenorrhea with Increased Androgen Secretion

- PCOS (Stein-Leventhal syndrome): See Chapter 18, Polycystic Ovary Syndrome.
- Nonclassic adrenal hyperplasia
- Masculinizing adrenal or ovarian tumors

PROGESTIN WITHDRAWAL TEST

- Indirectly reflects hypothalamic-pituitary-ovarian activity. Patients with adequate endogenous estrogen bleed within 3–5 days after medication, indicating adequate endogenous estrogen stimulation of the endometrium. However, this is an inaccurate test, as there may be enough extragonadal estrogen present to allow for endometrial growth and, hence, withdrawal bleed. High false-positive (Rarick et al., 1990) and false-negative (Nakamura et al., 1996) rates.

AMENORRHEA

AMERICAN SOCIETY FOR REPRODUCTIVE MEDICINE
CLASSIFICATION OF INTRAUTERINE ADHESIONS

Patient's Name _____ Date _____ Chart # _____

Age _____ G _____ P _____ Sp Ab _____ VTP _____ Ectopic _____ Infertile Yes _____ No _____

Other Significant History (i.e. surgery, infection, etc.) _____

HSG _____ Sonography _____ Photography _____ Laparoscopy _____ Laparotomy _____

Extent of Cavity Involved	<1/3	1/3 - 2/3	>2/3
	1	2	4
Type of Adhesions	Filmy	Filmy & Dense	Dense
	1	2	4
Menstrual Pattern	Normal	Hypomenorrhea	Amenorrhea
	0	2	4

Prognostic Classification   HSG*   Hysteroscopy   Additional Findings: _____
                     Score   Score

Stage I   (Mild)   1-4   _____   _____   _____

Stage II   (Moderate)   5-8   _____   _____   _____

Stage III   (Severe)   9-12   _____   _____   _____
*All adhesions should be considered dense

Treatment (Surgical Procedures): _____

_____

_____

_____

Prognosis for Conception & Subsequent Viable Infant*

_____ Excellent (> 75%)

_____ Good (50-75%)

_____ Fair (25%-50%)

_____ Poor (< 25%)

*Physician's judgment based upon tubal patency.

Recommended Followup Treatment: _____

_____

_____

DRAWING

HSG Findings

Hysteroscopy Findings

Source: Reproduced with permission from The American Fertility Society classifications of adnexal adhesions, distal tubal occlusion, tubal occlusion secondary to tubal ligation, tubal pregnancies, mullerian anomalies and intrauterine adhesions. *Fertil Steril* 49(6):944, 1988.

11. Exercise-Induced Amenorrhea

DEFINITION
* Hypothalamic amenorrhea arising from a combination of energy drain, caloric deprivation, and/or exercise intensity

PATHOPHYSIOLOGY

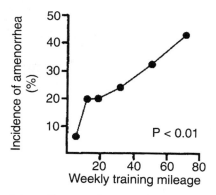

Correlation between training mileage and amenorrhea (Source: Reproduced with permission from Feicht CB, Johnson TS, et al. Secondary amenorrhoea in athletes. *Lancet* 2[8100]:1145, 1978.)

EXERCISE-INDUCED AMENORRHEA

- Hypogonadotropic hypoestrogenemia is often associated with the "female athlete triad" (Otis et al., 1997).

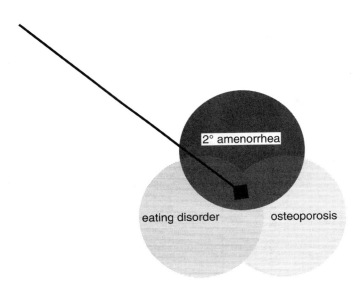

- The percentage contribution of weight loss and dietary restrictions to the syndrome of exercise-induced amenorrhea (EIA) is controversial:
  - EIA may occur with a relative caloric deficiency due to ↓ nutritional intake for the amount of energy expended (Laughlin and Yen, 1996).
  - A disrupted energy balance, accompanied by ↓ triiodothyronine (T_3) levels and loss of diurnal release of leptin from adipose cells, may lead to EIA (Laughlin and Yen, 1997).
- High-intensity exercise shifts estrogen metabolism from 16α to C-2 hydroxylation, which forms catecholestrogens that disrupt gonadotropin-releasing hormone (GnRH) pulsatility (i.e., ↓ GnRH secretion).

EXERCISE-INDUCED AMENORRHEA

- Likelihood of developing EIA:

HIGH

LOW

- Acute exercise
- Activities associated with low body weight (running, ballet, dancing)
- Sports with subjective scoring (figure skating, gymnastics)

- Swimming, biking

- Swimmers tend to have higher body weight and increased luteinizing hormone (LH) and dehydroepiandrosterone sulfate (DHEA-S) secretion (more polycystic ovary syndrome [PCOS]-like).
- In women who exercise at recreational levels (i.e., running ~12–15 miles/wk): 16% prevalence of anovulatory cycles despite regular (26–32 days) intervals of menses (De Souza et al., 1998).

CONSEQUENCES
- Menstrual disturbances
- Infertility
- Vaginal and breast atrophy
- ↓ Bone mineral density (lumbar spine)
- ↑ Total cholesterol

EVALUATION
- Diagnosis of exclusion
- Similar workup as for primary and/or secondary amenorrhea: human chorionic gonadotropin (hCG), prolactin (PRL), thyroid-stimulating hormone (TSH), follicle-stimulating hormone (FSH), anatomic evaluation, dual-energy x-ray absorptiometry (DXA) scan

EXERCISE-INDUCED AMENORRHEA

TREATMENT
General
1. ↓ Exercise
2. ↑ Caloric intake
3. Estrogen therapy (i.e., oral contraceptives [OCs]) (estradiol [E_2] will ↓ bone resorption) (Rickenlund et al., 2004)
4. Calcium: 1200–1500 mg/day (diet + 1 g supplemental calcium)
5. Vitamin D: 400 IU/day

- Although estrogen deficiency is the basis for the amenorrhea in EIA, nutritional factors may contribute. No randomized controlled study of estrogen treatment in athletes has been published.
- Recalcitrant low bone remodeling rate may explain the suboptimal response to antiresorptive agents such as estrogen and bisphosphonates (not recommended due to the unknown effects on a fetus from bisphosphonates residing in the bone for 10 yrs).

Infertility
1. ↓ Exercise
2. ↑ Caloric intake
3. Exogenous gonadotropins (FSH + LH)

- Clomiphene citrate or aromatase inhibitors tend to be ineffective due to a baseline hypoestrogenic state.

12. Ectopic Pregnancy

INCIDENCE (Lipscomb et al., 2000)
- 2% of pregnancies (1992); 9% of pregnancy-related deaths (5/10,000)
- Recurrence risk: approximately 15%

ETIOLOGY
- Tubal disease
  - In histologic sections of ectopic sites, there was a 45% incidence of pelvic inflammatory disease.
- Abnormal uterus
- Gonadotropin therapy
- Ratio of ectopic pregnancies (EPs) to all pregnancies:
  - All women—1:50
  - Copper intrauterine device (IUD)—1:16
  - Levonorgestrel IUD—1:2

DIAGNOSIS
- Signs and symptoms of eccyesis: severe abdominal pain (90%), vaginal spotting (80%), amenorrhea (80%), pelvic mass on examination (50%) (Pisarska et al., 1998)
- Most common location: ampullary region of tube (80%), isthmic (12%)

Human Chorionic Gonadotropin
- 0.79 mIU β-human chorionic gonadotropin (βhCG) per cell per day approximately 2 wks after fertilization (Braunstein et al., 1973)
- hCG produced 8–9 days after ovulation by cytotrophoblasts (for corpus luteum rescue)
- βhCG normally 100 mIU/mL at time of missed menses
- Levels rise in curvilinear fashion until plateau at 100,000 mIU/mL by 10 wks.
- βhCG 1000 mIU/mL at term

Gestational Age	↑ β-Human Chorionic Gonadotropin over 48 Hrs
<41 days	103%
41–56 days	33%
57–65 days	5%

- Linear increase early in pregnancy: mean doubling time for viable intrauterine pregnancy (IUP) = 48 hrs (only $\frac{1}{3}$ of EPs)
- hCG half-life ($t_{1/2}$) = 1 day

113

ECTOPIC PREGNANCY

- 90% of EPs have βhCG <6500 mIU/mL.
- Normal IUP should show at least **53% ↑ βhCG** in 48 hrs (Barnhart et al., 2004b).
- With suspected miscarriages, a rate of decline **<21% after 2 days** or 60% after 7 days suggests retained trophoblasts or an EP (Barnhart, 2004a).
- If βhCG <1000 mIU/mL → 88% of abnormal pregnancies (regardless of location) resolve without methotrexate (MTX).
- Note: Beware of the false-positive serum hCG due to heterophile antibodies (Cole, 1998).
- Of 18 brands, **First Response, Early Result** is the test most likely to detect a pregnancy at the time of the missed menses (best to include faintly discernible results and at extended reading time of 10 mins) (Cole et al., 2004).

Progesterone   (McCord et al., 1996)

- Serum progesterone (P_4) stays relatively constant from the 5th to 10th wk of pregnancy, then ↑ (Tulchinsky and Hobel, 1973).
- Single serum P_4 can be used as a screen for EP; it cannot be used to rule out an EP, however.

Progesterone (ng/mL)	Intrauterine Pregnancy (%)	Spontaneous Abortion (%)	Ectopic Pregnancy (%)
>25	—	—	2
20.0–24.9	—	—	4
<5.0	0.16	85	14
<2.5	0	—	—

Source: Adapted from McCord ML, Muram D, Buster JE, et al. Single serum progesterone as a screen for ectopic pregnancy: exchanging specificity and sensitivity to obtain optimal test performance. *Fertil Steril* 66:513, 1996.

Ultrasound

GS = 2 mm	28 days' estimated embryonic age
GS ≥10 mm	+ Embryo
GS ≥17 mm	+ Fetal cardiac activity (5 wks)

GS, gestational sac.

- Discriminatory βhCG value for transvaginal sonography (TVS) → >2000 mIU/mL

- Nonviability if (–) fetal cardiac activity associated with:
  - GS >17 mm or βhCG >30,000 mIU/mL
  - Presence of visible adnexal mass cannot be considered diagnostic of EP if βhCG <2000 mIU/mL unless a yolk sac, fetal pole, or FCA can be seen; otherwise, may just be a corpus luteum cyst.

Dilatation and Curettage

- If βhCG <2000 mIU/mL and abnormal βhCG rise, dilatation and curettage (D&C) eliminates the possibility of administering MTX unnecessarily to a patient with a nonviable IUP (Ailawadi et al, 2005).
- Rising or plateau of βhCG values 12–24 hrs after D&C is diagnostic of an EP.

Laparoscopy

- More of a therapeutic tool (linear salpingostomy vs. salpingectomy) rather than diagnostic at this time

Culdocentesis

- *Historical interest only at this time*
- Performed to establish the presence of intraperitoneal bleeding (ectopic/hemorrhagic corpus luteum)
- Contraindications: bleeding diathesis, large adnexal mass (carcinoma?)
- Secure posterior lip of the cervix with a tenaculum, use an 18-gauge spinal needle attached to a 20-mL syringe, insert into posterior cul-de-sac, inject 3–5 mL of saline to confirm placement, aspirate pooled peritoneal fluid.
- Normal peritoneal fluid = clear; nonclotting blood has undergone fibrinolysis and is a sign of intraperitoneal bleeding.
- Hematocrit of aspirate >15%, consistent with EP or hemorrhage from corpus luteum; if hematocrit <8%, this could be from a ruptured ovarian cyst or pelvic inflammation.

MEDICAL TREATMENT (Buster and Pisarska, 1999)

- MTX-folate antagonist that inactivates dihydrofolate reductase leading to ↓ tetrahydrofolate (essential cofactor in DNA and RNA synthesis during cell division).
- Single-dose MTX: 91.5% success (although ~20% require more than one course of treatment)
- History of a previous EP is an independent risk factor for failure (18.6%) of systemic MTX, but failure is not affected by previous treatment modality (salpingectomy, salpingostomy, MTX) (Lipscomb et al., 2004).
- Dose: MTX, 50 mg/m^2; m^2 = body surface area (BSA) (http://www.halls.md/body-surface-area/bsa.htm)

ECTOPIC PREGNANCY

Height	Surface area	Weight

Height (cm / in):
cm 200 — 79 in
78
195 — 77
76
190 — 75
74
185 — 73
72
180 — 71
70
175 — 69
68
170 — 67
66
165 — 65
64
160 — 63
62
155 — 61
60
150 — 59
58
145 — 57
56
140 — 55
54
135 — 53
52
130 — 51
50
125 — 49
48
120 — 47
46
115 — 45
44
110 — 43
42
105 — 41
40
cm 100 — 39 in

Surface area (m²):
2.80 m²
2.70
2.60
2.50
2.40
2.30
2.20
2.10
2.00
1.95
1.90
1.85
1.80
1.75
1.70
1.65
1.60
1.55
1.50
1.45
1.40
1.35
1.30
1.25
1.20
1.15
1.10
1.05
1.00
0.95
0.90
0.85 m²

Weight (kg / lb):
kg 150 — 330 lb
145 — 320
140 — 310
135 — 300
130 — 290
125 — 280
120 — 270
— 260
115 — 250
110 — 240
105 — 230
100 — 220
95 — 210
90 — 200
85 — 190
— 180
80 — 170
75 — 160
70 — 150
65 — 140
60 — 130
55 — 120
50 — 110
— 105
45 — 100
— 95
— 90
40 — 85
— 80
35 — 75
— 70
kg 30 — 66 lb

Body surface area nomogram. (Source: Reproduced with permission from DiSaia PJ, Creasman WT. Epithelial ovarian cancer. In *Clinical Gynecologic Oncology*. St. Louis: Mosby Year Book, 1997:529.)

116

- Indications/contraindications to MTX:

Indications		
Unruptured		
Ectopic mass <3.5 cm (exceptions noted)		
No FCA (exceptions noted)		
β-Human chorionic gonadotropin <6500 mIU/mL (exceptions noted)		
Contraindications		
Abnormal labs (creatinine [>1.3 mg/dL], liver function tests [>50 IU/L])		
Alcoholism, alcoholic liver disease, chronic liver disease		
Preexisting blood dyscrasias		
Active pulmonary disease		
Peptic ulcer disease		
Hepatic, renal, or hematologic dysfunction		

- Single dose protocol (stop prenatal vitamins [PNVs] and folate):

Day 0: MTX, 50 mg/m^2	βhCG, ALT, Cr, CBC, type and screen	Rh$_o$(D) immune globulin (RhoGAM; 300 µg IM) if Rh negative.
Day 4	βhCG	Usually > than day 0 βhCG.
Day 7	βhCG, ALT, Cr, CBC	If not ↓ by 15% from day 4, give 2nd MTX dose (50 mg/m^2) or laparoscopy.
Weekly	βhCG	Continue until <5 mIU/mL.[a]

ALT, alanine aminotransferase; βhCG, β-human chorionic gonadotropin; CBC, complete blood count; Cr, creatinine; MTX, methotrexate.
[a]If <15% decline in any follow-up week, protocol is repeated.

ECTOPIC PREGNANCY

- Multidose protocol (stop PNV and folate):

Day 0: MTX, 1 mg/kg IM or IV	βhCG, ALT, Cr, CBC, type and screen	RhoGAM (300 μg IM) if Rh negative.
Day 1: LEU, 0.1 mg/kg IM or IV	βhCG	If not ↓ by 15% from day 0, give 2nd MTX dose on day 2.
Day 2: MTX	—	—
Day 3: LEU	βhCG	If not ↓ by 15% from day 1, give 3rd MTX dose on day 4.
Day 4: MTX	—	—
Day 5: LEU	βhCG	If not ↓ by 15% from day 3, give 4th MTX dose on day 6.
Day 6: MTX	—	—
Day 7: LEU	βhCG, ALT, Cr, CBC	If not ↓ by 15% from day 5, laparoscopy.
Weekly	βhCG	Continue until <5 mIU/mL.[a]

ALT, alanine aminotransferase; βhCG, β-human chorionic gonadotropin; CBC, complete blood count; Cr, creatinine; LEU, leucovorin; MTX, methotrexate; RhoGAM, $Rh_o(D)$ immune globulin.
[a]Discontinue treatment when there is a decline in two consecutive βhCG titers or after four doses, whichever comes first.

- Average time to resolution (βhCG <15 mIU/mL) for those successfully treated with MTX = approximately 35 days, although it can take up to 109 days (Lipscomb et al., 1998).
- Longest interval between initial treatment and rupture = 42 days (Lipscomb et al., 2000)
- Pretreatment βhCG level is the only significant prognosticator of failure (Lipscomb et al., 1999a).
- Previous EP appears to be an independent risk factor for MTX failure (failure rate of 18.6% in those with a prior EP compared to a 6.8% failure rate for first-time EP) (Lipscomb et al., 2004).

β-Human Chorionic Gonadotropin Level (mIU/mL)	Failure Rate (%)
<1000	1.7
1000–9999	7–13
10,000–14,999	18
>15,000	32

Source: Adapted from Lipscomb GH, McCord ML, Stovall TG, et al. Predictors of success of methotrexate treatment in women with tubal ectopic pregnancies. N Engl J Med 341:1974, 1999.

- If the initial βhCG <1000 mIU/mL, 88% resolve without MTX (this is equivalent to MTX efficiency) (Trio et al., 1995).

ECTOPIC PREGNANCY

- After MTX, 56% of the masses increase in size (not necessarily treatment failures, but hematomas) (Brown et al., 1991).
- MTX complications:
  - Impaired liver function, stomatitis, gastritis-enteritis, bone marrow suppression
  - MTX leads to abdominal pain (tubal abortion or hematoma stretching tube-T11,12 [umbilical]).
  - ⇨ Treat with ibuprofen, 800 mg q6 hrs.
  - ⇨ Presence of blood in pelvis is not considered an absolute indication for surgical intervention if hemodynamically stable (Lipscomb, 1999a).

SURGICAL TREATMENT
- Linear salpingostomy reserved for nonisthmic EPs <5 cm in diameter (American Fertility Society, 1988).
  - **Ampullary** EPs usually grow outside of the lumen; postoperative patency expected.
  - **Isthmic** EPs usually grow within the lumen and destroy the tubal mucosa; segmental resection is the treatment of choice.
- 5–15% Chance of retained trophoblasts after surgery; some give one dose of MTX at time of surgery; more common with laparoscopic approach vs. laparotomy (Seifer et al., 1993)
- Use of hydrodissection to flush conceptus out the tube preferred to piecemeal removal

PROGNOSIS
- Risk of persistent EP after laparotomy = 5%, laparoscopy = 15%
- No difference in subsequent pregnancy rate for laparoscopic vs. laparotomy salpingostomy (~70%)
- Intrauterine conception rate similar for surgery vs. MTX (51% vs. 63%, $P = .37$) (Strobelt et al., 2000)
- Subsequent rate of EP for laparoscopic and laparotomy salpingostomy: 7% and 14%, respectively (Yao and Tulandi, 1997)
- Recurrent EP: ~15% salpingostomy vs. ~8% salpingectomy (Yao and Tulandi, 1997). Others note equal recurrent EP rates (Bateman and Taylor, 1991).
- After two EPs, the risk of a subsequent EP ↑ by tenfold.

ECTOPIC PREGNANCY

- Systemic MTX vs. laparoscopic salpingostomy:

Outcome Measure	Relative Risk (Confidence Interval)
Primary treatment success—ND	1.20 (0.93–1.40)
Tubal preservation—ND	0.98 (0.87–1.10)
Tubal patency—ND	0.93 (0.64–1.40)
Spontaneous IUP—ND	0.89 (0.42–1.90)
Spontaneous repeat ectopic—ND	0.77 (0.17–3.40)
Cumulative spontaneous IUP rates at 18 mos, 36% vs. 43%	

IUP, intrauterine pregnancy; ND, no difference.

Bottom line: Treatment with systemic methotrexate is not superior to laparoscopy based on effectiveness, side effects, burden to patients, and costs to society.

Source: Adapted from Dias Pereira G, Hajenius PJ, et al. Fertility outcome after systemic methotrexate and laparoscopic salpingostomy for tubal pregnancy. *Lancet* 353(9154):724, 1999.

A. Cornual vs. Angular vs. Interstitial Pregnancy

(Jansen and Elliott, 1983)

- **Cornual:** a pregnancy in one horn of a bicornuate uterus or in lateral half of a septate or subseptate uterus
- **Angular:** implantation just medial to the uterotubal junction, in the lateral angle of the uterine cavity; round ligament (*) is reflected upward and outward (see figure below); may be managed conservatively (i.e., expectant management) if there is no rupture or bleeding noted.
- **Interstitial:** implantation within interstitial portion of the tube reflecting the round ligament (*) medially so that the swelling is lateral to the round ligament (see figure below)

Angular   Interstitial

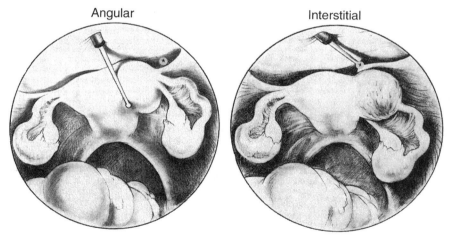

Source: Reproduced with permission from Jansen R, Elliott P. Angular intrauterine pregnancy. *Obstet Gynaecol* 58:167, 1981.

121

B. Approach to False-Positive Human Chorionic Gonadotropin Results

- Frequency of false-positive βhCG: between 1 in 10,000 and 1 in 100,000 tests
- False-positive βhCG usually <150 mIU/mL
- Most false positives are due to interference by non-hCG substances (i.e., anti–animal immunoglobulin antibodies).
- Characteristically, the serum is positive, but the urine is negative because the heterophilic antibodies are usually immunoglobulins G with a molecular weight of ~160,000 diopter and are not easily filtered through the renal glomeruli. In addition, serial dilutions of serum are not parallel to the hCG standard.

Causes of False-Positive Serum hCG

Interference by non-hCG substances
    Anti–animal heterophilic immunoglobulin antibodies
    hLH or hLHβ-subunit
    Rheumatoid factor
    Nonspecific serum factors
Injection of exogenous hCG
Pituitary hCG-like substance
Assay contaminants

---

hCG, human chorionic gonadotropin; hLH, human luteinizing hormone.

ECTOPIC PREGNANCY

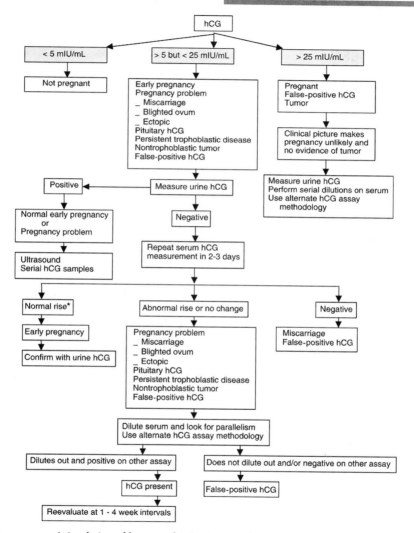

*Slowest or minimal rise of human chorionic gonadotropin (hCG) for a normal pregnancy: 1 day = 24%; 2 days = 53% (Barnhart et al., 2004a). (Source: Adapted from Braunstein, GD. False-positive serum human chorionic gonadotropin results: causes, characteristics, and recognition. *Am J Obstet Gynecol* 187[1]:217, 2002.)

13. Sheehan Syndrome

INCIDENCE
- 1/10,000 deliveries
- Hemorrhagic infarction usually occurs in the presence of a pituitary tumor.
- Ischemic infarction may occur after obstetric hemorrhage (Sheehan syndrome).

DEFINITIONS
- Postpartum pituitary necrosis is preceded by a history of massive obstetric hemorrhage, resulting in severe circulatory collapse, hypotension, and shock.
- Clinical manifestations may range from partial deficiency to panhypopituitarism.
- The posterior pituitary is usually spared.
- Return of normal fertility has been documented.

ETIOLOGY
- Anterior pituitary grows during pregnancy due to estrogenic stimulation, resulting in hyperplasia and hypertrophy of pituitary lactotropes: 500 mg → 1000 mg.
- Anterior pituitary insufficiency occurs when >75% of the gland has been destroyed.
- Severity of hemorrhage and occurrence of Sheehan syndrome may not correlate.
- Severe hypotension, in a setting of low portal vein pressure, leads to occlusive spasm of the arteries that supply the anterior pituitary and the stalk; when arteriospasm relaxes, blood flows into the damaged vessels, resulting in vascular congestion and thrombosis.
- Infarction with hemorrhage and edema may cause rapid expansion of the lesion, compressing surrounding structures with neurologic (visual) manifestations.

SHEEHAN SYNDROME

COURSE
- Classic progression of deficits:
  - Prolactin (PRL; 67–100%), growth hormone (GH; 88%), gonadotropins (58–76%), adrenocorticotropic hormone (ACTH; 66%), thyroid-stimulating hormone (TSH; 42–53%), diabetes insipidus (2%)

Acute form
- Hypotension
- Tachycardia
- Failure to lactate (breast involution)
- Hypoglycemia
- Extreme fatigue
- Nausea and vomiting
- Failure to regrow shaved pubic hair

Chronic form
- Light headedness
- Fatigue and cold intolerance
- Failure to lactate
- Scanty or absent menses
- ↓ Body hair
- Skin: dry, pale, and waxy
- Nausea and vomiting
- ↓ Melanin → pale areolae
- ↓ Libido

- ↓ ACTH signs and symptoms: fatigue, hypotension, poor tolerance to stress and infection, hypoglycemia, loss of pubic and axillary hair, ↓ body hair, ↓ pigment in skin, waxy skin
- ↓ TSH signs and symptoms: fatigue, slow speech, slow movements, cold intolerance, dry skin, constipation

DIAGNOSIS
- Magnetic resonance imaging (MRI) assesses the hemorrhage extension and need for ophthalmologic examination.
- Diagnostic tests:
  - Serum a.m. cortisol, ACTH, TSH, thyroxine (T_4), PRL, luteinizing hormone (LH), follicle-stimulating hormone (FSH), estradiol (E_2), insulin-like growth factor (IGF)-I
  - Metyrapone stimulation test: Metyrapone (2 g PO at 11 p.m.) blocks 11-deoxycorticosterone (DOC) → cortisol, which leads to ↑ ACTH (>100 pg/mL) and ↑ precursor 11-DOC (>7 µg/dL).

SHEEHAN SYNDROME

- Hormone deficits may be transient; therefore, function should be reevaluated several months after the event.
- May require pituitary reserve testing: draw blood (serum) samples at −30, 0, 30, and 60 mins, through an indwelling IV catheter; at time 0, give IV:
  1. Thyroid-releasing hormone (TRH), 200 μg → stimulates TSH and PRL release
  2. Gonadotropin-releasing hormone (GnRH), 100 μg → stimulates LH and FSH release
  3. Corticotropin-releasing hormone (CRH), 50 μg → stimulates ACTH release
  4. Growth hormone–releasing hormone (GHRH), 50 μg → stimulates GH release
     - Interpretation of results: All hormones should at least double above mean baseline values; pulsatile secretion necessitates several baseline values.
- No test for antidiuretic hormone (ADH) deficiency: urine specific gravity <1.005; symptoms are polyuria and polydipsia.
- After a full-term pregnancy without lactation, it takes 4 wks for the FSH pulsatility to return to normal (Liu et al., 1983).

TREATMENT
- Appropriate replacement of target hormones when needed (corticoid, thyroid, sex steroids, desmopressin acetate [DDAVP])
- Corticosteroids (usually aldosterone production is sufficient in the absence of ACTH, unlike in Addison's disease): dexamethasone, 2 mg q6 hrs
- Oral contraceptives (OCs) if necessary

PROGNOSIS
- Overall: excellent with correct diagnosis and treatment
- Fertility: Pregnancy can occur spontaneously in partial cases. Otherwise, human menopausal gonadotropin (hMG) induction of ovulation is necessary; if pregnancy ensues, hypoglycemia may occur due to ↓ GH and ACTH reserves.

14. Premenstrual Syndrome

HISTORY
- Dr. Frank at Mt. Sinai Hospital in New York City first defined premenstrual syndrome (PMS) in 1931 (Frank, 1931) as a " . . . Feeling of indescribable tension from 10 to 7 days preceding menstruation which in most instances continues until the time that the menstrual flow occurs."
- Drs. Greene and Dalton first used the phrase *premenstrual syndrome* in 1953 in a report of 84 cases (Greene and Dalton, 1953).

DEFINITIONS
- **PMS:** both physical and behavioral symptoms that occur repetitively in the 2nd 1/2 of the menstrual cycle to interfere with a woman's life followed by a period of time free of symptoms.
- **Premenstrual dysphoric disorder (PMDD):** American Psychiatric Association's *Diagnostic and Statistical Manual of Mental Disorders*, 4th Edition (*DSM-IV*), designation with prominence of anger, irritability, and internal tension; presumably the most severe form of PMS, although this designation is nonfunctional.

PREVALENCE (Rivera-Tovar and Frank, 1990; Raja et al., 1992)
- PMS: up to 75% in women with regular cycles
- PMDD: 3–8%
- No correlation with ethnicity
- Higher concordance rate in monozygotic twins compared with dizygotic twins (Condon, 1993), although role of genetic factors is far from certain (Glick et al., 1993).

PATHOGENESIS
Neurotransmitters
- Cyclic changes in ovarian steroids may influence central neurotransmitters (opioid, γ-aminobutyric acid, serotonin).
  - Women with PMS may be biochemically supersensitive to biologic challenges of the serotonergic system (Halbreich and Tworek, 1993).
  - PMS patients have lower serotonin and higher levels of serotonin metabolites during the luteal phase (Taylor et al., 1984; Steege et al., 1992).

PREMENSTRUAL SYNDROME

- Serotonin antagonist administration to women with PMDD → recrudescence of symptoms (Roca et al., 2002).
- PMS symptoms improved with serotonin agonists (Brzezinski et al., 1990) or serotonin reuptake inhibitors (e.g., fluoxetine).

Ovarian Steroids

- Gonadotropin-releasing hormone agonists used to induce hypoestrogenemia led to resolution of PMS symptoms (Muse et al., 1984).
  - The addition of estradiol (E_2) or progesterone (P_4) led to a recurrence of symptoms (Schmidt et al., 1998); however, the addition of a placebo in lieu of steroids also led to a return of symptoms.
- In contrast, there were no differences in serum E_2 and P_4 concentrations between women with PMDD and controls (Taylor, 1979).
- P_4 antagonist RU-486 did not ameliorate PMS symptoms (Chan et al., 1994).

Vitamins and Minerals

- No deficiencies in vitamin A, B_6, or E in women with PMS (Chuong et al., 1990a; Chuong et al., 1990b)
- One controlled study showed improved symptoms with magnesium pyrrolidone carboxylic acid (360 mg t.i.d.) given in the luteal phase (Facchinetti et al., 1991).

Psychosocial Factors

- Stress has little influence on PMS severity (Beck et al., 1990).

PREMENSTRUAL SYNDROME

SYMPTOMS

- 22 symptoms documented by Mortola et al. in 1990, occurring in the last 7–10 days of the cycle:

Symptom	Frequency (% of Cycles)
Fatigue	92
Irritability	91
Bloating	90
Anxiety/tension	89
Breast tenderness	85
Mood lability	81
Depression	80
Food cravings	78
Acne	71
↑ Appetite	70
Oversensitivity	69
Swelling	67
Expressed anger	67
Crying easily	65
Feeling of isolation	65
Headache	60
Forgetfulness	56
Gastrointestinal symptoms	48
Poor concentration	47
Hot flashes	18
Heart palpitations	14
Dizziness	14

Source: Data from Mortola JF, Girton L, Beck L, et al. Diagnosis of premenstrual syndrome by a simple, prospective, and reliable instrument: the calendar of premenstrual experiences. *Obstet Gynecol* 76(2): 302, 1990.

PREMENSTRUAL SYNDROME

DIAGNOSIS

- Symptoms, severity of symptoms, temporal relationship to luteal phase, absence of external factors (i.e., drugs) or other diagnoses
- Two established guidelines for diagnosing PMDD:
  1. *DSM-IV-TR* criteria

DSM-IV-TR Criteria for Diagnosis

A. Must occur during the week before menses and remit a few days after the onset of menses.

B. Five of the following 11 symptoms must be present and include at least one of the 1st four on the list:

1. **Markedly depressed mood or feelings of hopelessness**

2. **Marked anxiety or tension**

3. **Marked affective lability (i.e., sudden onset of being sad, tearful, irritable, or angry)**

4. **Persistent and marked anger or irritability or ↑ interpersonal conflicts**

5. ↓ Interest in usual activities

6. Marked lack of energy

7. Concentration difficulties

8. Changes in appetite, overeating, or food craving

9. Hypersomnia or insomnia

10. Feeling overwhelmed

11. Other physical symptoms, such as breast tenderness, headaches, bloating, or joint or muscle pain

C. Symptoms must interfere with work, school, or usual activities or relationships.

D. Symptoms must not be an exacerbation of another psychiatric disorder (major mental disorder, personality disorder, or general medical condition).

E. Criteria A, B, C, and D must be confirmed by prospective daily ratings ≥2 cycles.

Source: Reproduced with permission from American Psychiatric Association. *Diagnostic and Statistical Manual of Mental Disorders* (4th ed, text revision). Washington, DC: American Psychiatric Association, 2004.

2. **National Institute of Mental Health guidelines** (Osofsky and Blumenthal, 1985):

- Diagnosis requires the documentation of ≥30% ↓ severity of symptoms in the 5 days after menses (follicular phase) compared with the 5 days before menses (luteal phase) within a single cycle (using Prospective Record of the Severity of Menstruation [PRISM]).
- Calendar of premenstrual experiences: **PRISM**
  - Before recording in the calendar, the physician identifies the patient's chief complaints and the symptoms to be followed throughout treatment.

130

PREMENSTRUAL SYNDROME

- Scores for the symptoms of interest are added for 5 follicular days (cycle days 7–11) and 5 luteal days (−6 to −2), and these total phase scores are then compared.
- Within-cycle % change is calculated as follows:

$$\frac{\text{Luteal score} - \text{Follicular score}}{\text{Luteal score}} \times 100$$

PRISM calendar instructions:

1. Prepare the calendar on the first day of menses. Considering the first day of bleeding as day 1 of your menstrual cycle, enter the corresponding calendar date for each day in the space provided.

   e.g., Day of menstrual cycle. Month: _____ Date: _____

2. Each evening, at about the same time, complete the calendar column for that day as described below:

   Bleeding: Indicate if you have had bleeding by shading the box above that day's date; for spotting, use an (x).

   Symptoms: If you do not experience any symptoms, leave the corresponding square blank. If present, indicate the severity by entering a number from 1 (mild) to 7 (severe).

   Lifestyle impact: If the listed phrase applies to you that day, enter an (x).

   Life events: If you experienced one of these events that day, enter an (x).

   Experiences: For positive (happy) or negative (sad/disappointing) experiences unrelated to your symptoms, specify the nature of the events on the back of this form.

   Social activities: This implies such events as a special dinner, show, or party, etc., involving family or friends.

   Vigorous exercise: This implies participation in a sporting event or exercise program lasting >30 mins.

   Medication: In the bottom five rows, list medication used, if any, and indicate days when they were taken by entering an (x).

   Study number: _____ Baseline weight on Day 1 _____ lb or kg. (circle one)

Source: Reproduced with permission from Reid RL. Premenstrual syndrome. *Curr Probl Obstet Gynecol Fertil* 8:1–57, 1985.

PREMENSTRUAL SYNDROME

Study Number [ ][ ][ ][ ][ ]

Baseline weight on Day 1 _____ lbs. or kg.
(circle one)

Day of Menstrual Cycle Month: Date:	1	2	3	4	5	6	7	8	9	10	11	12	13	14	15	16	17	18	19	20	21	22	23	24	25	26	27	28	29	30	31	32	33	34	35
Bleeding																																			
SYMPTOMS																																			
Irritable																																			
Fatigue																																			
Inward anger																																			
Labile mood (crying)																																			
Depressed																																			
Restless																																			
Anxious																																			
Insomnia																																			
Lack of control																																			
Edema or rings tight																																			
Breast tenderness																																			
Abdominal bloating																																			
Bowels: const. (c) loose (l)																																			
Appetite: up ^ down ˅																																			
Sex drive: up ^ down ˅																																			
Chills (C)/sweats (S)																																			
Headaches																																			
Crave: sweets, salt																																			
Feel unattractive																																			
Guilty																																			
Unreasonable behavior																																			
Low self-image																																			
Nausea																																			
Menstrual cramps																																			
LIFESTYLE IMPACT																																			
Aggressive towards others — Physically																																			
Aggressive towards others — Verbally																																			
Wish to be alone																																			
Neglect housework																																			
Time off work																																			
Disorganized, distractible																																			
Accident prone/clumsy																																			
Uneasy about driving																																			
Suicidal thoughts																																			
Stayed at home																																			
Increased use of alcohol																																			
LIFE EVENTS																																			
Negative experience																																			
Positive experience																																			
Social activities																																			
Vigorous exercise																																			
MEDICATIONS																																			

PRISM survey. (Source: Reproduced with permission from Reid RL. Premenstrual syndrome. *Curr Probl Obstet Gynecol Fertil* 8:1–57, 1985.)

132

- Fine distinction between PMDD and PMS:
  - Women with PMDD meet criteria for PMDD by *DSM-IV* criteria.
  - Women with PMS do not meet all *DSM-IV* criteria for PMDD but do demonstrate symptom exacerbation premenstrually as calculated above.
  - In all practicality, this is a distinction that is best left in research papers, as either PMDD or PMS is a debilitating life stressor.

DIFFERENTIAL DIAGNOSIS
- Psychiatric disorders: major depression, anxiety disorders
- Perimenopause
- Medical disorders: migraine, irritable bowel syndrome, hyper- or hypothyroidism

DIAGNOSTIC TESTS
- History and physical examination (including past psychiatric history)
- Complete blood count, thyroid-stimulating hormone
- Record symptoms × 3 mos with a menstrual calendar (PRISM).

TREATMENT
Serotonin Reuptake Inhibitors
- Fluoxetine (Prozac): 20 mg/day (Steiner et al., 1995) for at least two cycles
  - U.S. Food and Drug Administration approved for PMDD
  - Approximately 75% overall response rate within 2–3 mos (Steiner et al., 2001)
  - Effect is maintained for many years (Pearlstein and Stone, 1994).
  - Some women may find that use is only required on cycle day 14 until menses (Halbreich and Smoller, 1997).
  - Side effects (15% incidence): headache, anxiety, nausea, anorgasmia
- Sertraline (Zoloft): 50–150 mg/day
- Paroxetine (Paxil): 10–30 mg/day
- Citalopram (Celexa): 20–30 mg/day
- Venlafaxine (Effexor): 50–200 mg/day
- Buspirone (BuSpar): 5 mg t.i.d. or 7.5 mg b.i.d., with maximum of 20 mg t.i.d. or 30 mg b.i.d. daily (12 days before menses)

Alprazolam (Xanax)
- 0.25 mg t.i.d. or q.i.d. in luteal phase only due to risk of dependence
- 2nd-line therapy

Ovulation Suppression
Gonadotropin-Releasing Hormone Agonists
- Limited efficacy with many disadvantages due to hypoestrogenemia

PREMENSTRUAL SYNDROME

- May be more effective for behavioral and physical symptoms and less effective for psychological symptoms
  - Leuprolide (Lupron): 3.75 mg IM each month
  - Nafarelin acetate (Synarel): 2 mg/mL daily, intranasally

Oral Contraceptives
- Most studies reveal ineffectiveness (Joffe et al., 2003).
- Possible utility as continuous oral contraceptives with drospirenone-containing (a progestin that is a spironolactone analog) contraceptive Yasmin (Freeman et al., 2001)

Debatable Treatment Approaches
- Magnesium, 360 mg/day, 14 days before menses (small trials) (Facchinetti et al., 1991; Walker et al., 1998)
- Calcium, 1 g/day (Thys-Jacobs et al., 1989)
- Regular exercise, relaxation, vitamin and mineral supplements, changes in work or recreation, changes in diet (small, frequent complex-carbohydrate meals; ↓ tobacco, chocolate, caffeine, alcohol, salt)

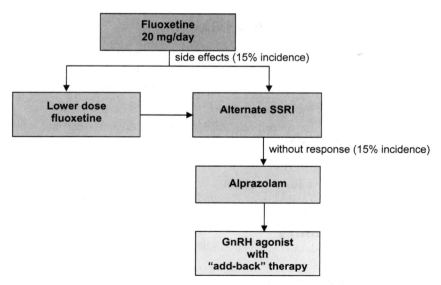

Treatment plan. GnRH, gonadotropin-releasing hormone; SSRI, selective serotonin reuptake inhibitor. (Source: Adapted from Casper RF. Treatment of premenstrual dysphoric disorder. UpToDate Patient Information Web site: http://www.utdol.com. Accessed February, 2005.)

15. Chronic Pelvic Pain

INCIDENCE
- Affects 15% of women in the United States (9 million)
- Accounts for 10% of gynecologist (GYN) visits
- Accounts for 40% of laparoscopies
- Accounts for ~12% of hysterectomies

HISTORY
- Menses; dysmenorrhea
- Dyspareunia (superficial suggests inflammatory process or introital muscle control; deep suggests endometriosis or pelvic adhesive disease)
- Sexually transmitted diseases (STDs); abnormal Pap smear
- Obstetric history
- Detailed social and family history
- Gastrointestinal (GI), urologic, and musculoskeletal review of symptoms (ROS)
- Past surgical history (abdominal or pelvic) → review old operative reports
- Past and current state of mental health
- History of sexual abuse; depression

Pain Inquiry
- Character
- Radiation
- Intensity
- Duration
- Location
- Associated events

Symptoms Suggestive of Irritable Bowel Syndrome
- Alternating constipation/diarrhea, abdominal distention, mucus per rectum, improvement in pain after a bowel movement, sensation of incomplete evacuation after defecation (Manning et al., 1978)

CHRONIC PELVIC PAIN

PHYSICAL EXAMINATION
- Observe posture and gait
- Back
- Skin
- Abdominal wall (single finger pointing by patient and examiner)
  - Evaluation with the patient's head raised off the table and rectus muscles tensed: Visceral origin pain usually diminishes with this, whereas myofascial pain or trigger points exacerbate.
- Pelvic:
  - Vulva: focal tenderness of the posterior vestibule may indicate vestibulodynia
  - Vagina, cervix, and paracervical tissues
  - Unimanual (single digit) followed by a bimanual examination: finger rotated anteriorly to palpate the anterior vaginal wall and base of the bladder; exquisitely painful bladder with interstitial cystitis

History	Examination Findings	Disease State
Progressively worsening dysmenorrhea; deep dyspareunia	Tenderness in implant areas; uterosacral ligament nodularity	Endometriosis
Symptom onset 3–6 mos after surgery; tugging and pulling sensation in abdomen or pelvis	Diminished mobility of the pelvic viscera	Pelvic adhesive disease
Abnormal uterine bleeding; dysmenorrhea	Enlarged, firm, irregular uterus	Leiomyoma or andenomyosis
Pain on arising, climbing stairs, driving car	Pain on external rotation of thigh, which is palpated transvaginally or externally	Piriformis muscle spasm
Frequency and urgency; urethral or bladder pain	Bladder tender to palpation	Interstitial cystitis

LABORATORY AND DIAGNOSTIC STUDIES
- Urine analysis (UA)/culture and sensitivity (C&S)
- Ultrasound
- Wet prep (saline and potassium hydroxide [KOH])
- Laparoscopy (pain mapping)
- Pelvic cultures (gonococcus [GC] and chlamydia)
- Cystoscopy and colonoscopy
- Psychometric instruments
- Trigger point injections

CHRONIC PELVIC PAIN

PROCEDURES
- Laparoscopic findings (for chronic pelvic pain [CPP]) in community survey (n = 1318):

Finding	%
No pathology	39
Endometriosis	28
Adhesions	25
Chronic pelvic inflammatory disease	6
Ovarian cyst	3
Leiomyomata	<1
Pelvic varicosities	<1
Other	4

Source: Adapted from Howard FM. The role of laparoscopy in chronic pelvic pain: promise and pitfalls. *Obstet Gynecol Surv* 48:357, 1993.

CAUSES OF CHRONIC PELVIC PAIN (Advincula and Song, 2004)

Extrauterine
- Endometriosis
- Adhesions
- Chronic pelvic infection
- Ovarian remnant syndrome
- Intrinsic vaginal apex pain
- Vulvar vestibulitis and vulvodynia

Gastrointestinal
- Irritable bowel syndrome
- Inflammatory bowel disease
- Chronic appendicitis
- Cancer
- Diverticular disease

Uterine
- Leiomyomata
- Adenomyosis
- Pelvic congestion
- Pelvic relaxation
- Uterine malposition

Musculoskeletal
- Levator ani syndrome

CHRONIC PELVIC PAIN

- Myofascial pain (trigger points, spasms)
- Hernias
- Low back pain and disc problems
- Scoliosis/lordosis/kyphosis

Urologic
- Chronic cystitis or calculi
- Interstitial cystitis
- Urethral syndrome
- Detrusor instability

Psychiatric
- Depression
- Hypochondriasis
- Somatization
- Somatic delusions

Neurologic
- Nerve entrapment syndrome
- Coccydynia
- Postherpetic neuralgia
- Incisional neuroma
- Visceral hyperalgesia
- Pudendal neuralgia

DYSMENORRHEA

Primary Dysmenorrhea: No Pelvic Pathology Evident
- Caused by the release of prostaglandins $F_{2\alpha}$ and E_2
- Other associated factors include family history, early menarche, increased duration of menses, and smoking
- Usually begins 6–12 mos after menarche at the initiation of ovulatory cycles
- Antiinflammatories: dosing for primary dysmenorrhea:
  - Nonsteroidal antiinflammatory drugs (NSAIDs):
    - ⇨ Ibuprofen, 400–800 mg PO q6–8 hrs
    - ⇨ Naproxen sodium, 275–500 mg PO q6–8 hrs
    - ⇨ Mefenamic acid, 250–500 mg PO q6–8 hrs

Secondary Dysmenorrhea: Pelvic Pathology Present
- Common causes include endometriosis, pelvic infections, cervical stenosis, adenomyosis, leiomyomas, congenital malformations (i.e., imperforate hymen), or intrauterine device (IUD).
- First-line medical management: oral contraceptives (and NSAIDs)

Residual Ovary Syndrome

- Occurs in 3% of women who have undergone hysterectomy with ovarian conservation
- Perioophoritis with a thickened ovarian capsule leading to pain from cyclical expansion of the ovary encased in adhesions

Ovarian Remnant Syndrome

- Follicle-stimulating hormone (FSH) in *pre*menopausal range
- Clomiphene citrate can assist in ultrasound diagnosis as well as surgical identification (100 mg/day for 7–10 days before the day of surgery; last dose, 1–2 days before surgery)

Vulvodynia

- Vulvar vestibulitis patients typically present with dyspareunia on entry, persistent yeast infection, soreness, burning, or rawness
- Tight clothing, prolonged sitting, or exercise may exacerbate these symptoms (itching is rarely a symptom).
- Treatment recommendations: Avoid soaps, douches, creams, or synthetic underwear; topical vegetable oil or zinc oxide or local anesthetic; low-dose tricyclic antidepressants or anticonvulsant, gabapentin (100 mg at bedtime, increasing by 100 mg every 2 days to 3 g/day in divided doses); surgical vestibulectomy may be effective in recalcitrant cases.

TREATMENT

- Integrated, either by an individual or an interdisciplinary/multispecialty team
- Set expectations early on.
- Medical and/or surgical management
- Low threshold for referral
- See respective entities in this manual (e.g., Chapter 16, Endometriosis; Chapter 17, Fibroids).
- Narcotics used in chronic pain management:

CHRONIC PELVIC PAIN

Drug	Usual Dose Range	Side Effects
Hydrocodone bitartrate with acetaminophen (all are scored tablets) Lorcet 10/650 Lorcet Plus 7.5/650 Lortab 2.5/500, 5/500, or 7.5/500 Vicodin 5/750	5–10 mg hydrocodone either q6 hrs or q8 hrs Can use additional acetaminophen between doses to potentiate effect	Lightheadedness, dizziness, sedation, nausea, vomiting, and constipation (these are all common side effects of all narcotics).
Oxycodone hydrochloride Percocet, 5 mg with 325 mg acetaminophen Percodan, 4.5 mg with 325 mg aspirin (also contains 0.38 mg oxycodone terephthalate)	1 tablet q6 hrs or q8 hrs Additional acetaminophen between doses may serve to potentiate effect	Common effects (see above).
Oxycodone controlled release OxyContin	10–40 mg q12 hrs	Common effects (see above).
Methadone hydrochloride Dolophine, 5- or 10-mg scored tablets	2.5 mg q8 hrs to 10 mg q6 hrs Commonly 15–20 mg q.d.	Common effects. Lower extremity edema or joint swelling may occur and require discontinuation. Cautious use in patients taking monoamine oxidase inhibitors.
Acetaminophen with codeine Tylenol No. 3, 300 mg acetaminophen with 30 mg codeine	1–2 tablets q6–8 hrs	Common effects. Constipation likely. Nausea and vomiting more common than with other narcotics. More common allergy rash.
Morphine sulfate MS Contin or Oramorph	15–60 mg q12 hrs; controlled-release tablets	Common effects. Higher doses increase risk of respiratory depression.
Fentanyl transdermal system Duragesic	25-μg patch, one q72 hrs; also available in 50 or 75 μg Always start with lowest dose	Common effects. Patch must be kept from heat sources, or dose may be increased. Extreme caution in patients taking other central nervous system medicines. Respiratory depression can result.

Source: Reproduced with permission from Steege JF. Chronic pelvic pain. In Curtis MG, Hopkins MP, eds. *Glass's Office Gynecology* (4th ed). Philadelphia: Lippincott Williams & Wilkins, 1999:330.

16. Endometriosis

DEFINITION
- Presence of functioning endometrial glands and stroma outside the usual location of the uterine cavity
- First described in 1860 by the Viennese pathologist Karl von Rokitansky

PREVALENCE
- 3–10% of reproductive-age group
- 25–35% of infertile women
- 39–59% of pelvic pain group
- Average age at diagnosis: 25–29 yrs; similar rates in the various races and socioeconomic backgrounds
- 7 million U.S. women are affected.
- Visualizing endometriosis:
  - 70% of women with pelvic pain (Koninckx et al., 1991)
  - 84% of women with pain and infertility (Koninckx et al., 1991)
  - 45% of women with no symptoms (Balasch et al., 1996)
  - 6% of biopsies of normal peritoneum in normal pelvis (Balasch et al., 1996)
  - 11–25% of biopsies of normal peritoneum in endometriosis patients (Murphy et al., 1986; Balasch et al., 1996)

RISKS OF CANCER

Cancer	Incidence Ratio	95% Confidence Interval
Overall	1.2	1.1, 1.3
Breast	1.3	1.1, 1.4
Ovarian	1.9	1.3, 2.8
Ovarian cancer with history of endometrioma	4.2	1.2, 7.7
Non-Hodgkin's lymphoma	1.8	1.2, 2.6

Source: Adapted from Brinton LA, Gridley G, et al. Cancer risk after a hospital discharge diagnosis of endometriosis. *Am J Obstet Gynecol* 176(3):572, 1997.

- Malignant neoplasms can arise in endometriotic tissue of the ovary.
  - Endometrioid: 57%
  - Other epithelial: 22.4%
  - Clear cell: 10%
  - Serous: 7%

...OMETRIOSIS

...SKS OF AUTOIMMUNE DISORDERS

Autoimmune Disorder	Prevalence in Women with Endometriosis vs. General U.S. Female Population (%)
Hyperthyroidism	6.6 vs. 1.50
Fibromyalgia	5.9 vs. 3.40
Chronic fatigue syndrome	4.6 vs. 0.03
Rheumatoid arthritis	1.8 vs. 1.20
Systemic lupus erythematosus	0.8 vs. 0.04
Sjögren's syndrome	0.6 vs. 0.03
Multiple sclerosis	0.5 vs. 0.07

Source: Adapted from Sinaii N, Cleary SD, et al. Autoimmune and related diseases among women with endometriosis: a survey analysis. *Fertil Steril* 77[Suppl 1]:S7, 2002.

PATHOGENESIS

Transplantation Theory (Sampson, 1927)

- Retrograde menstruation seeds the abdominal cavity.
- Prevalence of retrograde menstruation: 70–90%
- Higher incidence associated with outflow obstruction, shorter cycles, menorrhagia, delayed child-bearing
- A disease of menstruation; delaying childbirth has increased number of menstrual cycles (~450 cycles/lifetime).
- The sigmoid colon and filmy adhesions that frequently cover the left adnexa create an area isolated from the rest of the peritoneal cavity and, therefore, may be less exposed to the peritoneal current and thus clearance by the immune system. Cells regurgitated through the right tube are more exposed to the clockwise peritoneal current and may be removed by the macrophage disposal system (Rosenheim et al., 1979).

Coelomic Metaplasia

- Peritoneal mesothelium (from which the müllerian duct is derived) undergoes metaplastic transformation into endometrial tissue.
- Is this how endometriosis is formed in men treated with high doses of estrogens?
- Probable etiology of rectovaginal (RV) endometriotic nodules (Donnez et al., 1996)?
  - Lower mitotic activity
  - Smooth muscle and glandular elements
  - Decreased vimentin, estrogen receptors, progesterone receptors

142

ENDOMETRIOSIS

Induction Theory

- Unknown biochemical substances (from shed endometrium?) induce undifferentiated peritoneal cells to form endometriotic tissue.

Immunologic Theory (Halme et al., 1987; Lebovic et al., 2001)

- Alterations in cell-mediated immunity: natural killer (NK), macrophage, T- and B-cells
- Abnormal autoantibodies?
- Altered immune response → inhibited clearance of viable endometrial cells via immunosurveillance evasion:
  - Modification of human leukocyte antigen (HLA) class I antigen expression (related to immune recognition [Semino et al., 1995])
  - ↑ Soluble HLA or intercellular adhesion molecule (ICAM)-I that competes with surface antigens critical to immune recognition (Somigliana et al., 1996; De Placido et al., 1998)
  - ↑ Growth factors/cytokines that inhibit specific immune population functions (i.e., soluble tumor necrosis factor [TNF] receptor) (Hirata et al., 1994; Somigliana et al., 1996; Koga et al., 2000)
  - Induction of apoptosis in immune cells via Fas-mediated mechanisms (Garcia-Velasco et al., 1999)
  - ↑ Antiapoptotic factors (i.e., osteoprotegerin, Bcl-2 family) (Harada et al., 2004; Nishida et al., 2005)
  - Resistance to interferon (IFN)-γ–induced apoptosis (Nishida et al., 2005)
  - NK cell defect (D'Hooghe et al., 1995)

Genetic Predisposition

- Familial disposition (Simpson et al., 1980):
  - 1st degree relatives: 6.9% with endometriosis (controls at 1%)
  - Siblings: 5.8%
  - Mothers: 8.1%
- Multifactorial inheritance

Other

- Dioxin? The environmental pollutant dioxin was found in 18% of women with endometriosis vs. 3% of the controls (P <.05) (Mayani et al., 1997).
- Uncontrolled proliferation of the ectopic tissue is rarely seen; lack of proliferative activity, yet increased antiapoptosis?
- Peritoneal, ovarian, and RV endometriotic lesions are three separate entities with different pathogeneses: (a) peritoneal = retrograde effluent; (b) endometriomas = coelomic metaplasia; and (c) RV = müllerian remnants (Nisolle and Donnez, 1997).

143

ENDOMETRIOSIS

CLINICAL PRESENTATION

Pain
- Dysmenorrhea with premenstrual intensification
- Dyspareunia
- Chronic pelvic pain (>6 mos):
  - Peritoneum is richly supplied with afferent nerve fibers (Ottinger, 1974).
  - Criteria suggesting endometriosis as source of chronic pelvic pain (Hurd, 1998):
    ⇨ Cyclic pelvic pain (peritoneal irritation from intraabdominal menses?)
    ⇨ Surgically diagnosed endometriosis

Infertility
- Biased predilection for laparoscopy in infertile patients may overestimate the incidence of endometriosis in this group.
  - Prevalence in subfertile women vs. fertile women: 33% vs. 4%
- Severe endometriosis: adhesions
- Mild endometriosis is associated with a lower fecundity rate:
  - Cumulative pregnancy rate for minimal-mild endometriosis vs. unexplained subfertility: 15.7% (0.77; 95% confidence interval [CI], 0.52–1.15) vs. 23.6% (Berube et al., 1998)
  - Probability of pregnancy 3 yrs (untreated) after diagnostic laparoscopy for minimal-mild endometriosis vs. unexplained subfertility: 36% vs. 55% (P <.05) (Akande et al., 2004)
  - Probability of live birth 3 yrs (untreated) after diagnostic laparoscopy for minimal-mild endometriosis vs. unexplained subfertility: 33% vs. 48% (not significant [NS], although type II error) (Akande et al., 2004)

- Fertility for minimal-mild endometriosis vs. unexplained subfertility (Sung et al., 1997; Jensen et al., 1998; Hammond et al., 1986; Toma et al., 1992; Omland et al., 1998; Nuojua-Huttunen et al., 1999):

	Monthly Fecundity Rate after Expectant Management (%)	Monthly Fecundity Rate after Intrauterine Insemination (%)	Monthly Fecundity Rate after Therapeutic Donor Insemination (%)	Pregnancy Rate after Donor Oocyte (*In Vitro* Fertilization) (%)[a]
Minimal-mild endometriosis	2.5	9	4	28
Unexplained subfertility	3.5 NS[b]	19 $P <.01$	16 $P <.01$	29 NS

NS, not significant.

[a]Data in this column from Diaz I, Navarro J, Blasco L, et al. Impact of stage III-IV endometriosis on recipients of sibling oocytes: matched case-control study. *Fertil Steril* 74(1):31, 2000.

[b]Two caveats: (a) women with red/white/vesicular lesions considered as controls (may have lowered control group outcome); (b) underpowered to show smaller difference (Berube, 1998).

- ↑ Prostaglandins (PGs), cytokines, oligoovulation, luteal phase defect, autoimmune reaction
- Inhibitory effect of peritoneal fluid from women with moderate-severe endometriosis on sperm motility (Oral and Arici, 1996)
- Cumulative pregnancy rate after 5 yrs without therapy: 90% (minimal disease) (D'Hooghe et al., 2003)
- Comparison of pregnancy outcome after *in vitro* fertilization (IVF)/intra-cyloplasmic sperm injection (ICSI) for unexplained vs. endometrioisis (stage I) subfertility (Omland et al., 2005):
  - ↓ 1st cycle pregnancy rate (48.6% endometriosis vs. 58.8% unexplained; $P <.05$)
  - ↓ Live birth rate (66% endometriosis vs. 78.8% unexplained; $P <.05$)
  - ↑ Spontaneous abortion <6 wks estimated gestational age (19.3% endometriosis vs. 11.7% unexplained; $P <.05$)
- Women with stage III/IV endometriosis have diminished ovarian reserve (elevated basal follicle-stimulating hormone [FSH]) compared to age-matched controls undergoing IVF for male factor (Hock et al., 2001).

ENDOMETRIOSIS

Menstrual Irregularities (Vercellini et al., 1997)
- Premenstrual spotting (15–20%)
- Menorrhagia more common

Gastrointestinal Involvement (Weed and Ray, 1987)
- ~5% Gastrointestinal (GI) involvement:
  - Rectum/sigmoid (70%) > appendix > cecum > distal ileum > ascending colon > transverse/descending colon
- Only ~50% incidence of additional endometriotic lesions in such women
- Common symptoms: bloating, crampy abdominal pain, change in bowel habits, ↓ bowel movements, hematochezia, anorexia
- Serosa and muscularis most often affected, whereas the mucosa is rarely involved (Panganiban and Cornog, 1972).
- May be removed laparoscopically if located far enough from the anus and a skilled laparoscopic surgeon is present with the ability to do segmental colonic resection.

DIAGNOSIS
Examination
- Localized tenderness of cul-de-sac
- Nodularity of the uterosacral ligaments
- Obliteration of the cul-de-sac
- Fixed retroversion of the uterus
- Ovarian enlargement/transrectal ultrasound (for RV endometriosis) (Fedele et al., 1998)
- Lateral cervical displacement (resulting from uterosacral scarring) (Propst et al., 1998)

Transvaginal Sonography
- Useful in diagnosis of endometrioma → homogeneous hypoechoic carpet of low-level echoes or *ground-glass* appearance (Kupfer et al., 1992)

Laparoscopy
- Most common sites: ovary, post–cul-de-sac, broad ligament, uterosacral ligaments, rectosigmoid colon, bladder
- Endometriomas involve the *left* ovary more frequently than the *right* ovary (Jenkins et al., 1986).
  - Cells regurgitated through the right tube are more exposed to the clockwise peritoneal current and may be removed by the macrophage disposal system (Rosenheim et al., 1979).

146

ENDOMETRIOSIS

- Women with endometriotic lesions of the *left* hemipelvis have a greater risk of disease recurrence and delay of future pregnancy compared to those with disease confined to the *right* hemipelvis (Ghezzi et al., 2001).
- Blue-black "powder burn" lesion (older, enclosed implant?)
- Varied appearance: red, white, yellow, clear (active lesions? higher vascularity and mitotic activity)
- In women with no visible endometriosis, a biopsy of normal-appearing peritoneum shows evidence of endometriosis in 6% of cases (Balasch et al., 1996).
- Deep endometriosis when lesion penetrates through mesothelium (Koninckx et al., 1991)

RECTOVAGINAL ENDOMETRIOSIS CLASSIFICATION BASED ON LOCATION (Donnez et al., 2004)

- Type I/RV septum nodules (10% frequency): within the RV septum between the posterior wall of the vaginal mucosa and the anterior wall of the rectal muscularis
- Type II/posterior vaginal fornix nodules (65% frequency): posterior fornix (retrocervical) toward the RV septum
- Type III/hourglass-shaped nodules (25% frequency): posterior fornix lesions extending cranially to the anterior rectal wall; average size is 3 cm.

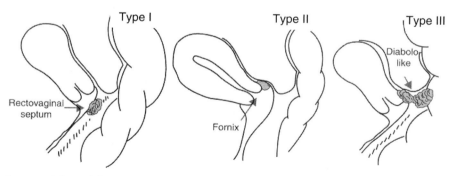

Source: Adapted from Donnez J, Pirard C, Smets M, et al. Surgical managment of endometriosis. *Best Practice Res Clin Obstet Gynecol* 18(2):329, 2004.

ENDOMETRIOSIS

AMERICAN SOCIETY FOR REPRODUCTIVE MEDICINE CLASSIFICATION

- American Society for Reproductive Medicine (ASRM) staging (American Society for Reproductive Medicine, 1997):

Patient's Name _____ Date_____

Stage I (Minimal) - 1-5   Laparoscopy_____ Laparotomy_____ Photography_____
Stage II (Mild)   - 6-15   Recommended Treatment_____
Stage III (Moderate) - 16-40
Stage IV (Severe)   -) 40
Total_____   Prognosis_____

PERITONEUM	ENDOMETRIOSIS		< 1cm	1-3cm	> 3cm
	Superficial		1	2	4
	Deep		2	4	6
OVARY	R	Superficial	1	2	4
		Deep	4	16	20
	L	Superficial	1	2	4
		Deep	4	16	20
	POSTERIOR CULDESAC OBLITERATION		Partial		Complete
			4		40
	ADHESIONS		< 1/3 Enclosure	1/3-2/3 Enclosure	> 2/3 Enclosure
OVARY	R	Filmy	1	2	4
		Dense	4	8	16
	L	Filmy	1	2	4
		Dense	4	8	16
TUBE	R	Filmy	1	2	4
		Dense	4*	8*	16
	L	Filmy	1	2	4
		Dense	4*	8*	16

*If the fimbriated end of the fallopian tube is completely enclosed, change the point assignment to 16.

Denote appearance of superficial implant types as red [(R), red, red-pink, flamelike, vesicular blobs, clear vesicles], white [(W), opacifications, peritoneal defects, yellow-brown], or black [(B) black, hemosiderin deposits, blue]. Denote percent of total described as R___%, W___% and B___%. Total should equal 100%.

Additional Endometriosis: _____   Associated Pathology: _____

_____   _____
_____   _____
_____   _____

To Be Used with Normal   To Be Used with Abnormal
Tubes and Ovaries   Tubes and/or Ovaries

L   R   L   R

EXAMPLES & GUIDELINES

STAGE I (MINIMAL)	STAGE II (MILD)	STAGE III (MODERATE)

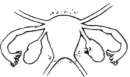 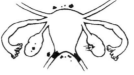 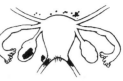

PERITONEUM
Superficial Endo — 1-3cm - 2
R. OVARY
Superficial Endo — < 1cm - 1
Filmy Adhesions — < 1/3 - 1
TOTAL POINTS 4

PERITONEUM
Deep Endo — > 3cm - 6
R. OVARY
Superficial Endo — < 1cm - 1
Filmy Adhesions — < 1/3 - 1
L. OVARY
Superficial Endo — < 1cm - 1
TOTAL POINTS 9

PERITONEUM
Deep Endo — > 3cm - 6
CULDESAC
Partial Obliteration - 4
L. OVARY
Deep Endo — 1-3cm - 16
TOTAL POINTS 26

STAGE III (MODERATE)	STAGE IV (SEVERE)	STAGE IV (SEVERE)

PERITONEUM
Superficial Endo — > 3cm - 4
R. TUBE
Filmy Adhesions — < 1/3 - 1
R. OVARY
Filmy Adhesions — < 1/3 - 1
L. TUBE
Dense Adhesions — < 1/3 - 16*
L. OVARY
Deep Endo — < 1 cm - 4
Dense Adhesions - < 1/3 - 4
TOTAL POINTS 30

PERITONEUM
Superficial Endo — > 3cm - 4
Deep Endo — 1-3cm - 32**
Dense Adhesions — < 1/3 - 8**
L. TUBE
Dense Adhesions — < 1/3 - 8**
TOTAL POINTS 52

*Point assignment changed to 16
**Point assignment doubled

PERITONEUM
Deep Endo — > 3cm - 6
CULDESAC
Complete Obliteration - 40
R. OVARY
Deep Endo — 1-3cm - 16
Dense Adhesions — < 1/3 - 4
L. TUBE
Dense Adhesions — > 2/3 - 16
L. OVARY
Deep Endo — 1-3cm - 16
Dense Adhesions — > 2/3 - 16
TOTAL POINTS 114

Determination of the stage or degree of endometrial involvement is based on a weighted point system. Distribution of points has been arbitrarily determined and may require further revision or refinement as knowledge of the disease increases.

To ensure complete evaluation, inspection of the pelvis in a clockwise or counterclockwise fashion is encouraged. Number, size and location of endometrial implants, plaques, endometriomas and/or adhesions are noted. For example, five separate 0.5cm superficial implants on the peritoneum (2.5 cm total) would be assigned 2 points. (The surface of the uterus should be considered peritoneum.) The severity of the endometriosis or adhesions should be assigned the highest score only for peritoneum, ovary, tube or culdesac. For example, a 4cm superficial and a 2cm deep implant of the peritoneum should be given a score of 6 (not 8). A 4cm

deep endometrioma of the ovary associated with more than 3cm of superficial disease should be scored 20 (not 24). In those patients with only one adnexa, points applied to disease of the remaining tube and ovary should be multiplied by two. **Points assigned may be circled and totaled. Aggregation of points indicates stage of disease (minimal, mild, moderate, or severe).

The presence of endometriosis of the bowel, urinary tract, fallopian tube, vagina, cervix, skin etc., should be documented under "additional endometriosis." Other pathology such as tubal occlusion, leiomyomata, uterine anomaly, etc., should be documented under "associated pathology." All pathology should be depicted as specifically as possible on the sketch of pelvic organs, and means of observation (laparoscopy or laparotomy) should be noted.

American Society for Reproductive Medicine revised classification of endometriosis. Endo, endometriosis. (Source: Reproduced with permission from Revised American Society for Reproductive Medicine classification of endometriosis: 1996. *Fertil Steril* 67(5):817, 1997.)

ENDOMETRIOSIS

TREATMENT

1. Expectant management
2. Surgical management
3. Medical treatment
4. Assisted reproductive technology
- Note: In >60% of cases, reappearance of lesions occurs within 1–5 yr (10% per yr) after hormonal and/or surgical treatment (Regidor et al., 1996).

Expectant Management

- Long-term pregnancy rate: 55–90% for stages I–III

Surgical Management

Conservative Surgery

- Regression of disease in 30–40% of women on second-look laparoscopy after initial surgery used to diagnose the disease (Harrison and Barry-Kinsella, 2000).
- Uterosacral nerve ablation:
  - Two randomized controlled trials (RCTs) reveal no evidence to support an additional laparoscopic uterine nerve ablation (LUNA) procedure for women undergoing surgical treatment for endometriosis pain (Johnson et al., 2004b; Vercellini et al., 2003a).
- No controlled trials have documented a benefit of preoperative or postoperative medical treatment to ↑ pregnancy rate over surgery alone.
- Metaanalysis regarding cyst recurrence rate (~10%) after cystectomy or drainage/coagulation (Vercellini et al., 2003b):
  - 21- to 36-mo common overall odds ratio (OR) = 3.09 (CI, 1.78–5.36) favoring cyst excision
  - It could be argued that a better outcome in terms of disease relapse after cystectomy may be counterbalanced by a worse postoperative pregnancy rate.
- In an RCT, laparoscopic cystectomy had a better 24-mo pregnancy rate than drainage and coagulation (67% vs. 24%, P <.05) (Beretta et al., 1998).
- Laparoscopic excision of endometriomas and ovarian reserve (Somigliana et al., 2003):
  - 32 patients over 46 cycles who had endometriomas removed from one ovary

- 53% ↓ in number of dominant follicles (IVF cycles) in ovary with prior endometriomas (P <.001):

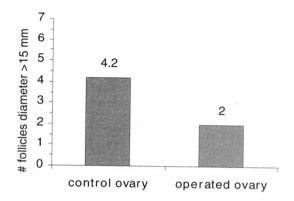

- Laparoscopic cystectomy for endometrioma (>3 cm) before an IVF cycle does not improve fertility outcomes; likewise, conservative surgical treatment of endometriomas does not impair IVF success rates (Garcia-Velasco et al., 2004).
- Evidence of enhanced fertility by conservative surgical treatment (minimal-mild):
  - **Marcoux, et al. (Marcoux et al., 1997) (Canadian study: ENDOCAN):**
    ⇨ RCT; data collected for 36 wks; stage I–II (30% stage II); infertility ~2 yrs

n = 341	Ablation (%)	Diagnostic Laparoscopy Only (%)
Cumulative pregnancy[a]	31.0[b]	18.0
Fecundity[c]	4.7	2.4

[a]>20 wks' gestation.
[b]P <.01.
[c]Rates of 20-wk pregnancies per 100 person-years.

   ❖ Eight women need surgery to achieve one additional pregnancy; however, because we cannot diagnose endometriosis preoperatively, the number may actually double to 16 surgeries for one pregnancy.
   ❖ Clear or pink vesicular lesions (may be *most active*!) not included
  - **Gruppo Italiano (Italian study) (Parazzini, 1999):**
    ⇨ RCT; data collected for 12 wks; stage I–II (60% stage II); unexplained infertility ≥2 yrs

ENDOMETRIOSIS

n = 96	Ablation	Diagnostic Laparoscopy Only
Spontaneous conceptions	24%	29%

⇨ Secondary finding:

n = 46	Adjuvant GnRH-a	No Adjuvant GnRH-a
Spontaneous conceptions	39%	18%

GnRH-a, gonadotropin-releasing hormone-agonist.

- Marcoux + Gruppo Italiano common odds ratio benefit:

	Common Odds Ratio Benefit
All conceptions	1.7 (95% CI, 1.1–2.6)
>20-wk pregnancy	1.6 (95% CI, 1.0–2.7)

CI, confidence interval.

⇨ Therefore, modest efficacy of endometriosis ablation in ↑ pregnancy rate in infertile women with minimal-mild endometriosis

Definitive Surgery
- Refractory to medicine/conservative surgery
- Hysterectomy with bilateral salpingo-oophorectomy: 90% rate of success
- Recurrence rate: 0–5% (same if patient taking estrogen treatment)
- Cohort study (138 women): Compared with women who had oophorectomy for endometriosis, patients who underwent hysterectomy with ovarian conservation had 6.1 times greater risk of developing recurrent pain and 8.1 times greater risk of reoperation (Namnoum et al., 1995).
- Posthysterectomy + oophorectomy estrogen replacement may start in the postoperative period without ↑ incidence of symptom recurrence (Hickman et al., 1998).

Postoperative Adjuvant Drug Therapy
- Six randomized trials:

Regimen	Length of Treatment (mos)	n	Results
Dz vs. medroxyprogesterone acetate vs. placebo	6	51	↓ Pain in treatment groups at 1 yr
GnRH-a vs. placebo	3	53	No difference in pain at 1 yr[a]
GnRH-a vs. placebo	6	93	↓ Pain at end of treatment but no difference at 1 yr[a]
Dz vs. no treatment	3	77	No difference in pain at 9 mos[a]
GnRH-a vs. no treatment	6	210	No difference in pain at 1 yr[a]
GnRH-a vs. no treatment	3	89	No difference in pain at 18 mos[a]

Dz, danazol; GnRH-a, gonadotropin-releasing hormone-agonist.
[a]Low statistical power to detect smaller, though clinically significant, differences.
Source: Adapted from Telimaa S, Ronnberg L, et al. Placebo-controlled comparison of danazol and high-dose medroxyprogesterone acetate in the treatment of endometriosis after conservative surgery. *Gynecol Endocrinol* 1(4):363, 1987; Parazzini F, Fedele L, et al. Postsurgical medical treatment of advanced endometriosis: results of a randomized clinical trial. *Am J Obstet Gynecol* 171(5):1205, 1994; and Hornstein MD, Hemmings R, et al. Use of nafarelin versus placebo after reductive laparoscopic surgery for endometriosis. *Fertil Steril* 68(5):860, 1997.

- Gonadotropin-releasing hormone (GnRH)-agonist + aromatase inhibitor (anastrozole, 1 mg/day): prospective, randomized trial:

Regimen × 6 Mos Postoperative	% Free of Recurrence at 24 Mos	Median Time to Recurrence
GnRH-a	10.4	17 mos
GnRH-a + aromatase inhibitor	54.7	>24 mos[a]

GnRH-a, gonadotropin-releasing hormone-agonist.
[a]$P < .01$.
Source: Adapted from Soysal S, Soysal ME, et al. The effects of post-surgical administration of goserelin plus anastrozole compared to goserelin alone in patients with severe endometriosis: a prospective randomized trial. *Hum Reprod* 19(1):160, 2004.

- No significant difference in climacteric symptoms or bone mineral density (at 24 mos), although low numbers of patients (40 in each group)

Medical Treatment (Dizerega et al., 1980)

Progestins
- Results in endometrial decidualization—atrophy and pseudodecidualization (Silverberg, 1986; Maruo et al., 2001).

ENDOMETRIOSIS

- 20–30 mg/day medroxyprogesterone acetate or progestin-only pill
- Levonorgestrel-intrauterine device (lng-IUD, Mirena) delivers 20 µg levonorgestrel/day over 5 yrs.
  - Pilot study using lng-IUD for 6 mos revealed statistically significant (P <.01) ↓ pain severity (7.7 → 4.6 on a visual analog scale) and ↓ % of moderate-to-severe dysmenorrhea (96% → 50%) (Lockhat et al., 2004).

Oral Contraceptives

- Continuously; 60–90% effective; 1st-yr recurrence = 17%, 5–10% annual recurrence rate
- 50 women who had surgery for endometriosis within 1 yr and experienced recurrent dysmenorrheal despite cyclic oral contraceptive (OC) use were treated with continuous OCs (ethinyl estradiol [EE] 20 µg + desogestrel 150 µg) for 2 yrs (Vercellini et al., 2003c):
  - ↓ 59% visual analog scale (dysmenorrhea) P <.001
  - ↓ 71% verbal rating scale (dysmenorrhea) P <.001

Gonadotropin-Releasing Hormone Agonist: Decapeptide

- To avoid flare effect, initiate GnRH-a at
  - Midluteal phase or
  - After 2 wks of OCs (started on cycle day 1 or 2) overlapping by 1 wk
- Side effects: breakthrough bleeding (BTB), vasomotor symptoms (2nd mo), vaginal dryness, mood alteration, insomnia, irritability, headache, depression, reversible bone mineral density loss (loss of 5% by dual-energy x-ray absorptiometry (DXA) at conclusion of 6 mos of therapy)

Leuprolide depot, 3.75 mg IM q28 days
Goserelin, 3.6 mg SC q28 days
Nafarelin, 400–800 mg/day intranasally in divided doses

Early-onset BTB
1. Rule out pregnancy.
2. Withdrawal bleed after 1st cycle is common.
3. Confirm adequate suppression (↓ E_2) if on GnRH-a.
4. Initiate GnRH-a closer to onset of menses.
5. Consider progestin or oral contraceptive pretreatment 2 wks pre–GnRH-a.

Late-onset BTB
1. Rule out pregnancy.
2. Confirm scheduling.
3. Confirm adequate suppression (↓ E_2).
4. Rule out atrophic bleeding (treatment: low-dose estrogen replacement therapy)

BTB, breakthrough bleeding; E_2, estradiol; GnRH-a, gonadotropin-releasing hormone-agonist.

ENDOMETRIOSIS

- 75–90% effective, pain symptoms return within 1 yr of treatment with GnRH-a, 20% having recurrent symptoms requiring retreatment (Hornstein et al., 1995).
- Time to pain recurrence after GnRH-a (Miller et al., 1998):
  - Stage I–II: 5.3 mos
  - Stage III–IV: 5.9 mos
- Add-back therapy:
  - Low-dose estradiol for vasomotor symptoms and bone preservation.
  - ⇨ Therapeutic window:

E_2 (pg/mL)	E_2-Dependent Ramification
<80	Lipid metabolism compromised
<60	Vaginal epithelial atrophy
<40	Vasomotor symptoms
<20	Bone density deterioration

E_2, estradiol.
Note: Optimal $[E_2]$ ≤30–50 pg/mL for endometriosis.
Source: Adapted from Barbieri RL. Hormone treatment of endometriosis: the estrogen threshold hypothesis. *Am J Obstet Gynecol* 166:740, 1992.

  - ⇨ **Estradiol, 25 μg transdermal patch each week**
  - ⇨ **Conjugated equine estrogen, 0.625 mg/day**
  - Progestins for vasomotor symptoms and bone preservation (Hornstein et al., 1998)
    - ⇨ **Norethindrone acetate, 5 mg PO/day**
  - Combined therapy for women unable to tolerate progestin-only add-back

Aromatase Inhibitor (Ailawadi et al., 2004)

- Regimen: letrozole (Femara), 2.5 mg/day; norethindrone acetate, 2.5 mg/day; vitamin D, 800 IU/day; calcium citrate, 1.25 g/day
- Nonrandomized pilot study on ten patients:
  - Pretreatment diagnostic laparoscopy (eight patients with stage III–IV) followed by 6 mos of treatment and posttreatment laparoscopy
    - ⇨ Significant ↓ ASRM endometriosis scores: 44.1 → 29.7
    - ⇨ Significant ↓ pain relief in nine of ten previously unresponsive

ENDOMETRIOSIS

Immunomodulators (Pentoxifylline, Trental) (Balasch et al., 1997)

- RCT: 29 treated with Trental, 400 mg PO b.i.d., and 27 treated with placebo
- 12-Mo overall pregnancy rate: 31% (Trental) vs. 18.5% (placebo), not statistically significant although there is a risk of type II error due to low number of patients

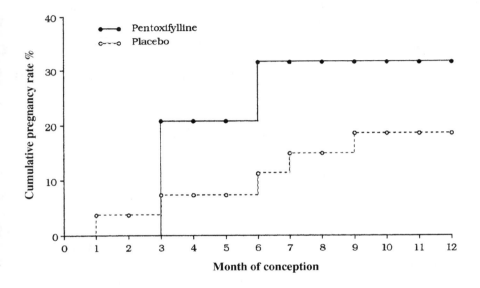

ENDOMETRIOSIS

SUMMARY OF MEDICAL AGENTS USED TO TREAT ENDOMETRIOSIS

Class	Drug	Dosage
Androgen	Danazol	400–800 mg/day PO for 4–6 mos
Gonadotropin-releasing hormone agonist	Leuprolide	500 µg/day SC
	Leuprolide depot	3.75 mg IM q28 days
	Buserelin	400 µg q.i.d. intranasally
	Goserelin	3.6 mg SC q28 days or 10.8 mg/3 mos
	Nafarelin	200 µg/day b.i.d. intranasally
Progestin	Gestrinone	2.5–5.0 mg/day
	Medroxyprogesterone acetate	20–30 mg/day PO for 6 mos, followed by 100 mg IM q2 wks × 2 mos, then 200 mg IM monthly × 4 mos
Oral contraceptive	Monophasic Estrogen/progestin	Ethinyl estradiol, 30–35 µg, plus a progestin; 1 tablet/day × 4–6 mos
Aromatase inhibitor	Letrozole (Femara) (Vit D, Ca^{2+}, NET-Acetate)	Femara, 2.5 mg PO/day; NET-Acetate, 2.5 mg/day; Vit D, 800 IU/day, + Ca^{2+}, 1.25 g/day
Immunomodulatory	Pentoxifylline	Trental, 400 mg PO b.i.d.

NET-Acetate, norethindrone acetate; Vit D, vitamin D.

Assisted Reproductive Technologies

• Fertility: No role for drug therapy (OC, progestins, GnRH-a) in the treatment of infertility associated with endometriosis

157

ENDOMETRIOSIS

- Induction of ovulation in women with endometriosis:

		Cycle Fecundity Rate (%)	
Regimen	n	Treatment Group	Expectant Group
Clomiphene citrate, IUI	67	9.5	3.3
Human menopausal gonadotropin, human chorionic gonadotropin, IUI	49	15.0	4.5
Follicle-stimulating hormone, IUI	103	11[a]	2[a]

IUI, intrauterine insemination.
[a]Live birth rate (%).
Source: Adapted from Deaton JL, Gibson M, et al. A randomized, controlled trial of clomiphene citrate and intrauterine insemination in couples with unexplained infertility or surgically corrected endometriosis. *Fertil Steril* 54(6):1083, 1990; Fedele L, Bianchi S, et al. Superovulation with human menopausal gonadotropins in the treatment of infertility associated with minimal or mild endometriosis: a controlled randomized study. *Fertil Steril* 58(1):28, 1992; and Tummon IS, Asher LJ, et al. Randomized controlled trial of superovulation and insemination for infertility associated with minimal or mild endometriosis. *Fertil Steril* 68(1):8, 1997.

- IVF outcome: endometriosis only vs. tubal factor only, metaanalysis:

	Pregnancy Rate		
Regimen	Stage I–II	Stage II–IV	Control Group
In vitro fertilization	21.1%	13.8[a]	27.7

[a]Odds ratio, 0.46 (0.28, 0.74).
Source: Adapted from Barnhart K, Dunsmoor-Su R, et al. Effect of endometriosis on in vitro fertilization. *Fertil Steril* 77(6):1148, 2002.

- GnRH-a pretreatment before IVF: *single* prospective, randomized trial:

Regimen	n	Cycle Pregnancy Rate (%)
No GnRH-a	26	55
GnRH-a × 3 mos	25	80[a]

GnRH-a, gonadotropin-releasing hormone-agonist.
[a]$P < .05$; NNT = 4.
Source: Adapted from Surrey ES, Silverberg KM, et al. Effect of prolonged gonadotropin-releasing hormone agonist therapy on the outcome of in vitro fertilization-embryo transfer in patients with endometriosis. *Fertil Steril* 78(4):699, 2002.

ENDOMETRIOSIS

Treatment Algorithms

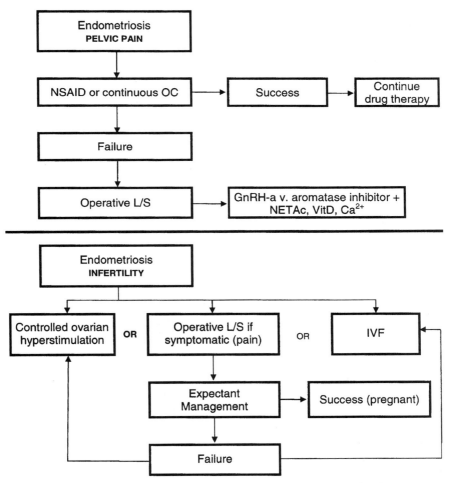

GNRH-a, gonadotropin-releasing hormone-agonist; IVF, *in vitro* fertilization; L/S, laparoscopy; NETAc, norethindrone acetate; NSAID, nonsteroidal antiinflammatory drug; OC, oral contraceptive; VitD, vitamin D.

17. Fibroids

PREVALENCE
• 20–50% (Novak and Woodruff, 1979)

CLASSIFICATION
Submucosal (Wamsteker et al., 1993)
• Fibroid distorts the uterine cavity.

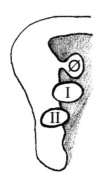

Type Ø	Pedunculated (intraluminal) without intramural extension
Type I	Sessile with intramural extension <50%
Type II	Sessile with intramural extension ≥50%

Intramural
• <50% protrudes into the serosal surface. >50% of the myoma is within the myometrium.

Subserosal
• >50% protrudes out of the serosal surface (sessile or pedunculated).

FIBROIDS AND BLEEDING
• Obstructive effect on uterine vasculature may lead to endometrial venule extasia → proximal congestion in the myometrium/endometrium → hypermenorrhea.
• ↑ Size of uterine cavity (sometimes appreciated on hysterosalpingogram) leads to greater surface area for endometrial sloughing.

FIBROIDS AND PAIN (Lippman et al., 2003)

- ↑ Severity of dyspareunia and noncyclic pelvic pain with the presence of fibroids
- Dysmenorrhea not more common in those with fibroids vs. those without fibroids
- Fibroids in the fundus may be associated with more severe dyspareunia and pelvic pain.

FIBROIDS AND INFERTILITY

- Sole factor for infertility in <10% of infertility cases (Wallach and Vu, 1995)
- Submucosal is most likely to cause infertility, then intramural, then subserosal (Farhi et al., 1995).
- Subserosal or intramural leiomyomas <4 cm not encroaching on the uterine cavity have *in vitro* fertilization (IVF)–intracytoplasmic sperm injection (ICSI) outcomes comparable to those of patients without such leiomyomas; patients with fibroids >4 cm may benefit from removal, but this remains to be determined (Note: underpowered study) (Oliveira et al., 2004).
- Submucosal mechanism of infertility:
  - Dysfunctional uterine contractility (Vollenhoven et al., 1990)
  - Focal endometrial vascular disturbance
  - Endometrial inflammation; endometritis
  - Secretion of vasoactive substances
  - Enhanced androgen environment (Buttram and Reiter, 1981)
- Patients are advised to wait 4–6 mos after myomectomy before attempting to conceive.
- Uterine artery embolization is not recommended in patients considering future fertility.

FIBROIDS

FIBROIDS AND REPRODUCTIVE OUTCOME

- 80% of fibroids remain the same size or diminish during pregnancy (Lev-Toaff et al., 1987).
- Complications: miscarriage, ectopic, preterm labor (15–20%), abdominal pain, abruption, intrauterine growth restriction (10%), obstructed labor, postpartum hemorrhage, malpresentation (20%) (Phelan, 1995)
- Five retrospective cohort studies:

	Pregnancy Rate (%)	Spontaneous Abortion (%)[a]
Submucosal	9	40
Intramural	37	33
Subserosal	16	33
Control	29	20

[a]Small numbers.
Source: Adapted from Bajekal N, Li TC. Fibroids, infertility, and pregnancy wastage. *Hum Reprod Update* 6:614, 2000.

- Recent review of 27 studies: no conclusive evidence on whether number, size, or location of fibroids before myomectomy influenced postoperative pregnancy (Vercellini et al., 1998).
- Ten retrospective studies, prognosis after myomectomy:

Pregnancy rate	50–68%
Spontaneous abortions	6–40%
Live births	57–93%

Source: Adapted from Bajekal N, Li TC. Fibroids, infertility, and pregnancy wastage. *Hum Reprod Update* 6:614, 2000.

Submucosal Fibroids

	Pregnancy Rate	Delivery Rate
Submucosal myoma	0.3 (CI, 0.1–0.7)	—
Submucosal myomectomy		
Compared with infertile control subjects with fibroids	1.7 (CI, 1.1–2.6)	—
Compared with infertile control subjects without fibroids	—	1.0 (0.5–2.4); no difference

CI, confidence interval.
Source: Adapted from Pritts EA. Fibroids and infertility: a systematic review of the evidence. *Obstet Gynecol Surv* 56(8):483, 2001.

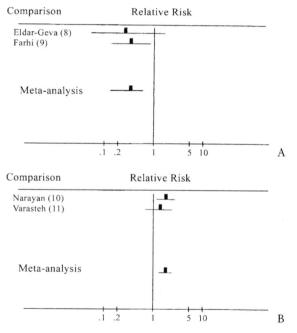

A: Metaanalysis of pregnancy rate for patients with submucosal fibroids compared with infertile controls (data from *in vitro* fertilization). **B:** Metaanalysis of pregnancy rate for submucosal myomectomy compared with controls (data from assisted reproductive technologies + spontaneous conceptions). (Reproduced with permission from Pritts EA. Fibroids and infertility: a systematic review of the evidence. *Obstet Gynecol Surv* 56:483, 2001.)

FIBROIDS

- The majority of women who conceive do so within the first year after a myomectomy.
- Many of the studies demonstrating a higher pregnancy rate after myomectomy are nonrandomized and suffer from an inherent selection bias. There is no datum addressing myomectomy outcomes for women with subserosal and/or intramural fibroids without intracavitary involvement. If there is no cavity distortion, then there are no data (Surrey et al., 2001).

RALOXIFENE VERSUS GONADOTROPIN-RELEASING HORMONE-AGONIST

- 3 Mos of raloxifene (120 mg/day) resulted in ↓ fibroid volume (~22%) compared with untreated controls, although less than expected for gonadotropin-releasing hormone-agonist (GnRH-a) alone; subjects asymptomatic before and after treatment (Jirecek et al., 2004).
- 6 Mos of raloxifene (60 or 180 mg/day) had no effect on fibroid size (Palomba, 2002a).
- 6 Mos of raloxifene (60 mg/day) + GnRH-a was more effective than GnRH-a alone (30% greater ↓ in fibroid size); no difference in fibroid-related symptoms (Palomba et al., 2002a), although the raloxifene group had no change in bone mineral density at the end of treatment whereas the GnRH-a group had significantly lower values compared with baseline and to the raloxifene group (P <.05) (Palomba, 2002b).

MIFEPRISTONE (RU-486) (Steinauer et al., 2004)

- Progesterone may stimulate fibroid growth.
- Metaanalysis of six clinical trials (no randomized controlled trials) using 5–50 mg/day mifepristone for 3–6 mos:
  - 27–49% ↓ in uterine volume
  - 26–74% ↓ in leiomyoma volume
  - ↓ Severity of dysmenorrhea, menorrhagia, and pelvic pressure
  - **Endometrial hyperplasia in 28%**

PREOPERATIVE GONADOTROPIN-RELEASING HORMONE-AGONIST
Background

- Greater potency and longer half-life ($t_{1/2}$) than native GnRH
- Analogs: decapeptide with substitutions at positions 6 and 10
- Initially stimulates gonadotropin release—lasts 1–2 wks
- Fibroid growth stimulated by estrogen and progesterone

FIBROIDS

- Down-regulation with GnRH-a induces a state of hypoestrogenism (<30 pg/mL) and anovulation.
- Long-term treatment with GnRH-a is limited due to side effects (bone mineral density loss and hot flashes)
- Myoma volume ↓ 30.4% using GnRH-a (leuprolide) in a double-blind, placebo-controlled study (Schlaff et al., 1989)
- Randomized, placebo-controlled study did not find that GnRH-a preoperative treatment led to ↓ size of small myomas, rendering them undetectable at surgery and early recurrence (Friedman et al., 1992).
- Fibroids regrow after discontinuing GnRH-a.
- Therefore, GnRH-a used mainly in preoperative setting for definitive therapy (hysterectomy) or conservative therapy (myomectomy).

Outcomes of Gonadotropin-Releasing Hormone-Agonist-Treated Groups versus Nontreated

Preoperative Gonadotropin-Releasing Hormone-Agonist Treatment × 3–4 Months

	Weighted Mean Difference	95% Confidence Interval
↑ Hematocrit	3.1%	1.8–4.5
↓ Uterine volume	−159 mL	−169 to −149
↓ Gestational size	−2.2 wks	−2.3 to −1.9
↓ Fibroid volume	−12 cc	−18.3 to −6.6
Pelvic symptom score	−2.1	−2.4 to −1.9

Source: Data from Lethaby A, Vollenhoven B, Sowter M. Efficacy of pre-operative gonadotropin hormone releasing analogues for women with uterine fibroids undergoing hysterectomy or myomectomy: a systematic review. *BJOG* 109:1097, 2002.

Intraoperative Outcomes

	Myomectomy	Hysterectomy
Blood loss	ND	↓ 58 mL (−76 to −40)
Duration of surgery	ND	↓ 5.2 mins (−8.6 to −1.8)
Hospital stay	ND	ND
Rate of blood transfusions	ND	ND
Proportion of vertical skin incisions	0.11 (0.1–0.8)	0.4 (0.2–0.6)

ND, no difference.
Source: Data from Lethaby A, Vollenhoven B, Sowter M. Efficacy of pre-operative gonadotropin hormone releasing analogues for women with uterine fibroids undergoing hysterectomy or myomectomy: a systematic review. *BJOG* 109:1097, 2002.

FIBROIDS

Postoperative Outcomes

	Myomectomy	Hysterectomy
Postoperative complications	ND	0.6% (0.4–0.9)
Postoperative hematocrit	ND	↑ 1.8% (1.1–2.4)
Fibroid recurrence[a]	4.0[b] (1.1–14.7)	Not applicable

ND, no difference.
[a]Only two published trials.
[b]May not see small fibroids at the time of surgery in pretreated women.
Source: Data from Lethaby A, Vollenhoven B, Sowter M. Efficacy of pre-operative gonadotropin hormone releasing analogues for women with uterine fibroids undergoing hysterectomy or myomectomy: a systematic review. *BJOG* 109:1097, 2002.

Laparoscopic Myomectomy: Outcomes of Gonadotropin-Releasing Hormone-Agonist–Treated Groups versus Nontreated (

Preoperative Gonadotropin Releasing Hormone-Agonist Treatment × 2 Months

	Value	*P* Value
Blood loss	↓ 60.3 mL	<.01
Duration of surgery[a]	↓ 14.8 mins	<.05
	↑ 13.4 mins	<.05

[a]Exception: hypoechoic fibroids
Source: Adapted from Zullo F, Pellicano M, et al. A prospective randomized study to evaluate leuprolide acetate treatment before laparoscopic myomectomy: efficacy and ultrasonographic predictors. *Am J Obstet Gynecol* 178(1 Pt 1):108, 1998.

18. Polycystic Ovary Syndrome

- ~10% of reproductive-aged women have polycystic ovary syndrome (PCOS)
- Genetics:

Affected 1st-Degree Relative	Risk of Polycystic Ovary Syndrome (%)
Mother	35
Sister	40

Source: Adapted from Kahsar-Miller MD, Nixon C, Boots LR, et al. Prevalence of polycystic ovary syndrome (PCOS) in first-degree relatives of patients with PCOS. *Fertil Steril* 75(1):53, 2001.

- PCOS patients frequently develop regular menstrual cycles when aging (Elting et al., 2000), due to ↓ size of the follicle cohort? Or due to ↓ inhibin?
- **Theory of etiology:** *enhanced serine phosphorylation unification theory* → ↑ CYP17 activity in the ovary (hyperandrogenism) and ↓ insulin receptor activity peripherally (insulin resistance [IR]) (Dunaif et al., 1995) lead to the endocrine dysfunction of PCOS.

PATHOPHYSIOLOGY OF POLYCYSTIC OVARY SYNDROME
Normal Ovulation Requirements
- Competent hypothalamus, pituitary, and ovary
- Coordinated activities of gonadotropins, steroids, inhibin, activin, insulin-like growth factor (IGF)-I, IGF-II, and their binding proteins, proteases, and prostaglandins

Endocrine Dysfunction
Hypersecretion/Elevation of Luteinizing Hormone
- ↑ Pulse amplitude and frequency, ↑ luteinizing hormone (LH) bioactivity (abnormal LH secretion is secondary to ovarian dysfunction):
  - Lack of negative feedback (↓ progesterone [P_4])?
  - Programming of the hypothalamic-pituitary axis by androgens?
  - ↓ Sex hormone–binding globulin (SHBG) from hyperinsulinemia and hyperandrogenemia leads to ↑ free estradiol levels, lowering follicle-stimulating hormone (FSH) relative to LH.
    ⇨ Insulin is the most potent inhibitor of SHBG (Nestler et al., 1991).

POLYCYSTIC OVARY SYNDROME

Hyperinsulinemia
- Hyperinsulinemia leads to ↓ SHBG, ↓ IGF-binding protein (IGFBP)-I and ↑ free androgens.
- Total serum IGF-I levels are normal in PCOS, but ↓ IGFBP-I concentrations can lead to ↑ **free IGF-I.**
- IGF-I and -II → ↑ LH stimulation of androgens in theca cells.
- Insulin may also ↑ androgen production directly or may ↑ LH secretion from the pituitary (Dorn et al., 2004).
- **Waist-hip ratio** >0.85 (central obesity) is significantly related to insulin sensitivity, but body mass index (BMI) is not.

Androgen Excess
- Ovarian production: ↑ LH results in theca hyperplasia (theca cell dysfunction), resulting in ↑ testosterone (T), androstenedione (A^4), dehydroepiandrosterone (DHEA), 17-hydroxyprogesterone (17-OHP), and estrone (E_1). Ovarian estradiol (E_2) production is unchanged.
- Adrenal is a secondary source of elevated serum androgens. Nonclassic adrenal hyperplasia (NCAH)—a genetic defect in either the 21-hydroxylase (*CYP21B*) or the 3β-hydroxysteroid dehydrogenase (*3βHSD*) genes, results in elevated levels of primarily adrenal androgens (i.e., DHEA-sulfate [DHEA-S]).
- ↓ SHBG leads to ↑ free androgen and estrogen (↓ SHBG from elevated insulin, hyperandrogenemia, hyperprolactinemia).
- 30% of patients with PCOS show mild hyperprolactinemia (Isik et al., 1997).

Organ Dysfunction
- **Pituitary:** Androgen excess may cause LH excess by counteracting the LH-suppressive effect of P_4 (Eagleson et al., 2000).
- **Ovary:** Functional ovarian hyperandrogenism (stromal hyperplasia, multicystic) may be a consequence or a **cause** of the endocrinopathy.
  - ↑ LH levels stimulate theca cells, thickening the ovarian stroma, and ↑ local androgen production within the ovary, which in turn prevents follicular maturation.
  - Low-normal circulating **FSH** levels maintain a continuous stimulation for follicular growth.
    - ⇨ The pool of preovulatory follicles is dynamic: atretic follicles continuously being replaced by new follicles of limited growth potential, none of which matures to become a dominant, ovulatory follicle
  - Hyperthecosis is an extreme variation of the syndrome: Nests of luteinized theca cells are seen throughout the ovarian stroma; hyperthecosis is almost always associated with IR.
  - High levels of local androgens may inhibit maturation of follicles.

168

POLYCYSTIC OVARY SYNDROME

- $\uparrow$ Expression of LH receptor, steroidogenic acute regulatory protein (*StAR*), *CYP11A*, and *CYP17* messenger RNAs (mRNAs) in theca cells from PCOS follicles versus size-matched control follicles (Jakimiuk et al., 2001)
- **Endometrium:** No ovulation $\rightarrow$ no P_4 production $\rightarrow$ proliferative endometrium $\rightarrow$ $\uparrow$ risk of endometrial hyperplasia and/or cancer
- **Adrenal gland:** Approximately one-half of patients with PCOS also have a characteristic type of adrenal dysfunction that consists of moderately excessive responses of 17-ketosteroids, particularly DHEA, to adrenocorticotropic hormone (ACTH) without evidence of a steroidogenic block.

Potential Long-Term Consequences of Polycystic Ovary Syndrome

Definite or Very Likely Consequences of Polycystic Ovary Syndrome	Possible Consequences of Polycystic Ovary Syndrome
Insulin resistance; type II diabetes mellitus (greater than weight-matched controls)	Hypertension
	Coronary heart disease
Endometrial hyperplasia/atypia	Dyslipidemia
Gestational diabetes	Ovarian cancer (conflicting data)
Sleep apnea (even when controlled for body mass index)	Spontaneous abortion (may not be greater than for subfertility population)

- Hyperlipidemia (Mahabeer et al., 1990; Orio et al., 2004) reported to elevate plasminogen activator inhibitor (PAI; major inhibitor of fibrinolysis); PAI is an independent risk factor for atherosclerosis.
- $\uparrow$ Left ventricular mass index among asymptomatic women with PCOS compared with controls (Orio et al., 2004).
- Studies showing no clear association between PCOS and cardiovascular events may be biased due to PCOS study patients having had wedge resection (Pierpoint et al., 1998; Wild et al., 2000).
- Type II diabetes mellitus (DM): $3-7\times \uparrow$ incidence in PCOS patients

POLYCYSTIC OVARY SYNDROME

CLINICAL SIGNS AND SYMPTOMS

Menstrual Dysfunction
- Onset at menarche: oligo/amenorrhea

Infertility
- Ovulatory dysfunction

Obesity
- Obesity occurs in 35–65% of women with PCOS (>80% are obese before puberty).
- Androgens converted to E_1 in peripheral fat and can contribute to endometrial hyperplasia.
- Fat contributes to insulin insensitivity.

Hirsutism
- Gradual onset over months to years; onset usually with puberty
- Dark, coarse hairs in androgen-dependent locations
- Associated with hyperandrogenemia (classic PCOS) and idiopathic increased end organ sensitivity
- *Ferriman-Gallway* scores (see Appendix B in this chapter) are used to quantify degree of hirsutism and grade responses to treatments (Ferriman and Gallway, 1961); on a day-to-day clinical basis, most endocrinologists rely on patient perceptions and frequency of waxing or electrolysis.

Variable Other Signs and Symptoms
- **Acne:** no known correlation between the severity of acne and plasma-free T (Slayden and Azziz, 1997)
- **Acanthosis nigricans:** usually seen with significant insulin resistance; called the *h*yper*a*ndrogenism, *i*nsulin *r*esistance–*a*canthosis *n*igricans (**HAIR-AN**) syndrome:
  - Dermal hyperkeratosis and papillomatosis presenting as a brown or gray, velvety, occasionally verrucous, hyperpigmented area over the vulva (most common), axillae, groin, umbilicus, and submammary areas
- **IR** (~30%) or overt non–insulin-dependent diabetes mellitus (NIDDM) (~8%) (Dunaif, 1997)
- Skin tags

POLYCYSTIC OVARY SYNDROME

- **Polycystic-appearing ovaries** (PCAOs) not necessarily a prerequisite for diagnosis (see criteria below); present in 30% of population:

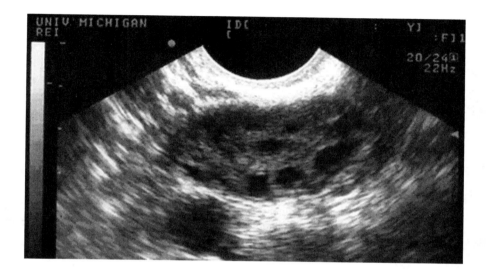

CLINICAL EVALUATION OF POLYCYSTIC OVARY SYNDROME/HIRSUTISM

- Dr. Andrea Dunaif (*personal communication*): "PCOS is like pornography: It's hard to define, but when you see it, you recognize it."
- Revised 2003 Rotterdam European Society for Human Reproduction and Embryology (ESHRE)/American Society for Reproductive Medicine (ASRM)–sponsored PCOS consensus on diagnostic criteria for PCOS (**two out of three**) (Rotterdam ESHRE/ASRM-Sponsored PCOS Consensus Workshop Group, 2004):

1. Oligo- and/or anovulation
2. Clinical and/or biochemical (total T >70 ng/dL; A^4 >245 ng/dL; DHEA-S >248 μg/dL) signs of hyperandrogenism
3. Polycystic ovaries (≥12 follicles [2–9 mm diameter] in each ovary)
   Exclusion of other etiologies (e.g., nonclassic congenital adrenal hyperplasia [NCAH], hyperprolactinemia, Cushing's syndrome, and androgen-secreting tumors)

POLYCYSTIC OVARY SYNDROME

- In most cases, the diagnosis can be made on history and physical examination (H&P) alone; ~10% incidence

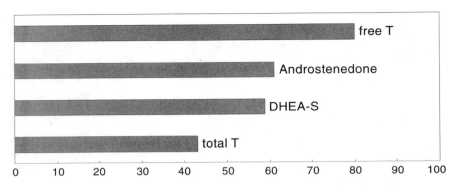

Frequency of elevation of each of the androgens in 138 women with polycystic ovary syndrome (Wild et al., 1983), listed as a percentage. DHEA-S, dehydroepiandrosterone sulfate; T, testosterone. (Source: Adapted from Wild RA, Umstot ES, Andersen RN, et al. Androgen parameters and their correlation with body weight in one hundred thirty-eight women thought to have hyperandrogenism. *Am J Obstet Gynecol* 146[6]:602, 1983.)

Diagnostic Studies (Phipps, 2001)

Testosterone
- Total T upper limit = 200 ng/dL; 6.9 nmol/L; free T upper limit = 2.2 pg/mL
- Rule out ovarian androgen-producing tumor if T levels >200 ng/dL; 6.9 nmol/L.

Estradiol and Follicle-Stimulating Hormone
- Exclude hypogonadotropic hypogonadism ($\downarrow$ E$_2$, $\downarrow$ FSH) and premature ovarian failure (POF) ($\downarrow$ E$_2$, $\uparrow$ FSH).

Dehydroepiandrosterone Sulfate
- Upper limit = 430 µg/dL; 11.7 µmol/L
- Rule out adrenal androgen-producing tumor if >700 µg/dL; 19 µmol/L.
- Note: may not be of benefit if T is normal

17-Hydroxyprogesterone (in Follicular Phase, 8:00 a.m.) + Progesterone
- 17-OHP upper limit = 2 ng/mL; 69 pmol/L; if P$_4$ <3 ng/mL; 104 pmol/L, this signifies follicular phase
- Rule out nonclassic 21-hydroxylase deficiency.
- P$_4$ is drawn to be sure that the patient is not in the luteal phase when 17-OHP is naturally elevated; want P$_4$ <3 ng/mL; 104 pmol/L

POLYCYSTIC OVARY SYNDROME

24-Hr Urinary Cortisol
- Cortisol usually <50 µg/24 hr (<135 nmol/24 hr)
- Rule out Cushing's syndrome if patient is hypertensive.

Prolactin
- Upper limit = 30 ng/mL
- Rule out hyperprolactinemia as cause of ovulatory dysfunction.
- Also check thyroid-stimulating hormone (TSH) to rule out hyperprolactinemia from hypothyroidism.

Thyroid-Stimulating Hormone
- Rule out thyroid disease as cause of ovulatory dysfunction.

Oral Glucose Tolerance Test versus Fasting
Glucose to Insulin Ratio (glucose:mg/dL; insulin:µU/mL) (Rotterdam ESHRE/ ASRM-Sponsored PCOS Consenses Workshop Group, 2004)
- If BMI >27 kg/m² or family history of diabetes → oral glucose tolerance test (OGTT)
- If BMI <27 kg/m² and no family history of diabetes → glucose to insulin ratio to assess for hyperinsulinemia (if the ratio is <4.5, follow up with secondary OGTT)
- Values <4.5 are abnormal (sensitivity = 95%; specificity = 84%) (Legro et al., 1998); follow up with 2-hr OGTT (75-g oral glucose): ≥200 ng/dL indicates DM.
- Used to identify those at greater risk of developing diabetes and hyperlipidemia

	Fasting Plasma Glucose (mg/dL)	2-hr Plasma Glucose (mg/dL)
Normal	≤ 99	≤139
Impaired	100–125	140–199
Type II diabetes mellitus	≥126 mg/dL	≥200

- Incidence of IR or NIDDM in women with PCOS (Legro et al., 1999):
  - IR: 30%
  - Type II DM: 8%

Lipid Profile
- Cholesterol, high-density lipoprotein (HDL), low-density lipoprotein (LDL), tri-glycerides (Orio et al., 2004)

Androgens
- Unbound (free) T (uT), total T, 17-OHP, DHEA-S
- % Free T of total T:

POLYCYSTIC OVARY SYNDROME

- Men: 3%
- Women: 1%
- Hirsute women: 2% (ovary is major source of $\uparrow$ T and A^4)
- A single androgen level may not be representative of the average because the secretion is pulsatile; a single serum T level may differ by 38% from the 24-hr mean.
- Measure free T by (a) equilibrium dialysis or (b) ammonium sulfate precipitation.

Follicle-Stimulating Hormone and Estradiol
- May be helpful to exclude hypogonadotropic hypogonadism ($\downarrow$ FSH and E_2) and POF ($\uparrow$ FSH, $\downarrow$ E_2).

Adrenocorticotropic Hormone Stimulation Test
- For those with moderately elevated 17-OHP (2–4 ng/mL), in setting of normal P_4, in whom NCAH is suspected (see section Nonclassic Congenital Adrenal Hyperplasia)

Pelvic Ultrasound
- For PCAO (polycystic-appearing ovaries) and endometrial thickness
- **PCAO** in ~30% of all reproductive-aged women
  - May occur from a variety of causes (Givens, 1984)
  - Ovarian volume may be proportional to the level of circulating insulin (Pache et al., 1993)
- **Endometrium:** Incidence of endometrial abnormalities in 56 obese women with PCOS (Cheung, 2001):
  - Hyperplasia: 36%
  - Atypia: 9%
    - ⇨ Progression to carcinoma (Kurman et al., 1985):
      - ❖ 2% of untreated hyperplasia without atypia
      - ❖ 23% untreated hyperplasia with atypia
  - Evidence for $\uparrow$ risk of endometrial carcinoma in PCOS is incomplete and contradictory; it may apply only to the subgroup who are obese (BMI >27) (Hardiman et al., 2003)

POLYCYSTIC OVARY SYNDROME

RULE OUT OTHER DIAGNOSES

Virilizing Ovarian or Adrenal Tumor

- *Rapid* onset and *progressive* course of virilizing symptoms
- *Severe* hirsutism: male pattern balding, clitoromegaly, weight gain
- Total T >200 ng/dL or DHEA-S >700 µg/dL
  - Positive predictive value of a repeat total T >250 ng/dL → 9%; negative predictive value of 100% (Waggoner et al., 1999)

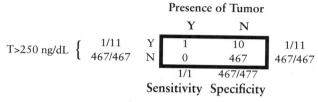

Presence of Tumor

		Y	N	
T>250 ng/dL { 1/11 467/467	Y	1	10	1/11
	N	0	467	467/467
		1/1	467/477	
		Sensitivity	Specificity	

- Computed tomography (CT) of pelvis and adrenals with contrast if tumor suspected (may require selective venous catheterization of ovarian/adrenal veins)
  - Most common virilizing ovarian tumor: *arrhenoblastoma*
  - **Adrenal tumor:** suspect if DHEA-S >700 µg/dL
    - ⇨ Diagnosis: Dexamethasone, 0.5 mg PO q6 hr × 2 days
      - ❖ DHEA-S and 17-OHP, before and after
        If no decrease to normal → virilizing adrenal tumor (Cushing's syndrome), although some tumors may suppress DHEA-S.
        If levels decrease → NCAH vs. PCOS; need to check 17-OHP

Cushing's Syndrome

- If patient is hypertensive, assess 24-hr free urinary cortisol; >50 µg consistent with Cushing's syndrome

Idiopathic Hirsutism

- Clinical hyperandrogenism with normal androgen levels and regular ovulatory cycles
  - Women with PCOS have greater 5α-reductase activity than healthy women (Fassnacht et al., 2003).
  - The enzyme responsible for the degradation of dihydrotestosterone (DHT) (3α-hydroxysteroid dehydrogenase, type III) may be deficient in some hirsute women (Steiner et al., 2004).

Nonclassic Congenital Adrenal Hyperplasia

- Measure 17-OHP and P_4 to discriminate between PCOS and NCAH:
  - a.m. follicular phase, due to circadian variability

175

POLYCYSTIC OVARY SYNDROME

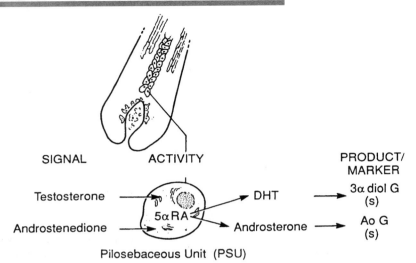

SIGNAL	ACTIVITY		PRODUCT/ MARKER
Testosterone	→	→ DHT	→ 3α diol G (s)
	5αRA		
Androstenedione	→	→ Androsterone	→ Ao G (s)

Pilosebaceous Unit (PSU)

Ao G, androstenediol glucuronide; 3α diol G, 3α-androstenediol glucuronide; 5α-RA, 5α-reductase; DHT, dihydrotestosterone. (Source: Reproduced with permission from Lobo RA. Androgen excess. In Michell DR Jr., Davajan V, Lobo RA, eds. *Infertility, Contraception and Reproductive Endocrinology* [3rd ed]. Cambridge, MA: Blackwell Scientific Publications, 1991:426.)

- 50% of those with NCAH have elevated DHEA-S.

17-Hydroxyprogesterone (17-OHP) (ng/mL)	Diagnosis
<2	Polycystic ovary syndrome
2–4	Cortrosyn stimulation test[a]
>4	Nonclassic congenital adrenal hyperplasia

[a]Cortrosyn stimulation test: Measure 17-OHP at t = 60 after 0.25 mg IV adrenocorticotropic hormone administration (see list below).

t = 60 17-Hydroxyprogesterone (ng/mL):
>15 = NCAH
>10 = Likely NCAH
<10 = Polycystic ovary syndrome

- **21-Hydroxylase deficiency** (gene: *CYP21A2*) (20–50% enzyme activity) is an autosomal-recessive trait with variable genotype-phenotype patterns. More than 40 CYP21A2 mutations have been found in association with NCAH due to 21-hydroxylase deficiency.
  - Incidence: 1/1000
  - Treatment: 5.0–7.5 mg prednisone in two divided doses
    - ⇨ May restore ovulation but relatively ineffective for existing hirsutism; monitor for iatrogenic Cushing's syndrome (rapid weight gain, hypertension, pigmented striae, and osteopenia).
    - ⇨ Treatment efficacy is considered a target 17-OHP between 1 and 10 ng/mL measured at the nadir of steroid blood levels.
  - Treatment during pregnancy:
    - ⇨ **Pregnant women with NCAH** should have A⁴, T, and 17-OHP measured q2 wks, and the glucocorticoid dose (prenatal dexamethasone, 20 μg/kg body weight per day, in three divided doses) should be increased, if necessary, to maintain the concentrations within the normal ranges for the stage of pregnancy and ameliorates genital ambiguity* in affected female fetuses. Begin at the time of a positive pregnancy test and continue only if chorionic villus sampling shows a female with affected *CYP21* genotype (Speiser and White, 2003). Even if androgen production cannot be suppressed to normal, placental aromatase activity protects the fetal genitalia and, presumably, the brain from masculinization (Lo et al., 1999).
- **3β-Hydroxysteroid dehydrogenase deficiency** (gene: *HSDB2*) (less common and no consensus on this diagnosis)

---

*At <12 wks of gestation, high fetal androgen levels lead to a varying degree of labioscrotal fusion and clitoral enlargement in the female fetus; exposure to androgen at >12 wks induces clitoromegaly alone.

POLYCYSTIC OVARY SYNDROME

- Diagnosis with ACTH stimulation test (0 and 60 min) (Lutfallah et al., 2002):

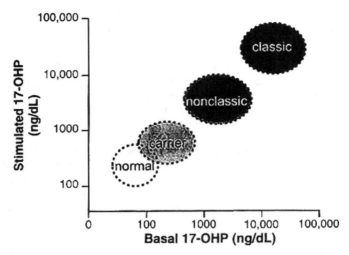

Nomogram for comparing 17-hydroxyprogesterone (17-OHP) ratio before and after administration of 0.25-mg IV cosyntropin (carriers = heterozygotes). (Source: Reproduced with permission from White PC, Speiser PW. Congenital adrenal hyperplasia due to 21-hydroxylase deficiency. *Endocr Rev* 21[3]:2454, 2000.)

TREATMENT
Goals
- Prevent endometrial hyperplasia/cancer
- Restore normal menstruation; resolution of anovulation/infertility
- Improve hirsutism and acne

Weight Reduction
- As little as 5–7% of body weight reduction can reduce hyperandrogenism, improve insulin sensitivity, and restore spontaneous ovulation and fertility in 75% of women with PCOS (Kiddy et al., 1992).
  - Low-calorie diet (1000–1500 kcal/day)
  - Waist-hip ratio >0.85 at greater risk for morbidity
  - Metformin may stimulate weight loss.

POLYCYSTIC OVARY SYNDROME

Oral Contraceptives

- 1st line of drug treatment (i.e., **Yasmin** [ethinyl estradiol, 30 µg; drospirenone, 3 mg]; avoid norgestrel and levonorgestrel)
- Method of action: ↑ SHBG, suppression of LH, inhibition of 5α-reductase and androgen receptor binding
- Greatest efficacy against acne (hirsutism usually requires the addition of antiandrogens)
- Avoid levonorgestrel-containing oral contraceptives (OCs), due to the androgenic properties of the progestin (e.g., Alesse, Levlen, Nordette, Triphasil).
- OCs ↓ LH but not to normal levels (Polson et al., 1988).
- Gonadotropin-releasing hormone (GnRH)-agonist plus add-back no better than OCs alone (Carr et al., 1995).

Progestins

- Give progestins q month or q 2–3 mos to prevent endometrial hyperplasia.

Antiandrogens

- Antiandrogens are effective in the treatment of hirsutism after 6–9 mos; however, cessation of antiandrogen therapy is followed by recurrence (Yucelten et al., 1999).
  - **Spironolactone** (Aldactone, 100–200 mg/day) plus OCs (Lobo et al., 1985; Young et al., 1987). *Contraception is mandatory* with the use of spironolactone, as incomplete virilization of a male fetus may occur. Should wait ≥2 mos after discontinuance of spironolactone to begin attempts at conception.
    ⇨ Aldosterone antagonist, K⁺-sparing diuretic:
      - ❖ Inhibits steroidogenic enzymes and binds the DHT receptor at the hair follicle
      - ❖ Can cause irregular uterine bleeding
      - ❖ 25-mg tablets are generic and inexpensive
  - **Finasteride** (Proscar, 5 mg/day), type II 5α-reductase inhibitor; shows signs of being an excellent and safe antiandrogen
    ⇨ ↓ Circulating DHT levels; not effective topically (Price et al., 2000); not approved by the U.S. Food and Drug Administration (FDA) for this purpose
    ⇨ Low dose (2.5 mg) every 3 days is as effective as continuous administration in ↓ hirsutism (Tartagni et al., 2004).
    ⇨ *Contraception is mandatory* (Ciotta et al., 1995; Wong et al., 1995; Fruzzetti et al., 1999) because its use during the late first trimester may ↑ risk of hypospadias and other genital abnormalities in male fetuses.
  - **Cyproterone acetate** (Androcur), not approved in the United States (used extensively in Europe [Diane 35] and Israel for hirsutism)
    ⇨ Androgen receptor antagonist, decreases 5α-reductase activity, impairs androgen synthesis

POLYCYSTIC OVARY SYNDROME

⇨ Reports of liver tumors in beagles have kept this effective drug from the U.S. market.
- **Eflornithine** (Vaniqa, 13.9% topical cream b.i.d.)
  ⇨ Irreversibly inhibits ornithine decarboxylase (ODC) to inhibit follicle polyamine synthesis necessary for hair growth
  ⇨ Effect seen over 4–8 wks; *reversible* if medicine stopped
  ⇨ <1% systemic absorption, skin irritation may occur.
  ⇨ Category C drug

Hair Removal Systems
- Systemic treatment of hyperandrogenism and hirsutism should be combined with hair removal (shaving, waxing, depilatories [short-acting], or electrolysis or laser [long-acting]) for maximum effect on existing hair.

Electrolysis
- Electric current (through needle in hair follicle) destroys hair follicle.
- Blend most effective: galvanic electrolysis and thermolysis most effective
- Expensive, painful, and time-consuming but can be permanent
- Scarring if not done correctly

Laser-Assisted Hair Removal
- Thermal injury targeted to follicular melanin ("selective photothermolysis") destroys hair follicle (Hobbs et al., 2000).
- Works best for those with light skin and dark hair, although newer lasers are better at light hair.
- May cause pigment changes: hypo- or hyperpigmentation
- Requires multiple (4–6) treatments; effect may be improved by waxing before procedure.
- Avoid in patients who form keloids or hypertrophic scars or who are on retinoids.
- For dark skin, choose longer wavelength: Nd:YAG, Diode; avoid long-pulsed Ruby (Lanigan, 2003).
- Types of Lasers
  - **Nd:YAG:** 1064 nm, Q-switched or long-pulsed, temporary hair loss, uses carbon solution massaged into hair follicles
  - **Ruby:** 694 nm, long-pulsed, long-term reduction in hirsutism, pigment changes can occur
  - **Alexandrite:** 755 nm, long-pulsed, may have fewer pigment changes, long-term reduction
  - **Diode:** 800 nm, long-term hair loss, fewer pigment changes, works less well on fine hair

POLYCYSTIC OVARY SYNDROME

Insulin Sensitizing Drugs
Metformin (Glucophage)
- Biguanide oral hypoglycemic agent
- ↓ Hepatic gluconeogenesis; ↓ intestinal glucose absorption; ↑ peripheral glucose uptake and utilization; no change in insulin secretion but ↓ fasting insulin levels; ↓ LH, free T, and PAI-I
  - 50% have improved menstrual function.
- Commonly used *whether or not* the insulin to glucose ratio reflects IR.
- If glucose to insulin ratio is <4.5, patient needs further testing to rule out diabetes:
  - 1st check a 2-hr GTT to rule out overt diabetes.
  - Avoid metformin if creatinine >1.2 mg/dL or liver function tests (LFTs) are elevated → ↑ risk of lactic acidosis.
  - Metformin may cause dizziness and/or gastrointestinal (GI) discomfort and should not be taken with IV contrast dye (e.g., hysterosalpingogram [HSG]); it is recommended to stop the drug 1 day before a contrast study.
  - Metformin XR regimen (no consensus regarding optimal dose [Nestler, 2001]):

500 mg —1 week→ 1000 mg —1 week→ 1500 mg metformin XR QHS

  - Stop after 1st trimester, although preliminary studies suggest no teratogenicity.
- Effectiveness of metformin alone for ovulation induction vs. placebo—Cochrane database: overall odds ratio = 3.91 (2.20, 6.95) (Lord et al., 2003)
- Single randomized, placebo-controlled study (abstract) showing that lean women with PCOS and no insulin resistance respond favorably to metformin (Baillargeon et al., 2002)
- Higher LH to FSH ratios (>2.5) may predict greater success with metformin (Kriplani and Agarwal, 2004).
- How long to give metformin before concluding that there is no effect? Unknown but likely 3–4 mos
- Velazquez et al. (1997) found that
  - Metformin therapy (500 mg PO t.i.d.) restored menstrual cyclicity in 21 of 22 (96%).
  - Most studies on *ovulatory rate*, not pregnancy rate

POLYCYSTIC OVARY SYNDROME

- Can metformin ↓ early pregnancy loss (EPL; 1st trimester)? All prospective/historical studies, some with suspect methodology.

Reference	Pregnancies (No.)	Spontaneous Abortion Rate (%)	
		Historical Controls	Metformin-Treated
Glueck et al., 2002b	46	62	26
Jakubowicz et al., 2002	65	42	9
Heard et al., 2002	20	Not available	35

- Metformin and the incidence of preeclampsia and perinatal mortality—single study with unsubstantiated results (Hellmuth et al., 2000):
  - Metformin vs. insulin-treated: 32% vs. 10% incidence of preeclampsia ($P <.001$)
  - Metformin vs. insulin- or sulfonylurea-treated: 11.6% vs. 1.3% incidence of perinatal mortality ($P <.02$)
- In a randomized, controlled trial, metformin reduced the incidence of diabetes in persons at high risk (↓ 31%/3 yrs; number needed to treat = 14) (Jakubowicz et al., 2002):

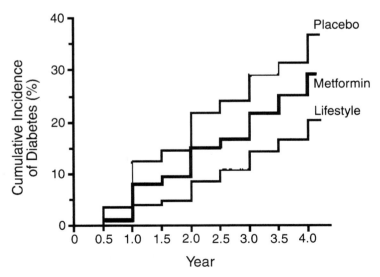

Source: Reproduced with permission from Knowler WC, Barrett-Connor E, Fowler SE, et al. Reduction in the incidence of type 2 diabetes with lifestyle intervention or metformin. *N Engl J Med* 346(6):393, 2002.

POLYCYSTIC OVARY SYNDROME

Rosiglitazone and Pioglitazone (Avandia and Actos)
- Class C
- Peroxisome proliferator-activated receptor (PPAR)-γ receptor agonists used to treat type II diabetes
- ↓ Fasting plasma glucose, fasting insulin, and glycosylated hemoglobin (HbA1c)
- Prospective studies using rosiglitazone (4 mg/day) in PCOS show benefit, few randomized studies using rosiglitazone + clomiphene (CC) citrate vs. CC citrate show improved outcomes (Belli et al., 2004; Ghazeeri et al., 2003; Shobokshi and Shaarawy, 2003).
- Check LFTs, as these drugs are contraindicated if LFTs are >2.5× normal values.

TREATMENT OF ANOVULATION AND INFERTILITY
- **Weight loss** (5%): A recent study by Guzick et al. (1994) compared weight loss to no weight loss in obese, hyperandrogenic, anovulatory women. Women in the treatment group displayed ↑ SHBG, ↓ free T, and ↓ fasting insulin levels. Four of six spontaneously ovulated. As little as a 7% ↓ in body weight significantly improves hyperandrogenism (Kiddy et al., 1992). 5–10% ↓ in body weight is enough to restore ovulation in 55–100% within 6 mos (Kiddy et al., 1992).
- **Metformin:** See Metformin section.
- **Aromatase inhibitor**
- **CC:** treatment of choice (after starting metformin) for anovulatory patient
  - CC-resistant, anovulatory, PCOS patients given metformin *in conjunction with* CC.
    - ⇨ ↑ Ovulation rate (threefold: 27% vs. 75%) and ↑ conception rate (eightfold: 7% vs. 55%) (Vandermolen et al., 2001)
- Ovulatory rates of ~80%
- Pregnancy rates of 60–70% within the first 6 mos
- Monitor with ovulation predictor kits + midluteal progesterone (8 days after positive LH kit)
- Rule of five 5s:
  - Oral progestin, 10 mg q day × 5 days (after negative β-human chorionic gonadotropin [β-HCG])
  - Begin CC on day 5 of bleeding.
  - 50 mg CC q day × 5 days
  - Timed coitus 5 days later and for 5 days every other day (vs. intrauterine insemination [IUI])
- Women who require doses of CC >150 mg/day for 5 days may benefit from an extended CC regimen, supplemental FSH, or adjunctive oral dexamethasone (0.25 mg/day) or prednisone (5.0–7.5 mg/day) (McKenna and Cunningham, 1995). Glucocorticoids are stopped when positive for pregnancy.

183

POLYCYSTIC OVARY SYNDROME

- Gonadotropins: PCOS patients are highly susceptible to hyperstimulation; start with low doses.
- Glucocorticoids
  - Steroid treatment appears to be related to the suppression of excessive androgen levels (Steinberger et al., 1979).
  - Two randomized trials revealed ↑ pregnancy rates (40–75% vs. 5–35%) in CC-resistant women (Daly et al., 1984; Parsanezhad et al., 2002).
- **Treatment algorithm for anovulatory PCOS** (see Appendix A in this chapter)
- **Metformin + ovulation induction** (Nestler et al., 1998):
  - 90% of obese women with PCOS responded to CC + metformin.
  - No data on pregnancy rate

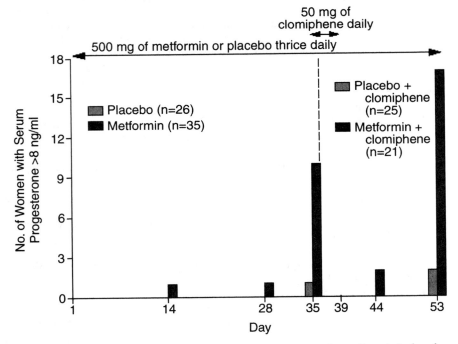

Number of women with a serum progesterone concentration >8 ng/mL by day. (Source: Reproduced with permission from Nestler JE, Jakubowicz DJ, et al. Effects of metformin on spontaneous and clomiphene-induced ovulation in the polycystic ovary syndrome. *N Engl J Med* 338[26]:1876-80, 1998.)

POLYCYSTIC OVARY SYNDROME

- Laparoscopic ovarian cautery/drilling:
  - Restores spontaneous ovulation in ~50% of CC-resistant hyperandrogenic women (Gjønnæss, 1984; Daniell and Miller, 1989; Abdel Gadir et al., 1990; Gjønnæss, 1998; Lazovic et al., 1998; Vegetti et al., 1998).
  - Consider the balance between reducing androgen levels and potential negative effects:
    ⇨ Postoperative adhesion formation
    ⇨ General endotracheal anesthesia
    ⇨ Iatrogenic diminished ovarian reserve
  - Spontaneous abortion (SAB) rate may be lower for ovarian cautery compared with medical induction of ovulation (Abdel Gadir et al., 1992).
  - Predictors of success:
    ⇨ Good responders:
      ❖ Women with hyperinsulinemia respond better to ovarian drilling than do those with normoinsulinemia with respect to lowered glucose and insulin values (Saleh et al., 2001).
      ❖ LH >10 IU/L (Amer et al., 2004)
    ⇨ Poor responders (Amer et al., 2004):
      ❖ BMI ≥35 kg/m^2
      ❖ Total T ≥4.5 nmol/L or 1.3 ng/mL
      ❖ Duration of infertility >3 yrs
- In women with PCOS, the pregnancy rate at 12 and 18 mos after drilling is 55% and 70%, respectively (Felemban et al., 2000).
- Randomized, controlled trial for CC-resistant women with PCOS: ovarian cauterization or recombinant FSH:

Technique	Pregnancies (%)	Live Births (%)
r-hFSH	67	60
Ovarian cauterization	34	34
Ovarian cauterization → anovulatory women given CC	29	29
Ovarian cauterization → anovulatory women given r-hFSH after failed CC	65	52

CC, clomiphene citrate (Clomid); r-hFSH, recombinant human follicle-stimulating hormone.
Source: Adapted from Bayram N, van Wely M, et al. Using an electrocautery strategy or recombinant follicle stimulating hormone to induce ovulation in polycystic ovary syndrome: randomised controlled trial. *BMJ* 328(7433):192, 2004.

POLYCYSTIC OVARY SYNDROME

- Randomized, double-blind, placebo-controlled trial for CC-resistant women with PCOS: laparoscopy + metformin vs. laparoscopic ovarian cautery + placebo:

Outcome	Laparoscopy + Metformin	Cautery + Placebo
Ovulation rate (%)	54.8	53.3
Pregnancy rate (%)	18.6[a]	13.4
Spontaneous loss rate (%)	15.4[a]	29.0
Live birth rate (%)	82.1[a]	64.5

[a]$P < .05$.

Source: Adapted from Palomba S, Orio F, Jr., et al. Metformin administration versus laparoscopic ovarian diathermy in clomiphene citrate-resistant women with polycystic ovary syndrome: a prospective parallel randomized double-blind placebo-controlled trial. *J Clin Endocrinol Metab* 89(10):4801, 2004.

COCHRANE LIBRARY REVIEW CONCLUDING STATEMENT

There is a lack of controlled data, and relatively few RCTs of this surgical technique have been carried out. With such a small number of patients studied in a controlled way and underpowered studies, conclusions about the effectiveness of laparoscopic treatment of the polycystic ovarian syndrome remain uncertain. Although observational data show that it is likely that ovarian drilling has a beneficial effect on ovulation and pregnancy rates for anovulatory PCOS patients wishing to conceive, more data on the short- and long-term safety of the procedure are required.

TREATMENT SUMMARY

	Dose/ Technique	Mechanism of Action	Side Effects
Spironolactone	100–200 mg b.i.d.	Aldosterone antagonist Competitive AR blockage 5α-Reductase and CYP17 inhibitor Inhibits androgen synthesis	DUB, headaches, mastalgia, ambiguous genitalia in male offspring
Finasteride	5 mg q.d.	Azasteroid 5α-Reductase inhibitor	Ambiguous genitalia in male offspring
Metformin XR	1500 mg q.d.	Biguanide oral hypoglycemic Reduces ovarian cytochrome p450c17α; ↑ sex hormone–binding globulin	Gastrointestinal: nausea, vomiting, flatulence, diarrhea
D-*chiro*-inositol (experimental)	1200 mg q.d.	Enhanced insulin sensitivity ↓ Serum androgens	Not reported
Ovarian drilling	5–8/ovary (electro-cauterization) (Gjønnæss, 1998) 25–40/ovary (laser) (Daniell and Miller, 1989)	Alteration of the intraovarian steroid environment and, in turn, the feedback to the hypothalamic pituitary axis May last >18 yrs (Gjønnæss, 1998)	Adhesion formation; ?premature ovarian failure; ?ovarian epithelial tumors

A. Treatment Algorithm for Anovulatory Polycystic Ovary Syndrome

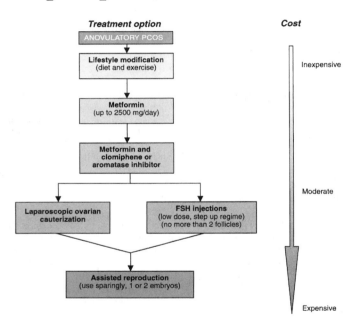

FSH, follicle-stimulating hormone; PCOS, polycystic ovary syndrome. (Source: Adapted from Norman RJ. Metformin—comparison with other therapies in ovulation induction in polycystic ovary syndrome. *J Clin Endocrinol Metab* 89[10]:4797, 2004.)

B. Ferriman-Gallway Scores

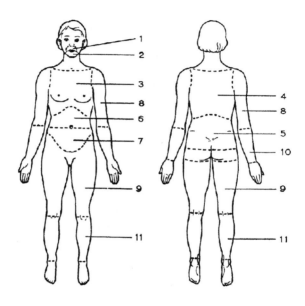

POLYCYSTIC OVARY SYNDROME

Site	Grade	Definition
Upper lip	1	Few hairs at outer margin
	2	Small moustache at outer margin
	3	Moustache extends halfway from outer margin
	4	Moustache extending to midline
Chin	1	Few scattered hairs
	2	Scattered hairs with small concentrations
	3, 4	Complete cover, light and heavy
Chest	1	Circumareolar hairs
	2	With midline hair in addition
	3	Fusion of these areas, with $3/4$ cover
	4	Complete cover
Upper back	1	Few scattered hairs
	2	Rather more, still scattered
	3, 4	Complete cover, light and heavy
Lower back	1	Sacral tuft of hair
	2	With some lateral extension
	3	$3/4$ Cover
	4	Complete cover
Upper abdomen	1	Few midline hairs
	2	Rather more, still midline
	3, 4	Half and full cover
Lower abdomen	1	Full midline hairs
	2	Midline streak of hair
	3	Midline band of hair
	4	Inverted V-shaped growth
Arm	1	Sparse growth affecting $\leq 1/4$ limb surface
	2	More than this; cover still incomplete
	3, 4	Complete cover, light and heavy
Forearm	1, 2, 3, 4	Complete cover of dorsal surface; two grades of light and two grades of heavy growth
Thigh	1, 2, 3, 4	As for arm
Leg	1, 2, 3, 4	As for arm
Total Score:	____	

Source: Reproduced with permission from Ferriman D, Gallway JD. Clinical assessment of body hair growth in women. *J Clin Endocrinol Metab* 21:1440, 1961.

C. Steroid Hormone Synthesis

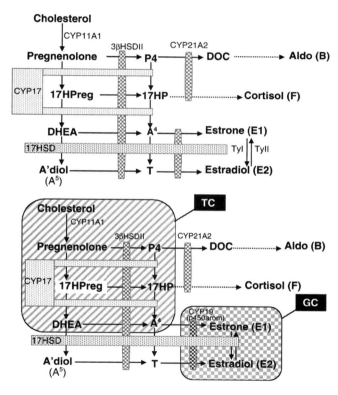

A^4, androstenedione; A'diol, androstenediol; Aldo (B), aldosterone; DHEA, dehydro-epiandrosterone; DOC, deoxycorticosterone; 17HP, 17OH-progesterone; GC, granulosa cell; HSD, hydroxysteroid dehydrogenase; 17-HPreg, 17OH-pregnenolone; P$_4$, progesterone; T, testosterone; TC, theca cell; TyI, type I; TyII, type II.

continued

POLYCYSTIC OVARY SYNDROME

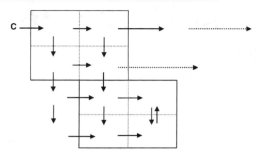

Steroid biosynthesis worksheet.

19. Female Subfertility

- 12% of all couples are childless.
  - Monthly pregnancy rate (PR) in couples with unexplained subfertility after 18 mos' duration → 1.5–3.0%
  - Cumulative PRs for couples with unexplained subfertility 1 yr and 3 yrs after the first visit are 13% and 40%, respectively.
- Approximately 50% of healthy women become clinically pregnant during the first two cycles, and between 80% and 90% during the first 6 mos (Gnoth et al., 2003; Wang et al., 2003).

DEFINITIONS
- **Subfertility:** failure to conceive after 1 yr of unprotected intercourse (IC)
- **Fecundability:** conception rate, usually *per month*
  - Normal → 20%
  - 38-yr-old with 3-yr history of infertility → 2%
- **Fecundity:** birth rate per 1 mo

ETIOLOGY

Cause of Infertility	%
Female factors (single)	36
Tubal factor	14
Endometriosis	6
Ovulatory dysfunction	6
Diminished ovarian reserve	9
Uterine factor	1
Male factor (single)	17
Other causes(s)[a]	7
Unexplained cause[b]	10
Multiple factors (female only)	13
Multiple factors (female + male)	17

[a]Includes immunologic problems, chromosomal abnormalities, cancer chemotherapy, and serious illness.
[b]No cause of infertility found in either partner.
Source: Adapted from the Centers for Disease Control and Prevention. 2001 Assisted Reproductive Technology Success Rates, December 2003.

FEMALE SUBFERTILITY

MATERNAL AGE
• Fertility decreases with maternal age.

Age	Subfertile (%)
≤30 yrs old	25
30–35 yrs old	33
35–40 yrs old	50
>40 yrs old	>90

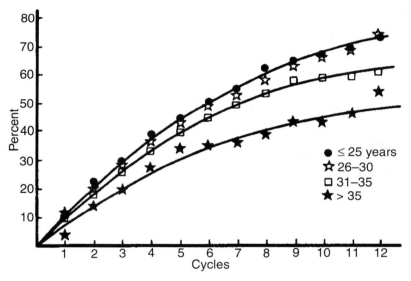

Effect of age on the cumulative pregnancy rate in a donor insemination program. The younger age groups (<31 yrs) were significantly different from the older groups. (Source: Reproduced with permission from Schwartz D, Mayaux MJ. Female fecundity as a function of age: results of artificial insemination in 2193 nulliparous women with azoospermic husbands. Federation CECOS. *N Engl J Med* 306:404, 1982.)

FEMALE SUBFERTILITY

EVALUATION OF THE FEMALE
Family History
- Endometriosis
- Recurrent spontaneous abortions

Past Medical History
- Infections, sexually transmitted diseases, pelvic inflammatory disease (PID)
- Postpartum or postabortion infections
- Appendicitis (ruptured?)

Surgery
- Ovarian cysts
- Appendectomy

Menstrual History
- Length of cycles: normal = 24–35 days
- Flow: Hypermenorrhea suggests fibroids or anovulation.
- Cramps: Ovulation is often associated with some dysmenorrhea.

Coital History
- Dyspareunia suggests salpingitis or endometriosis.
- Frequency is important:
  - More than q.o.d. may cause a ↓ count
  - Infrequent coitus ↓ fecundity
  - Must antecede ovulation

Physical Examination
- Body hair distribution; breast development; galactorrhea; clitoromegaly; male escutcheon; adnexal mass; uterosacral nodularity
- Vagina: with amenorrhea, women with **polycystic ovary syndrome (PCOS)** are well estrogenized, whereas **hypothalamic amenorrhea** is associated with vaginal atrophy

Evaluation of Specific Functions
- Timing of diagnostic tests

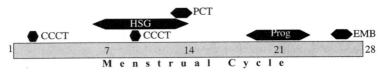

CCCT, clomiphene citrate challenge test; EMB, endometrial biopsy (historical purposes only); HSG, hysterosalpingogram; PCT, postcoital test (historical purposes only); Prog, progesterone.

FEMALE SUBFERTILITY

- *Chlamydia trachomatis* titers if subfertile <1 yr (controversial):
  - ≥1:256 immunoglobulin G serum antibody titers → treat with doxycycline (both partners)
  - Associated with tubal occlusion, odds ratio (OR), 2.4 (confidence interval [CI], 1.7–3.2) (comparing fertile control subjects to infertile control subjects) (Hubacher et al., 2001)
- Ovulation
  - Basal body temperature (BBT) chart: normal → biphasic, 12- to 14-day luteal phase
  - Luteinizing hormone (LH) stimulates resumption of meiosis (germinal vesicle [GV] → meiosis II [MII])
  - LH urine detection kits: ovulation occurs ~20–24 hrs after LH rise (95% CI, 14–26 hrs) in urine or ~16 hrs after LH peak (Miller and Soules, 1996)
    - ⇨ The rise in **serum** LH occurs ~36 hrs before ovulation
    - ⇨ The LH surge appears in **urine** 12 hrs after it appears in serum
    - ⇨ Therefore, **a positive urine LH kit occurs ~24 hrs before ovulation**
    - ⇨ Note: ovulation occurs ~36 hrs after human chorionic gonadotropin (hCG) administration
  - What is the best way to time the IUI?

Type of Study (Using Clomiphene Citrate [Clomid])	No Difference in Pregnancy Rate
Retrospective (Awonuga and Govindbhai, 1999)	LH-timed hCG-timed hCG-boost (after positive LH)
Randomized, cross-over (Zreik et al., 1999)	LH-timed hCG-timed

hCG, human chorionic gonadotropin; LH, luteinizing hormone.

  - Key points on **ovulation predictor kits** (from Fertility Plus Web Site: http://www.fertilityplus.org/faq/opk.html):
    1. Best time to test → 2 p.m.; anytime between noon and 8 p.m. is fine; first morning urine is not recommended because most women experience a surge in the morning, but it can take 4 hrs to show up in the urine.
    2. Clomiphene citrate (CC; Clomid) can cause a false-positive result if tested too soon; should wait at least 3 days (3–7 regimen → start on day 10; 5–9 regimen → start on day 12) after finishing the CC.
    3. Most kits do not show a full positive result until ≥25–40 mIU, but many will show a faint line with LH >10 mIU.
    4. The BBT thermal shift occurs **after ovulation** in response to ↑ progesterone (P_4) production; positive kits allow timing **before ovulation**.

FEMALE SUBFERTILITY

5. False-negative results can occur if peak LH concentrations are <40 IU/I, and this may occur in up to 35% of ovulatory cycles (Arici et al., 1994).

- **Fertility monitors** assess LH, estrogen, and P_4 levels.
- Serum P_4: mid-luteal (8 days post-LH surge)
  - ⇨ **≥5 ng/mL** → ovulatory
  - ⇨ **≥10 ng/mL** → adequate P_4 production
- hCG has ~4× the receptor affinity and 3× the $t_{1/2}$ compared with LH
- PRL: normal <20 mg/mL; if magnetic resonance imaging reveals an adenoma, need to check insulin-like growth factor-1 for growth hormone tumor (acromegaly), 25% of which will produce PRL as well
- TSH: >10 mIU/mL = hypothyroid
- Hirsutism laboratory tests: (a.m. follicular phase) **free testosterone; total testosterone; dehydroepiandrosterone sulfate; 17-hydroxyprogesterone;** P_4 (if unsure of time of cycle); **fasting glucose/insulin** (insulin resistant if <4.5); **24-hr urinary cortisol** if patient hypertensive
- TSH: >5 mIU/mL = hypothyroidism
- Ovarian reserve testing: **day 3 (D3) FSH/E_2 or CC challenge test**
  - Variability does not affect the prognostic category (Scott et al., 1990).
  - Basal FSH screening retains its predictive value in women with one ovary (Khalifa et al., 1992)
  - If D3 value is >25 mIU/mL, there is a **<4% chance of conception with IVF or FSH/IUI** (Scott, 1989).
    - ⇨ Variability in different months is just as bad (Buyalos et al., 1998)

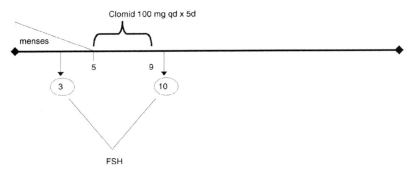

FSH, follicle-stimulating hormone.

FEMALE SUBFERTILITY

	Follicle-Stimulating Hormone (mIU/mL)[a] D3 or D10 via Chemiluminescence Assay
Gray zone	15–25
<4% pregnancy rate	≥25

[a]Chemiluminescence assay.

- Women with diminished ovarian reserve have a higher pregnancy loss rate compared to patients with normal ovarian reserve (Levi et al., 2001).

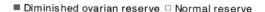

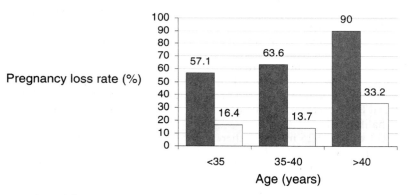

Source: Adapted from Levi AJ, Raynault MF, et al. Reproductive outcome in patients with diminished ovarian reserve. *Fertil Steril* 76(4):666, 2001.

- ↑ In mean FSH for Down's syndrome mothers compared with a control group

	Down's Syndrome Mothers (n = 118)	Control Subjects (n = 102)	P
Age (yrs)	33.8	34.2	NS
Single FSH >11.5 IU/L	16 (18.9%)	5 (5.1%)	.03
Mean FSH concentration (IU/L)	6.9 ± 2.1	6.3 ± 1.7	.02

FSH, follicle-stimulating hormone; NS, not significant.
Source: Adapted from van Montfrans JM, Dorland M, et al. Increased concentrations of follicle-stimulating hormone in mothers of children with Down's syndrome. *Lancet* 353(9167):1853, 1999.

- Nearly all pregnancies can be attributed to IC during a 6-day period ending on the day of ovulation (Wilcox et al., 1995).

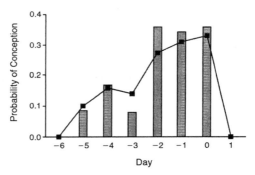

"O" denotes the day of ovulation. (Source: Reproduced with permission from Wilcox AJ, et al. Timing of sexual intercourse in relation to ovulation. Effects on the probability of conception, survival of the pregnancy, and sex of the baby. *N Engl J Med* 333:1517–1521, 1995.)

- The 6 consecutive days with the highest frequency of IC corresponded exactly with the 6 fertile days in a study of women with an intrauterine device or tubal ligation (Wilcox et al., 2004).

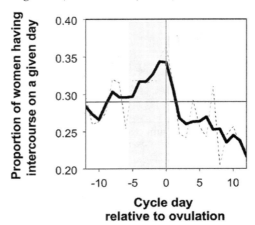

Source: Reproduced with permission from Wilcox AJ, et al. On the frequency of intercourse around ovulation: evidence for biological influences. *Hum Reprod* 19(7):1539, 2004.

FEMALE SUBFERTILITY

- Tubal patency and uterine abnormalities
  - Ultrasound: look for fibroids/polyps; location of ovaries; hydrosalpinx (Boer-Meisel et al., 1986; Jansen, 1980)
  - Sonohysterogram or flexible hysteroscopy: assess uterine cavity
  - Hysteroscopy: most accurate assessment of uterine cavity
  - Diagnostic laparoscopy:
    ⇨ Pelvic adhesions
- Endometriosis: 25–35% of infertile women (~10% of fertile women)
- Cervical mucus: postcoital test (no longer performed, no correlation found)
  - Postcoital (Simms-Huhner) test performed preovulatory once LH kit is positive; 2–18 hrs postcoital
    ⇨ Normal: **1 motility sperm/3-of-5 hpf**; copious mucus; Spinnbarkeit, 8–10 cm; acellular
    ⇨ Poor validity, lack of standard methodology, and unknown reproducibility (Griffith and Grimes, 1990)
    ⇨ No significant effect on PR (Oei and Helmerhorst, 1998)

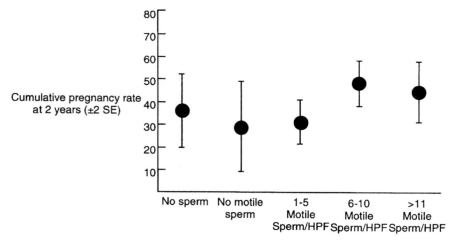

Cumulative pregnancy rates by number of sperm per high-power field (HPF) on postcoital test. (Source: Reproduced with permission from Griffith CS, Grimes DA. The validity of the postcoital test. *Am J Obstet Gynecol* 162:615, 1990.)

FEMALE SUBFERTILITY

TREATMENT

Abnormal Semen Analysis

- See Chapter 20, Male Subfertility.

Ovulatory Dysfunction

- Treat endocrine abnormalities:
  - Bromocriptine; thyroid replacement
- Induce ovulation: CC, recombinant human FSH, hCG
- βhCG 8–11 days after injection of 10,000 mIU/mL should be <50 mIU/mL (Liu et al., 1988)
- Ovarian cancer risk → pooled data from eight case-control studies (Ness et al., 2002)
  - Fertility drug use in nulligravid women is associated with borderline serous tumors (OR = 2.4; 95% CI, 1.01–5.88) but not with invasive histologic subtypes
- CC:
  - Available as ~3 to 2 ratio of two triphenylethylene derivative geometric isomers: enclomiphene (62% inactive isomer) and **zuclomiphene** (38% active isomer)
  - $t_{1/2}$ = 5 days
  - Body weight and hyperandrogenemia are the predominant predictors for **ovulation** after CC, whereas age and cycle history dictate **pregnancy** chances in **ovulatory women** (Imani et al., 1998; Imani et al., 1999).
  - Ovulation rate by dose: 50 mg (52%), 100 mg (22%), 150 mg (12%), 200 mg (7%), 250 mg (5%) (Gysler et al., 1982)
  - CC failure vs. conceptions (Imani et al., 1999):
    - ⇨ Age (<30 ↑ fecundity by 10%)
    - ⇨ Cycle history (amenorrhea ↑ fecundity by 46%)
    - ⇨ Baseline pregnancy rates of **1–2%** in patients with **unexplained infertility** may be enhanced to **2–4%** per cycle with CC (Hughes et al., 2000).
  - 2/3 of patients who conceived reached this endpoint within the 1st three ovulatory CC treatment cycles

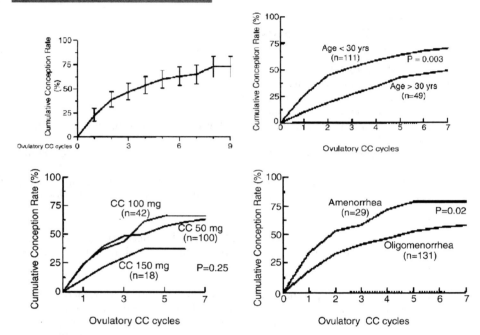

CC, clomiphene citrate. (Source: Reproduced with permission from Imani B, et al. Predictors of chances to conceive in ovulatory patients during clomiphene citrate induction of ovulation in normogonadotropic oligoamenorrheic infertility. *J Clin Endocrinol Metab* 84:1617–1622, 1999.)

- Rare visual changes (palinopsia = prolonged afterimages or shimmering of the peripheral field) that may be irreversible (Purvin, 1995)
- **Letrozole (Femara®):** Letrozole reduces FSH dose and eliminates antiestrogenic effect of CC on the endometrium; PR equivalent to FSH-only (Mitwally and Casper, 2003)
  - Letrozole's terminal elimination half-life is approximately 2 days
  - Letrozole, 5 mg/day, days 3–7, and FSH injection (50–150 IU/day starting on day 7 until the day of hCG [10,000 IU])
  - Clinical studies:
    ⇨ Prospective: Ten PCOS women (four failed to ovulate with CC; six ovulatory but lining 5 mm with CC) (Mitwally and Casper, 2000)

FEMALE SUBFERTILITY

- ❖ Letrozole → 70% ovulatory; 20% clinical PR
- ⇨ Prospective randomized clinical trial (RCT): CC vs. letrozole (Sammour et al., 2001)
  - ❖ CC → 5.6% PR vs. letrozole → 16.7% ($P = .55$, type II error)
- ⇨ Prospective trial: 12 PCOS women with inadequate CC response (Mitwally and Casper, 2001)
  - ❖ Letrozole → 75% ovulatory; 25% clinical PR
- ⇨ Prospective: 324 treatment cycles

Method	Cycles (n)	Chemical Pregnancy Rate (%)
CC	80	12.5
Letrozole	33	18.2
CC + FSH	33	12.1
FSH	110	13.6
AI + FSH	30	6.7

AI, aromatase inhibitor; CC, clomiphene citrate; FSH, follicle-stimulating hormone.
Source: Adapted from Mittwally MF, Casper RF. P-486: Pregnancy outcome after the use of an aromatase inhibitor for ovarian stimulation. *Fertil Steril* 78(3, S1):S278, 2002.

⇨ Prospective trial: unexplained infertility or mild male factor

Method (+ Intrauterine Insemination)	Clinical Pregnancy Rate (%)[a]
FSH	21.4
FSH + CC	11.1
Letrozole + FSH	22.2

CC, clomiphene citrate; FSH, follicle-stimulating hormone.
[a]$P <.05$.
Source: Adapted from Mitwally MF, Casper RF. Aromatase inhibition reduces gonadotrophin dose required for controlled ovarian stimulation in women with unexplained infertility. *Hum Reprod* 18(8):1588, 2003.

Drug	Half-Life (Days)	Pregnancy Category
Clomiphene citrate (Clomid)	5	X
Aromatase inhibitor (Femara)	2	D

- Glucocorticoids
  - Steroid treatment appears to be related to the suppression of excessive androgen levels (Steinberger et al., 1979).
  - Two randomized trials revealed ↑ pregnancy rates (40–75% vs. 5–35%) in CC-resistant women (Daly et al., 1984; Parsanezhad et al., 2002).

FEMALE SUBFERTILITY

Tubal Disease

- Operative laparoscopy
- Hydrosalpinx: remove or clip hydrosalpinx; Strandell et al. (1999) maintain that if found on hysterosalpingogram, recheck with ultrasound at mid-cycle.
  - Occlusion secondary to PID, appendicitis, endometriosis
  - Meta-analysis: hydrosalpinx $\downarrow$ PR by 50% and $\uparrow$ spontaneous abortion ×2 (Camus et al., 1999)
  - Mechanism of adverse effect (Strandell and Lindhard, 2002)
    - $\Rightarrow$ $\downarrow$ Nutrients in hydrosalpinx fluid
    - $\Rightarrow$ Toxic effect of fluid on embryos (Sachdev et al., 1997) and/or sperm (Ng et al., 2000)
    - $\Rightarrow$ $\downarrow$ Expression: $\alpha_v\beta_3$, LIF, HOXA10 (Meyer et al., 1997)
    - $\Rightarrow$ Wash-out effect from fluid
    - $\Rightarrow$ $\uparrow$ Endometrial peristalsis due to hydrosalpinx fluid
  - Ligation of the hydrosalpinx or salpingectomy restores normal PR (Johnson et al., 2002; Strandell et al., 2001a)
  - Number needed to treat calculation: Seven to eight women would need to have a salpingectomy before IVF to gain one additional live birth (Johnson et al., 2002).
  - Salpingectomy if hydrosalpinx seen on ultrasound:
    - $\Rightarrow$ No compromise of ovarian stimulation (Strandell et al., 2001b)
    - $\Rightarrow$ RCT (192 patients; outcome = birth rate after first embryo transfer):

	Birth Rate (%)[a]
Salpingectomy	28.6
No intervention	16.3

[a]P <.05.
Source: Adapted from Strandell A, Lindhard A, et al. Hydrosalpinx and IVF outcome: a prospective, randomized multicentre trial in Scandinavia on salpingectomy prior to IVF. *Hum Reprod* 14:2762–2769, 1999.

- $\Rightarrow$ RCT (186 patients; outcome = birth rate for cumulative cycle data; 452 transfers):
  - ❖ OR, 3.8; 95% CI, 1.5–9.2; P <.05 (Strandell et al., 2001a)
  - Laparotomy with microsurgical techniques (tubal reversal—tubal length after reanastomosis is most important, need ≥4 cm length; duration of sterilization not important); laparoscopic tubal anastomosis has a 50% PR at 6 months (Bissonnette et al., 1999)
  - IVF

Uterine Abnormalities

- Hysteroscopic resection of septum, submucosal leiomyoma, polyp (if >0.5 cm)
- Laparotomy for removal of multiple leiomyoma

Endometriosis

- Medical therapy: suppressive not curative
- Surgical therapy: recurrence, 5–20% per year; 40% after 5 yrs

Cervical Problems

- Infection: antibiotics
- Poor mucus: IUI
- Stenosis: IUI

Unexplained Infertility

- IC, IUI, CC, CC/IUI, FSH, FSH/IUI, IVF
  - Retrospective analysis of 45 reports (Guzick et al., 1998)

Method	Pregnancy Rate (%)
Intercourse	4
IUI	4
CC	5.6
CC + IUI[a]	8
FSH	7.7
FSH + IUI[a]	17
In vitro fertilization[a]	21

CC, clomiphene citrate; FSH, follicle-stimulating hormone; IUI, intrauterine insemination.
Note: No randomized control trial: CC vs. CC/IUI; CC vs. FSH.
[a]Statistically significant difference.
Source: Adapted from Guzick DS, et al. Efficacy of treatment for unexplained infertility. *Fertil Steril* 70:207, 1998.

- IUI vs. FSH/IUI (randomized) (Guzick et al., 1999)

Method	Pregnancy Rate (%)	LB/Couple (%)	LB/Cycle (%)
IUI	18	13	4
Follicle-stimulating hormone/IUI[a]	33	22	8

IUI, intrauterine insemination; LB, live birth.
[a]Statistically significant difference.
Source: Adapted from Guzick DA, et al. Efficacy of superovulation and intrauterine insemination in the treatment of infertility. National Cooperative Reproductive Medicine Network. *N Engl J Med* 340:177, 1999.

FEMALE SUBFERTILITY

- Treatment of infertility usually does not make the difference between conceiving and not conceiving; the difference lies in conceiving sooner rather than later. The risks of the "sooner" option in terms of multiple pregnancy, ovarian hyperstimulation syndrome, emotional stress, and financial costs may be unacceptably high. (te Velde and Cohlen, 1999)

MULTIPLE PREGNANCY RISKS
- Cerebral palsy incidence in multiple pregnancies

0.15%	Singletons (general prevalence)
1.5%	Twins
8%	Triplets
43%	Quadruplets

Source: Adapted from Yokohama Y, Shimizu T, et al. Prevalence of cerebral palsy in twins, triplets and quadruplets. *Int J Epidemiol* 24(5):943, 1995.

INTERPREGNANCY INTERVAL
- Infants **conceived 18–23 months after a live birth** had the lowest risk of delivering low-birth-weight, preterm, and/or small size for gestational age (Zhu et al., 1999)

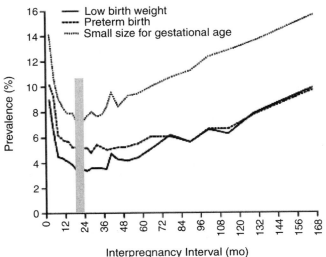

Source: Adapted from Zhu BP, et al. Effect of the interval between pregnancies on perinatal outcomes. *N Engl J Med* 340(8):589, 1999.

A. Non-Assisted Reproductive Technology Treatment Outcomes

Diagnostic Group	Treatment (Unit)	Live Birth Rate (%)
Amenorrhea	None (3 yrs)	6
	Clomid (cycle)	19
	Gns (cycle)	21
Oligomenorrhea	None (3 yrs)	46
	Clomid (cycle)	9
	Gns (cycle)	21
	Metformin + Clomid (cycle)	11
	Ovarian cauterization (1 yr)	38
Hyperprolactinemia	None (3 yrs)	30
	Bromocriptine (1 yr)	31
Tubal obstruction	None (3 yrs)	5
	Tubal surgery (1 yr)	18
Other tubal disease	None (3 yrs)	22
	Tubal surgery (1 yr)	28
	Gns + IUI (cycle)	8
Endometriosis, I–II	None (3 yrs)	25
	Laparoscopic ablation (1 yr)	18
	CC + IUI (cycle)	5
	Gns + IUI (cycle)	8
Endometriosis, III–IV	None (3 yrs)	10
	Surgery (1 yr)	30
	Gns + IUI (cycle)	8
Azoospermia	None (3 yrs)	5
	Therapeutic donor insemination (cycle)	13
Oligospermia	None (3 yrs)	32
	IUI (cycle)	5
	Gns + IUI (cycle)	5
Unexplained infertility	None (3 yrs)	36
	CC + IUI (cycle)	5
	Gns + IUI (cycle)	8

CC, clomiphene citrate; Gns, gonadotropins; IUI, intrauterine insemination.
Source: Adapted from Collins JA, Van Steirteghem A. Overall prognosis with current treatment of infertility. *Hum Reprod Update* 10:309–316, 2004.

20. Male Subfertility

- A male factor is solely responsible in approximately 20% of subfertile couples and contributory in another 17%.
- Causes of male factor subfertility can be divided into four main areas:
  - Idiopathic (40–50%)
  - Testicular (30–40%)
  - Posttesticular (10–20%)
  - Pretesticular (1–2%)

EVALUATION OF THE MALE PATIENT
- At a minimum, evaluation should include reproductive history and two semen analyses.

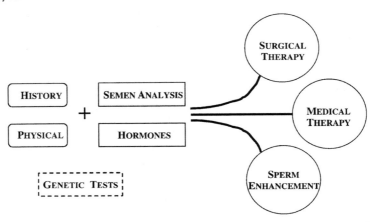

Source: Adapted from Howards SS. Treatment of male infertility. *N Engl J Med* 332(5):312, 1995.

- Goals are to identify:
  - Potentially correctable conditions
  - Irreversible conditions that are amenable to assisted reproductive technologies (ARTs) using the sperm of the male partner
  - Irreversible conditions that are not amenable to ART, and for which adoption or donor insemination is an option.
  - Life- or health-threatening conditions that may underlie the subfertility and require medical attention

MALE SUBFERTILITY

- Genetic abnormalities that may affect the health of offspring if ART is used

Semen Analysis

- Collect × 2 if 1st one is abnormal, one test is not enough. Patient must be abstinent for 2–3 days before collection of semen.
- Collected by masturbation or by intercourse using special semen collection condoms that do not contain substances detrimental to sperm
- Collected at home or in the laboratory; should be kept at room temperature during transport and examined within 1 hr of collection
- Parameters can vary widely over time, even among fertile men, and exhibit seasonal variation.

Parameter	Reference Value	Possible Pathologies
Volume	1.5–5.0 mL (pH, 7.2)	Low: ejaculatory dysfunction, hypogonadism, poor collection technique. Acidic semen: ejaculatory duct obstruction, congenital absence of the vasa deferentia
Concentration	>20 million/mL	Azoospermia or oligospermia: varicocele, genetic, cryptorchidism, endocrinopathy, drugs, infections, toxins or radiation, obstruction, idiopathic
Total motile count	≥10 million	—
Motility	>50%	Asthenospermia: prolonged abstinence, antisperm antibodies, partial obstruction, infection, sperm structural defects, idiopathic
Normal morphology	>30% normal (World Health Organization, 1999) >14% normal (Kruger and Coetzee, 1999)	Teratospermia: varicocele, genetic, cryptorchidism, drugs, infections, toxins or radiation, idiopathic
Indirect immunobead assay (sperm antibodies)	≥20%	Ductal obstruction, prior genital infection, testicular trauma, and prior vasovasostomy or vasoepididymostomy (50–70% incidence)

Source: Adapted from World Health Organization. *WHO Laboratory Manual for the Examination of Human Semen and Semen-Cervical Mucus Interaction.* New York: Cambridge University Press, 1999.

MALE SUBFERTILITY

Total Motile Count
- Total motile count (TMC) *before processing* (million = volume × concentration × .% motility):
  - 10–20 million: intrauterine insemination (IUI) helpful
  - 5–10 million: *in vitro* fertilization (IVF)
  - <5 million: intracytoplasmic sperm injection (ICSI)

Morphology
- If abnormal (<14% normal Kruger) → urology consultation (Kruger et al., 1987)
  - 4–14% intermediate rates of fertilization (Guzick et al., 2001)
  - Sperm morphology and IUI: metaanalysis (Van Waart, 2001)

Morphology	Other	Recommendation
>4%	Irrespective	IUI
≤4%	IMC >1 million Motility >50% ≥2 follicles	4 IUI cycles
≤4%	IMC <1 million Motility <50%	Intracytoplasmic sperm injection/*in vitro* fertilization

IMC, inseminating motile count; IUI, intrauterine insemination.
Source: Adapted from Van Waart J, Kruger TF, Lombard CJ, et al. Predictive value of normal sperm morphology in intrauterine insemination (IUI): a structured literature review. *Hum Reprod Update* 7(5):495, 2001.

Motility
- <50% bad (longer abstinence may result in higher density and lower motility)

Antisperm Antibodies
- spermMAR ≥20% necessitates obtaining immunobead testing wherein head-binding antibodies are worse than tail, and >50% head-binding antibodies are worrisome (Clarke et al., 1985).
- Pregnancy rates are lower when >50% of sperm are antibody-bound (Ayvaliotis et al., 1985).
- ICSI can circumvent adverse effects of antisperm antibodies (ASAs).
- Screen for ASA when there is isolated asthenospermia with normal sperm concentration, sperm agglutination, or an abnormal postcoital test.
- ASAs found on the surface of sperm by direct testing are more significant than ASAs found in the serum or seminal plasma by indirect testing.
- ASA testing is not needed if sperm are to be used for ICSI.

Round Cells
- Leukocytes and immature germ cells appear similar and are properly termed *round cells.*

- When >5 million/mL or >10/hpf (hpf = 40× magnification), must differentiate using cytologic staining and immunohistochemical techniques.
- Mild prostatitis, epididymitis? (Treatment: ciprofloxacin [Cipro])

Postejaculatory Urinalysis

- Perform in patients with volumes <1 mL, unless patient has bilateral vasal agenesis, clinical signs of hypogonadism, collection problems, or short abstinence interval: All offer an explanation.
- Centrifuge for 10 mins at a minimum of 300 g and inspect at 400× magnification.
- Presence of *any sperm* in a patient with azoospermia or aspermia is suggestive of retrograde ejaculation.

Specialized Clinical Tests on Semen and Sperm

- Not required for diagnosis
- May be useful in a small number of patients for identifying a male factor contributing to unexplained infertility or for selecting therapy such as ART.

Sperm Viability Tests

- Assessed by mixing fresh semen with a supravital dye, such as eosin or trypan blue, or by the use of the hypoosmotic swelling (HOS) test
- Determine whether nonmotile sperm are viable by identifying which sperm have intact cell membranes.
- Nonmotile but viable sperm, as determined by the HOS test, may be used successfully for ICSI.

Sperm Penetration Assay

- Removal of the zona pellucida from hamster oocytes allows human sperm to fuse with hamster ova (hamster egg penetration assay [HEPA]).
- Number of penetrations per egg by the sperm of the test subject is compared to that observed using sperm from a known fertile individual.
- Evaluates capacitation, the acrosome reaction, fusion with the oocyte, and ability to penetrate membrane
- Results are sensitive to culture conditions and difficult to standardize.
- Not widely available, costly, time-consuming
- Sperm function can also be evaluated using human zona pellucida–binding tests; not often used

Computer-Assisted Sperm Analysis (Davis and Katz, 1993)

- Computer-assisted sperm analysis requires sophisticated instruments to generate digitized video images for quantitative assessment of sperm motion characteristics: Kinematics may be more specific.
- May be important factors in determining sperm fertility potential.

MALE SUBFERTILITY

Acrosome Reaction
- Acrosome reaction: fusion of acrosome and plasma membrane → release of acrosomal enzymes and exposure of sperm head
- Infertile men have increased prevalence of spontaneous acrosome loss and decreased acrosome reactivity assessed by fluorescein-labeled pea or peanut agglutinins and specific monoclonal antibodies in response to challenge by calcium ionophore.
- Not necessary for routine evaluation because uncommon problem

Biochemical Tests
- Measurements of sperm creatine kinase and reactive oxygen species (ROS) (Aitken et al., 1989)
  - May detect a probable cause for low fertilization rates or failed IVF
  - Sperm creatine phosphokinase enzyme is involved in generation, transport, and use of energy within the sperm.
  - ROS interfere with sperm function by peroxidation of sperm lipid membranes and creation of toxic fatty acid peroxides.
  - Studies have yielded conflicting results.

History
- Focus on potential causes (Speroff and Fritz, 2005).

Medical History
- Childhood illnesses and developmental history, including testicular descent, pubertal development, loss of body hair or decreased shaving frequency, school performance
  - Systemic illness: diabetes, cancer, upper respiratory diseases, infection
  - Surgical history: cryptorchidism, herniorrhaphy, trauma, torsion
  - Medication use: nitrofurantoin, cimetidine, sulfasalazine, spironolactone, α-blockers

Fertility History
- Duration of subfertility and prior fertility; previous infertility treatments

Sexual History
- Sexually transmitted infections; coital frequency and timing; lubricants

Family History
- Cryptorchidism, midline defects (Kallmann syndrome), hypospadias, primary ciliary dyskinesia (immotile cilia syndrome)

Social and Occupational History
- Gonadal toxin exposure:
  - Ethanol, cocaine, anabolic steroids

MALE SUBFERTILITY

- Exposure to ionizing radiation, chronic heat exposure → ↓ count and motility
- Aniline dyes, pesticides, heavy metals (lead)
- Tobacco → ↓ motility
- Marijuana → ↓ count, motility, testosterone, and acrosome reaction; cannabinoid-binding sites found on human sperm (Rossato et al., 2005)

Physical Examination
- Focus on finding evidence of androgen deficiency.

Penis Examination
- Including the location of the urethral meatus

Palpation of the Testes and Measurement of Their Size
- In normal men, testes are firm and measure 15–25 mL in volume.
- Small soft testes suggest testicular failure.

Presence and Consistency of Both the Vas Deferens and Epididymis
- Diagnosis of congenital bilateral absence of the vas deferens is made by physical examination alone and does not require scrotal sonography or exploration.

Presence of a Varicocele
- Incidence:
  - 11%: Normal semen analysis
  - 25%: Abnormal semen analysis
  - 35%: Infertile men with primary infertility
  - Up to 80%: Men with secondary infertility
  - 53%: Sons of fathers with a varicocele
- Mechanism of injury to sperm is inconclusive:
  - Impaired blood drainage from testis leading to ↑ stromal temperature, hypoxia, ↑ testicular pressure, and reflux of adrenal metabolites
- Associated with ↓ testosterone (statistically significant but not necessarily clinically significant); ↓ total sperm count, morphology, and motility
  - No consistent semen analysis pattern distinguishes men with a varicocele.
- Repair improves testosterone deficit, although change may not be clinically significant.
- Unilateral grade I varicoceles may not cause subfertility, as there is no improvement with varicocele repair in this setting (Sandlow et al., 2000).
- Outcome after subclinical (detected by ultrasound, not clinical examination) varicocelectomy is significantly less beneficial than after repair of clinical varicocele (Jarow et al., 1996).
- Factors associated with improved outcomes after varicocelectomy:
  - Grade III varicocele

213

MALE SUBFERTILITY

- Lack of testicular atrophy
- Normal follicle-stimulating hormone (FSH)
- TMC >5 million
- Motility >60%
- There are few adequately controlled, prospective trials of the effect of varicocele repair on fertility, and those that have been reported give conflicting results (Redmon et al., 2002).

Secondary Sexual Characteristics

- Body habitus, hair distribution, and breast development
  - Men with Klinefelter's syndrome (47,XXY) are classically tall and eunuchoid, with gynecomastia and small testes.

Digital Rectal Examination

- Defines size and symmetry of the prostate and may reveal the presence of midline cysts or dilated seminal vesicles suggesting ejaculatory duct obstruction.

Hormones

- Evaluation of the pituitary-gonadal axis (1.7% incidence of abnormalities); evaluate if <10 million/mL sperm concentration, impaired sexual function, or other clinical findings suggestive of a specific endocrinopathy.
  - Testosterone: ↓ if prolactinoma or hypogonadotropism
    ⇒ If low, obtain a repeat measurement of total and free testosterone.
  - FSH: ↑ in germ cell aplasia
  - Prolactin (PRL): ↓ libido/impotence
  - Thyroid-stimulating hormone (TSH): leads to hyperprolactinemia

Clinical Condition	Follicle-Stimulating Hormone	Luteinizing Hormone	Testosterone	Prolactin
Normal spermatogenesis	Normal	Normal	Normal	Normal
Hypogonadotropic hypogonadism	Low	Low	Low	Normal
Abnormal spermatogenesis[a]	High/normal	Normal	Normal	Normal
Complete testicular failure/ hypergonadotropic hypogonadism	High	High	Normal/low	Normal
Prolactin-secreting pituitary tumor	Normal/low	Normal/low	Low	High

[a]Many men with abnormal spermatogenesis have a normal serum follicle-stimulating hormone, but a marked elevation of serum follicle-stimulating hormone is clearly indicative of an abnormality in spermatogenesis.

Urologic Evaluation

- *Transrectal ultrasonography indicated in azoospermic patients with palpable vasa and low ejaculate volumes to determine if ejaculatory duct obstruction is present.*
  - Findings of dilated seminal vesicles, dilated ejaculatory ducts, and/or midline prostatic cystic structures are suggestive of complete or partial ejaculatory duct obstruction.
  - Complete ejaculatory duct obstruction: low-volume, fructose-negative, acidic, azoospermic ejaculates
  - Partial ejaculatory duct obstruction: low volume, oligoasthenospermia, and poor forward progression
  - Transscrotal ultrasonography may be useful to clarify ambiguous findings on examination or in patients in whom a testicular mass is suspected.
  - May identify nonpalpable varicoceles, but these have not been shown to be clinically significant.

GENETICS OF MALE SUBFERTILITY

Cystic Fibrosis Gene Mutations (Autosomal Recessive)

- Strong association between CBAVD (congenital bilateral absence of vas deferens) and mutations of the CFTR gene on chromosome 7.
  - CBAVD is associated with mutations within the CF gene in 70–80% of men.
  - CBAVD in 1% of infertile males
- Besides CF gene mutations, a second genetic etiology involves abnormal differentiation of the mesonephric ducts.
- One of the more common diagnoses in patients with obstructive azoospermia
- Seminal volume low (<1 cc), pH <7.0
- Important to test patient's partner before performing a treatment that uses his sperm, because of the risk that his partner may be a CF carrier.

Chromosomal Abnormalities Resulting in Impaired Testicular Function

- Prevalence of karyotypic abnormalities in infertile men: 7%
- Frequency is inversely proportional to sperm count.
  - 10–15% in azoospermic men
  - 5% in oligospermic men
  - <1% in normospermic men
- Klinefelter's syndrome (47,XXY or 46XY/47XXY) accounts for $2/3$ of the chromosomal abnormalities observed in subfertile men.
- Structural abnormalities of the autosomal chromosomes, such as inversions and translocations, are also observed at a higher frequency in infertile men than in the general population.

MALE SUBFERTILITY

- Couple is at increased risk for miscarriages and children with chromosomal and congenital defects when the male has gross karyotypic abnormalities.
- Karyotyping should be offered to men who have nonobstructive azoospermia (NOA) or severe oligospermia (<5 million/mL) before IVF with ICSI.
- Genetic counseling should be provided whenever a genetic abnormality is detected.

Y-Chromosome Microdeletions Associated with Isolated Spermatogenic Impairment

- Y-chromosome analysis should be offered to men who have NOA or severe oligospermia (<1 million/mL) before ICSI.
- Found in approximately 10% of men with azoospermia or severe oligospermia
- Too small to be detected by standard karyotyping but can be found by using polymerase chain reaction
- The intervening large segment of the Y chromosome, known as the *male specific Y*, contains many genes involved in spermatogenesis.
- Regions prone to microdeletion: *AZFa, AZFb,* and *AZFc.*

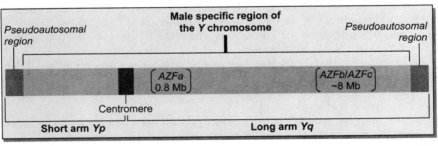

Source: Adapted from Oates RD. The genetics of male reproductive failure: what every clinician needs to know. *Sexuality, Reproduction and Menopause* 2(4):213, 2004.

- Microdeletion in *AZFc* region in 1 in 4000 men; most common molecular cause of NOA
  - Approximately 70% of men with an *AZFc* microdeletion possess sperm.
  - 13% of men with NOA are *AZFc* microdeleted.
  - Approximately 6% of men with severe oligospermia, <5 million/mL, are *AZFc* microdeleted.

CAUSES OF MALE FACTOR SUBFERTILITY (Turek, 2004)
- Four main areas:
  1. Pretesticular (hypothalamic disease) (1–2%)
  2. Testicular (primary hypogonadism) (30–40%)
  3. Posttesticular (disorders of sperm transport) (10–20%)
  4. Idiopathic (40–50%)

Hypothalamic Disease

Gonadotropin Deficiency (Kallmann Syndrome)
- Rare (1 in 50,000 persons) disturbance of neuron migration from the olfactory placode during development
- Two most common clinical deficits: anosmia and absence of GnRH
- Other signs and symptoms:
  - Facial asymmetry, color blindness, renal anomalies, microphallus, cryptorchidism, and, the hallmark of the syndrome, → delay in pubertal development
- Low testosterone, low luteinizing hormone (LH), and low FSH levels
- Men can be fertile when given FSH and LH to stimulate sperm production. Virilization with testosterone or human chorionic gonadotropin.

Isolated Luteinizing Hormone Deficiency ("Fertile Eunuch")
- Rare; due to partial gonadotropin deficiency
- Enough LH is produced to stimulate intratesticular testosterone production and spermatogenesis, but insufficient testosterone to promote virilization. Eunuchoid body proportions, variable virilization, and often gynecomastia.
- Normal testis size, but the ejaculate contains reduced numbers of sperm.
- FSH levels are normal, but serum LH and testosterone levels are low-normal.

Isolated Follicle-Stimulating Hormone Deficiency
- Extremely rare; insufficient FSH
- FSH levels are uniformly low and do not respond to stimulation with GnRH. Sperm counts range from azoospermia to severely low numbers (oligospermia).

Congenital Hypogonadotropic Syndromes
- Prader-Willi syndrome (1 in 20,000 persons): genetic obesity, retardation, small hands and feet, and hypogonadism
- Caused by a deficiency of hypothalamic GnRH
- Single-gene deletion associated with this condition is found on chromosome 15.
- Spermatogenesis can be induced with exogenous FSH and LH.
- Bardet-Biedl syndrome: rare, autosomal recessive, results from GnRH deficiency: retardation, retinitis pigmentosa, polydactyly, and hypogonadism
- The hypogonadism can be treated with FSH and LH.

MALE SUBFERTILITY

Pituitary Disease

Pituitary Insufficiency
- Tumors, infiltrative processes, operation, radiation, deposits

Hyperprolactinemia
- Systemic diseases and medications should be ruled out.
- PRL-secreting pituitary adenoma
- Elevated PRL usually results in decreased FSH, LH, and testosterone levels and causes infertility.
- Associated symptoms include loss of libido, impotence, galactorrhea, and gynecomastia.
- Signs and symptoms of other pituitary hormone derangements (adrenocorticotropic hormone, TSH) should also be investigated.

Exogenous Hormones
- Estrogen-androgen excess, glucocorticoid excess, hyper- and hypothyroidism
- Excessive obesity, adrenocortical tumors, Sertoli cell tumors, and interstitial testis tumors may produce estrogens.
- Congenital adrenal hyperplasia, in which the enzyme 21-hydroxylase is most commonly deficient: abnormally high production of androgenic steroids by the adrenal cortex
- Hormonally active adrenocortical tumors or Leydig cell tumors of the testis.
- Sources of exogenous glucocorticoids include chronic therapy for ulcerative colitis, asthma, or rheumatoid arthritis.
- Cushing's syndrome is a common reason for excess endogenous glucocorticoids.
- Thyroid abnormalities are a rare cause (0.5%) of male infertility.
- Some infertile men have deficient responses to growth hormone challenge tests and may respond to growth hormone treatment with improvements in semen quality.

Testicular (Primary Hypogonadism) Effects
- Testicular (primary hypogonadism) effects are, at present, largely irreversible.
- **Chromosomal** (Klinefelter's syndrome [47,XXY], 46,XX sex reversal, 47,XYY syndrome)
- **Noonan's syndrome** (male Turner syndrome): 75% have cryptorchidism.
- **Myotonic dystrophy:** testis atrophy; fertility has been reported.
  - Testis biopsies show seminiferous tubule damage in 75% of cases.
- **Vanishing testis syndrome** (bilateral anorchia): rare, occurring in 1 in 20,000 males
- **Sertoli-cell–only syndrome** (germ cell aplasia)
- **Y chromosome microdeletions**

- **Gonadotoxins** (radiation, drugs)
  - Ketoconazole, spironolactone, and alcohol inhibit testosterone synthesis; cimetidine is an androgen antagonist.
  - Marijuana, heroin, and methadone are associated with lower testosterone.
  - Pesticides are likely to have estrogen-like activity.
- **Systemic disease** (renal failure, liver failure, sickle cell anemia)
- **Defective androgen activity**
  - 5α-Reductase deficiency
    - ⇨ Normal development of the testes and wolffian duct structures (internal genitalia) but ambiguous external genitalia
  - Androgen receptor deficiency: X-linked
- **Testis injury (orchitis, torsion, trauma)**
- **Cryptorchidism**
- **Varicocele** (also see discussion of varicocele in the Physical Examination section above)
  - Objectives of repair:
    - ⇨ Relieve pain
    - ⇨ Improve semen parameters
    - ⇨ Studies have shown that repair improves semen parameters in up to 60–70% of cases, with natural pregnancy rates up to 50% (Nagler et al., 1997). However, Cochrane review of several randomized controlled trials did not show sufficient evidence regarding the treatment to warrant repair (Evers and Collins, 2003).
    - ⇨ Enhance testicular function
    - ⇨ Improve pregnancy rates in couples with male factor infertility associated with varicocele

Posttesticular Causes of Infertility
Reproductive Tract Obstruction
Congenital Blockages
- Congenital absence of the vas deferens
- Young syndrome: triad of chronic sinusitis, bronchiectasis, and obstructive azoospermia. The obstruction is in the epididymis.
- Idiopathic epididymal obstruction
- Polycystic kidney disease: usually secondary to obstructing cysts in the epididymis or seminal vesicles
- Ejaculatory duct obstruction: Transurethral resection of an obstruction results in increased semen volume in approximately $2/3$ of affected men and returns sperm to the ejaculate in approximately $1/2$ of azoospermic men.

MALE SUBFERTILITY

Acquired Blockages
- **Vasectomy:** 5% of men have the vasectomy reversed, most commonly because of remarriage.
  - Overall pregnancy rate: 50%
  - Choice may also depend on presence of female factors.
  - Pregnancy rate decreases as the time passes since the vasectomy:

Years since Vasectomy	Pregnancy Rate (%)
2	77
5	49
10	43
15	30

Source: Adapted from Belker AM, Thomas AJ, Jr., et al. Results of 1,469 microsurgical vasectomy reversals by the Vasovasostomy Study Group. *J Urol* 145(3):505, 1991.

- **Groin surgery** can result in inguinal vas deferens obstruction in 1% of cases.
- **Infection** *may* involve the epididymis, with scarring and obstruction.

Functional Blockages
- **Sympathetic nerve injury:** In men with spinal cord injuries, demyelinating neuropathies, or diabetes, and in those who have had retroperitoneal lymph node dissections, ejaculation can be achieved with vibratory stimulation, and in those who do not respond, electroejaculation.
- **Pharmacologic:** Antihypertensives, antipsychotics, antidepressants

Disorders of Sperm Function or Motility
- **Immotile cilia syndromes:** Kartagener syndrome is a subset of this disorder (1 in 40,000 males) that presents with the triad of chronic sinusitis, bronchiectasis, and situs inversus. Most immotile cilia cases are diagnosed in childhood with respiratory and sinus difficulties.
- **Maturation defects:** seen in vasectomy-induced blockage
- **Immunologic infertility:** Autoimmune infertility has been implicated as a cause of infertility in 10% of infertile couples.
- **Infection**
- **Age-related effects:** Several studies show that semen volume and sperm motility may decrease continuously between 22 and 80 yrs of age (Eskenazi et al., 2003).

Disorders of Coitus
- **Impotence**
- **Hypospadias** can cause inappropriate placement of the seminal coagulum too distant from the cervix.
- Timing and frequency: Appropriate frequency is every 2 days, within the periovulatory period.
- Avoid lubricants if at all possible (see Appendix B).

MALE SUBFERTILITY

TREATMENT
Abnormal Semen Analysis
Antibiotics
- Culture for urethritis; empiric therapy for epididymitis, prostatitis

Surgery
- Varicocele repair: ↑ motility, not count

Intrauterine Insemination

Total Motile Count (Million)	Live Birth Rate (%)
<10	1.4
>10	6.0

Source: Adapted from Van Voorhis BJ, Sparks AE. Semen analysis: what tests are clinically useful? *Clin Obstet Gynecol* 42(4):957, 1999.

Therapeutic Donor Insemination
- Frozen to prevent human immunodeficiency virus transmission

In Vitro Fertilization with Intracytoplasmic Sperm Injection (Bonduelle et al., 1998a; Bonduelle et al., 1998b)
- Indications: morphology ≤1%; motility <10%; TMC <5 million
- No correlation between chromosomal anomalies and a normal semen analysis specimen used for ICSI
- Major malformations: same rate as for IVF (approximately 2.3%)
- Can use testicular or epididymal sperm for ICSI

Aberration	General Public (%)	ICSI (%)
Autosomal	0.020 (2 in 1000)	0.83 (8 in 1000)
Sex chromosomal	0.25 (1 in 400)	0.83 (1 in 125)
Structural *de novo* (i.e., non-balanced)	0.07	0.36

Source: Adapted from Bonduelle M, Aytoz A, et al. Incidence of chromosomal aberrations in children born after assisted reproduction through intracytoplasmic sperm injection. *Hum Reprod* 13(4):781, 1998a.

221

MALE SUBFERTILITY
A. Approach to Diagnosis of Male Subfertility

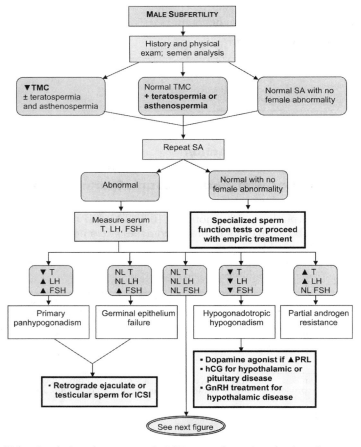

FSH, follicle-stimulating hormone; GnRH, gonadotropin-releasing hormone; hCG, human chorionic gonadotropin; ICSI, intracytoplasmic sperm injection; LH, luteinizing hormone; NL, normal; PRL, prolactin; SA, semen analysis; T, testosterone; TMC, total motile count. (Adapted from Swerdloff RS, Wang C. Evaluation of male infertility. UpToDate Patient Information Web site: http://www.utdol.com. Accessed February, 2005.)

MALE SUBFERTILITY

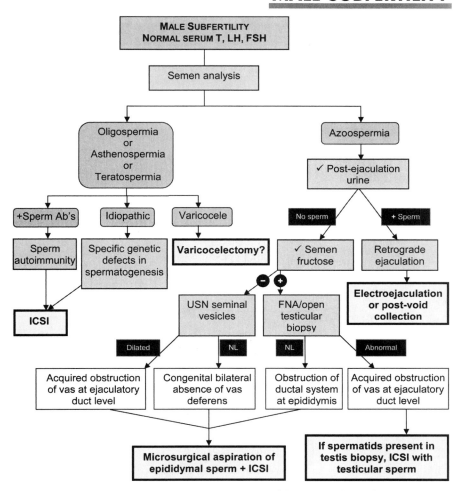

Ab's, antibodies; FNA, fine-needle aspiration; FSH, follicle-stimulating hormone; ICSI, intracytoplasmic sperm injection; LH, luteinizing hormone; NL, normal; T, testosterone; USN, ultrasound. (Adapted from Swerdloff RS, Wang C. Evaluation of male infertility. UpToDate Patient Information Web site: http://www.utdol.com. Accessed February, 2005.)

B. Lubricants and Sperm

VAGINAL LUBRICANTS: EFFECT ON SPERM

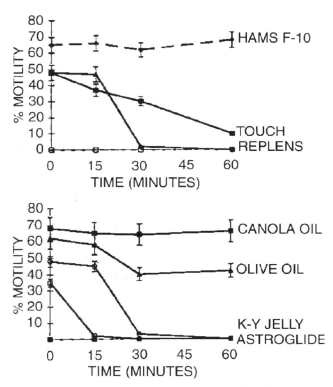

Motility determined by computer-assisted semen analysis of various sperm-lubricant treatments at 1, 15, 30, and 60 mins. Control media (Hams F-10) shown in the top graph had minimal effect on sperm motility. A spermicidal agent with nonoxynol 9 had immediate and prolonged inhibitory effects on sperm motility (shown as a *dashed line* at the bottom of each graph). (Source: Reproduced with permission from Kutteh WH, Chao CH, et al. Vaginal lubricants for the infertile couple: effect on sperm activity. *Int J Fertil Menopausal Stud* 41[4]:400, 1996.)

21. Diminished Ovarian Reserve

DEFINITION
- *Diminished ovarian reserve* (DOR) refers to the condition of having a low number of normal oocytes or having poor quality oocytes (Scott et al., 1995)

BACKGROUND
- ↑ Age is associated with ↓ fecundity (ability to get pregnant), ↓ live birth rate, ↑ early follicular phase follicular-stimulating hormone (FSH) levels, ↑ miscarriage rates, and ↑ *in vitro* fertilization (IVF) cancellation rates due to poor stimulation (Pearlstone et al., 1992; Pellestor et al., 2003; Stein, 1985).
- Despite age, some young, normally cycling women do not become pregnant with repetitive cycles of IVF, experience frequent miscarriage, or do not respond well to exogenous gonadotropins.
- From 1969 to 1994, the number of women older than 30 yrs having their first child ↑ from 4.1% to 21.2% (Heck et al., 1997)
- Donor insemination recipients' 1-year pregnancy rate (Schwartz and Mayaux, 1982):
  - <31 yrs old = 74%
  - 31–35 yrs old = 62%
  - >35 yrs old = **54%**

IMPLICATIONS
- Women with low ovarian reserve have ↓ fecundity with IVF cycles and natural cycles.
- Some of these women should be offered donor eggs and counseled about adoption.
- This **does not mean** that they do not ovulate, that they will not respond to gonadotropins or oral ovulation induction, or that there are **no** good eggs remaining within the ovary.
- It **does** mean, however, that **there are no means by which to selectively stimulate the good eggs to ovulate.**
- Before embarking on aggressive surgery or infertility treatment to enhance fertility, it is a good idea for some patients to undergo ovarian reserve testing.
- ↑ Incidence of Down syndrome in women with ↑ FSH, regardless of age (van Montfrans et al., 1999)

DIMINISHED OVARIAN RESERVE

HORMONAL TESTS
Caveats
- Different assays may report varying hormone levels from the same serum samples; it is important to calibrate the assay to that in the original studies (Sharara et al., 1998)
- Valid to test basal FSH on CD 2–5 but estradiol (E_2) only CD 2–3 (Hansen et al., 1996)
- Nocturnal pulses begin 4 wks postpartum (Liu et al., 1983)
- Studies have equal validity in women who have just one ovary (Khalifa et al., 1992)
- A normal FSH does not improve a woman's age-related $\downarrow$ fecundity (Sharara et al., 1998)
  - Dr. Toner's rule of thumb (Toner, 2003):

Age = egg quality, whereas CD 3 FSH = egg quantity

Hormones
Day 3 Follicle-Stimulating Hormone (Scott et al., 1989)
- Most centers consider CD 3 FSH ≤ 10 mIU/mL as normal and ≥ 20 mIU/mL as abnormal.
- When CD 3 FSH >25 mIU/mL, ongoing pregnancy rate is 2%.
- CD 3 FSH is more predictive of outcome than is age (Toner et al., 1991).
- If a single CD 3 FSH is abnormal, the pregnancy rate is 5%; with two abnormal CD 3 FSHs (≥ 20 mIU/mL) the IVF pregnancy rate is 0% (Martin et al., 1996).
- Variability does not affect the prognostic category (Buyalos et al., 1998; Scott et al., 1990).
- Many prospective studies report that CD 3 FSH is equally predictive of outcome regardless of age; however, a prospective study showed no statistical difference in live birth rates in women <38 yrs old who completed IVF cycles (Abdalla and Thum, 2004).
- Basal FSH screening may not be of value in the general subfertility population with ovulatory menstrual cycles (van Montfrans et al., 2000).

Day 3 Estradiol
- Levels typically nadir at CD 3 (Sharara et al., 1998).
- Elevated E_2 levels on CD 3 indicates advanced follicular phase; this is due to a premature rise in FSH in the luteal phase and reflects DOR (Sharara et al., 1998).
- Inappropriately high E_2 can suppress FSH back into the normal range by CD 3, and therefore may mask DOR.
- E_2 >80 pg/mL have higher cancellation rates with IVF (Smotrich et al., 1995).

DIMINISHED OVARIAN RESERVE

- CD 3 E_2 <20 pg/mL or ≥80 pg/mL have an ↑ risk for canceled IVF cycles, but these levels do not seem to predict pregnancy outcome nor correlate with ovarian response in those patients not canceled (Frattarelli et al., 2000).

Clomiphene Citrate Challenge Test (Navot et al., 1987)

- Steps: Measure CD 2–3 FSH, give patient clomiphene citrate (Clomid), 100 mg, CD 5–9, measure FSH on CD 10–11
- This test unmasks DOR, sensitivity of the clomiphene citrate challenge test (CCCT) to identify depletion of the primordial follicle pool is higher than that of screening for elevated CD 3 FSH (26% vs. 8%) (Barnhart and Osheroff, 1998)
- Incidence of abnormal CCCT:
  - <30 yrs old = 3%
  - >30 yrs old = 26%
  - Unexplained subfertility = 38%
- Any abnormal value indicates poor prognosis.
  - Initial study: 51 patients 35 yrs old or older with normal CD 3 FSH; 18 had abnormal levels on CD 10; none of these 18 patients conceived (Navot et al., 1987)
  - Multiple retrospective studies show that CCCT is highly predictive of poor outcome with IVF (<10%), regardless of age.
- Understanding how the CCCT works:
  - Clomid blocks the effects of E_2 at the hypothalamus and pituitary, mimicking a hypoestrogenic state; the hypothalamic-pituitary (HP) axis responds by releasing a flood of FSH.
    ⇨ A woman with a normal, healthy cohort of follicles will produce enough E_2 and inhibin B to dislodge the Clomid and suppress FSH.
    ⇨ A woman with a poor cohort and aging follicles cannot generate enough E_2 or inhibin B to clear the Clomid or suppress FSH, respectively; therefore, FSH stays high.

Day 3 Inhibin B

- ↓ Inhibin B levels lead to ↑ FSH levels; ↓ inhibin B levels precede increases in FSH (Seifer et al., 1999).
- Women with inhibin B ≤45 pg/mL have 1/3 the pregnancy rate and 3× the cancellation rate in IVF than women with higher levels.
- Most data do not support using this test because it is not as predictive as CD 3 FSH for outcome (Creus et al., 2000; Parinaud and Lesourd, 2002).

DIMINISHED OVARIAN RESERVE

OTHER TESTS

Ultrasound
- Performed on CD 3
- Data inconsistent (Bancsi et al., 2002; Frattarelli et al., 2003; Hansen et al., 2003)
- Fewer than five total follicles predicts higher gonadotropin dose and cancellation rates; pregnancy rates lower (23% with IVF) but still adequate (Frattarelli et al., 2003)

Ovarian Volume
- Predictive of ovarian responsiveness
- Pregnancy rates are ↓ with small volume, but studies have not been done prospectively for predictive value (Syrop et al., 1995, 1999)

Ovarian Biopsy
- Not reliable; oocytes are heterogeneously located throughout ovarian cortex (Sharara and Scott, 2004)

RECOMMENDATIONS FOR DIMINISHED OVARIAN RESERVE SCREENING
- Age >35 yrs
- Unexplained subfertility
- Family history of early menopause
- Smoking
- Previous ovarian surgery
- History of radiation or chemotherapy
- Previous poor response to gonadotropins

22. Assisted Reproductive Technologies

- *Assisted reproductive technologies* (ART) by definition are any fertility treatments in which **both egg and sperm** are handled. Accordingly, ART procedures involve the surgical removal of eggs, known as *egg retrieval.*
- *In vitro* fertilization (IVF) is the most common ART procedure; IVF has been used in the United States since 1981, and data are collected by the Centers for Disease Control and Prevention and published annually (http://www.cdc.gov/reproductivehealth/art.htm).
  - In 2002, 115,392 ART cycles were performed in 391 fertility clinics.
    - ⇨ 33,141 live births yielding 45,751 babies

DEFINITIONS

- *In vitro* **fertilization** (IVF): ovulation induction, oocyte retrieval, and fertilization of the oocytes in the laboratory; embryos are then cultured for 3–5 days with subsequent transfer transcervically under abdominal ultrasound guidance into the uterine cavity.
- **Gamete intrafallopian transfer** (GIFT): ovarian stimulation and egg retrieval along with laparoscopically guided transfer of a mixture of unfertilized eggs and sperm into the fallopian tubes
- **Zygote intrafallopian transfer** (ZIFT): ovarian stimulation and egg retrieval followed by fertilization of the eggs in the laboratory and laparoscopic transfer of the day 1 fertilized eggs (*zygotes*) into the fallopian tubes
- **Donor egg IVF:** used for patients with poor egg numbers or egg quality; involves stimulation of an egg donor with typical superovulation followed by standard egg retrieval; eggs are then fertilized by the sperm of the infertile woman's partner, and embryos are transferred to the infertile woman in a standard IVF-like process.
- **Intracytoplasmic sperm injection** (ICSI): developed in the early 1990s to help couples with severe male factor infertility; one sperm is injected directly into each mature egg, typically resulting in a 50–70% fertilization rate.

ASSISTED REPRODUCTIVE TECHNOLOGIES

EVALUATION BEFORE ASSISTED REPRODUCTIVE TECHNOLOGIES

Ovarian Reserve (see Chapter 21, Diminished Ovarian Reserve)

- Ovarian reserve testing determines the number and quality of eggs present before infertility treatment:

Day 3 FSH, E_2	FSH on day 3 of <10 is normal. Levels between 10 and 14 are a gray zone with decreasing fertility as levels rise. FSH >14 results in a <1% chance of a live birth per cycle (Levi et al., 2001). E_2 should be <60 on day 3. Higher levels suggest early follicular recruitment, which results in a poor prognosis.
Clomiphene citrate challenge test	A more extensive test of ovarian reserve. Indicated for women ≥35 yrs old, smokers, those with one ovary or unexplained infertility, and patients in whom decreased ovarian reserve is suspected. Involves standard day 3 laboratory tests, as described above, along with the administration of clomiphene citrate, 100 mg days 5–9, and a repeat FSH on day 10. Day 10 FSH thresholds should be the same as those on day 3.

E_2, estradiol; FSH, follicle-stimulating hormone.

Evaluation of Tubal Status

- Patients with a hydrosalpinx on ultrasonography (Camus et al., 1999):
  - 50% ↓ pregnancy rate
  - Twofold ↑ miscarriage rate
- Mechanism of adverse effect (Strandell and Lindhard, 2002):
  1. ↓ Nutrients in hydrosalpinx fluid
  2. Toxic effect of fluid on embryos (Sachdev et al., 1997) and/or sperm (Ng et al., 2000)
  3. ↓ Expression: $\alpha_5\beta_3$, LIF, HOXA10
  4. Wash-out effect from fluid
  5. ↑ Endometrial peristalsis due to hydrosalpinx fluid
  - Ligation of the hydrosalpinx or salpingectomy restores normal pregnancy rate (Strandell et al., 2001a; Johnson et al., 2002).

Evaluation of the Uterine Cavity

- Significantly lower clinical pregnancy rates with IVF–embryo transfer (IVF-ET) occur if uterine cavity abnormalities are present (8.3% vs. 37.5%) (Shamma et al., 1992).
- Evaluation techniques: sonohysterogram, hysterosalpingogram, hysteroscopy

ASSISTED REPRODUCTIVE TECHNOLOGIES

Trial Transfer

- Trial transfer is performed before ovulation induction with the same type of catheter used for embryo transfer to help ensure atraumatic transfer of the embryos into the uterine cavity.

Evaluation of Male Factor Infertility

- Semen analysis: Basic semen analysis should include volume of ejaculate, concentration, motility, and morphology using the Kruger strict criteria.
- Antisperm antibody testing: When present, they can significantly ↓ fertilization rates when standard insemination is performed. This can be corrected with ICSI (Kutteh, 1999).

OVULATION INDUCTION MEDICINES

- Fresh cycle IVF pregnancy rates relative to patient age tend to peak after ten mature eggs are retrieved. Gonadotropin-releasing hormone agonists (GnRH-as) or antagonists are used to prevent a woman from ovulating on her own before egg retrieval (40% incidence without such medicines).
- Low-dose aspirin (80 mg/day) may improve IVF outcome as assessed by a prospective, randomized study of 1380 women → odds ratio, 1.2 (95% confidence interval [CI], 1.0–1.6) (Waldenstrom et al., 2004).

Gonadotropin Preparations

Trade Name, Manufacturer	Source
FSH/LH-containing preparations	
Pergonal, Serono[a]	Urine of menopausal women
Repronex, Ferring	Urine of menopausal women
Menopur, Ferring	Urine of menopausal women
Humegon, Organon[a]	Urine of menopausal women
FSH-containing preparations	
Bravelle, Ferring	Urine of menopausal women
Fertinex, Serono[a]	Urine of menopausal women
Gonal-F, Serono	Recombinant, Chinese hamster ovary cells
Follistim, Organon	Recombinant, Chinese hamster ovary cells
LH-only–containing preparation	
Luveris, Serono	Recombinant

FSH, follicle-stimulating hormone; LH, luteinizing hormone.
[a]Drug has been discontinued.

ASSISTED REPRODUCTIVE TECHNOLOGIES

Human Chorionic Gonadotropin Preparations

Trade Name, Manufacturer	Source	Formulations
Profasi, Serono[a]	Urine of pregnant females	10,000 IU IM
Pregnyl, Organon	Urine of pregnant females	10,000 IU IM
Novarel, Ferring	Urine of pregnant females	10,000 IU IM
Chorex, Hyrex	Urine of pregnant females	10,000 IU IM
Ovidrel, Serono	Recombinant, Chinese hamster ovary cells	250 µg SC

[a]Drug has been discontinued.

Gonadotropin-Releasing Hormone Agonist/Antagonist Preparations

Trade Name, Manufacturer	Formulations
Lupron Depot, TAP	1 mg/0.2 mL = 20 U SC
Synarel, Searle	2 mg/mL intranasal
Zoladex, AstraZeneca	3.6 mg SC
Antagon, Organon	250 µg/0.5 mL SC
Cetrotide, Serono	250 µg/1 mL SC

Gonadotropin-Releasing Hormone Agonists
- Agonists bind to and stimulate the pituitary GnRH receptor (GnRH-R) and have a long half-life. They ultimately down-regulate the GnRH-R, thereby decreasing follicle-stimulating hormone (FSH) and luteinizing hormone (LH) secretion. This eliminates the possibility of an LH surge with continued GnRH-a administration. The first injection is usually administered in the luteal phase of a natural cycle to help prevent cysts from forming.

Advantages
- More eggs retrieved
- Elimination of LH surge
- ↑ Cohort synchronization

Disadvantages
- ↑ Costs
- ↑ Gonadotropin medication requirement
- Possible administration during an early conception

232

ASSISTED REPRODUCTIVE TECHNOLOGIES

Gonadotropin-Releasing Hormone Antagonists
- Newly developed synthetic GnRH molecule that has antagonist properties on the GnRH-R. Immediately binds to and blocks GnRH binding to the receptor. Typically administered late in ovarian stimulation once the follicular size is 14 mm.

Advantages
- Immediate onset of action
- ↓ Number of injections

Disadvantages
- ↑ Costs
- ↑ Gonadotropin medication requirement
- Possible administration during an early conception
- Possible reduction in implantation rates

STIMULATION PROTOCOLS AND DOSES
- Estimating the patient's responsiveness to the fertility agents:
  - Age, body mass index, day 3 FSH/estradiol (E_2), ovarian volume, antral follicle count, response to prior ovarian stimulation

Oral Contraceptive–Gonadotropin-Releasing Hormone Agonist Stimulation Protocol
- Oral contraceptives (OCs) can help with scheduling of IVF cycles and may help synchronize the ovary and result in a better cohort size. OCs typically increase the amount of medications required during stimulation and may decrease the number of eggs in older women.

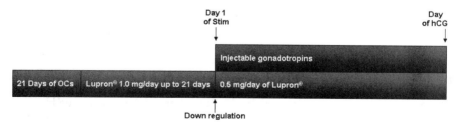

Oral contraceptive (OC)/gonadotropin-stimulating hormone agonist stimulation (Stim). hCG, human chorionic gonadotropin.

1. Start OCs between days 1 and 3 of menstrual cycle. Typically administer for 15–21 days.

233

ASSISTED REPRODUCTIVE TECHNOLOGIES

2. Start GnRH-a 3–5 days before the completion of the OCs. This overlap of OCs and GnRH-as helps to prevent ovarian cyst formation.
3. Spontaneous menses expected 10–12 days after the 1st day of GnRH-a.
4. Start ovarian stimulation and continue GnRH-a. Stimulation is typically a step-down protocol, using a higher dose of medicine early in the stimulation and gradually decreasing the dose. Stimulation can be with FSH, human menopausal gonadotropin (HMG), or a combination of FSH and HMG.
5. Serial ultrasounds and E_2 levels monitor follicular development; E_2 should ↑ by 50% each day of stimulation.
6. Once follicular size reaches 18–22 mm, administer hCG, typically 5000–10,000 U SC or IM.
7. Oocyte retrieval 34–35 hrs after hCG

Luteal Gonadotropin-Releasing Hormone Agonist Stimulation Protocol

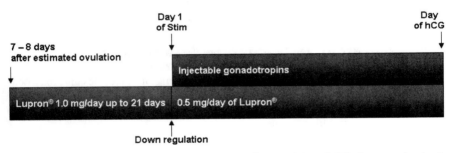

Gonadotropin-releasing hormone agonist stimulation (Stim). hCG, human chorionic gonadotropin.

1. Start GnRH-a on day 21 of menstrual cycle. The luteal start is typically confirmed by a serum progesterone level >4 ng/mL. The luteal start of GnRH-as helps to prevent ovarian cyst formation.
2. Spontaneous menses expected 10–12 days after the 1st day of GnRH-a.
3. Start ovarian stimulation and continue Lupron at lower dose. Stimulation is typically a step-down protocol, using a higher dose of medicine early in the stimulation and gradually decreasing the dose. Stimulation can be with FSH, HMG, or a combination of FSH and HMG.
4. Serial ultrasounds and E_2 levels monitor follicular development; E_2 should ↑ by 50% each day of stimulation.

ASSISTED REPRODUCTIVE TECHNOLOGIES

5. Once follicular size reaches 18–22 mm, administer hCG, typically 5000–10,000 U SC or IM.
6. Oocyte retrieval 34–35 hrs after hCG

Microdose Gonadotropin-Releasing Hormone Agonist Flare Stimulation Protocol

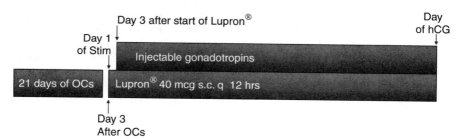

Microdose gonadotropin-releasing hormone agonist flare stimulation (Stim). hCG, human chorionic gonadotropin; OCs, oral contraceptives.

1. Start of OCs between days 1 and 3 of menstrual cycle and administer for 21 days. (Note: Many programs do not use OCs at all for this protocol.)
2. Start Lupron, 40 μg SC q12 hrs, 3 days after the end of the OC course (i.e., day 24).
3. Start ovarian stimulation with FSH, HMG, or a combination of FSH and HMG 3 days after the start of Lupron (i.e., day 27) and continue Lupron. (Note: Many programs start the gonadotropins on the same day as the microdose Lupron.)
4. Serial ultrasounds and E_2 levels monitor follicular development; E_2 should ↑ by 50% each day of stimulation.
5. Once follicular size reaches 18–22 mm, administer hCG, typically 5000–10,000 units SC or IM.
6. Oocyte retrieval 34–35 hrs after hCG

ASSISTED REPRODUCTIVE TECHNOLOGIES

Oral Contraceptive–Gonadotropin-Releasing Hormone Antagonist Stimulation Protocol

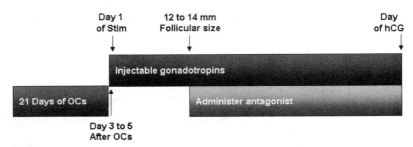

Gonadotropin-releasing hormone antagonist stimulation (Stim). hCG, human chorionic gonadotropin; OCs, oral contraceptives.

1. Start of OCs between days 1 and 3 of menstrual cycle. Typically, administer for 15–21 days.
2. Start ovarian stimulation 3–5 days after discontinuing OCs. Stimulation is typically a step-down protocol, using a higher dose of medicine early in the stimulation and gradually decreasing the dose. Stimulation can be with FSH, HMG, or a combination of FSH and HMG.
3. Serial ultrasounds and E_2 levels to monitor follicular development; E_2 should rise 50% per day.
4. Once a follicular size of 14 mm is reached, start GnRH antagonist. Administration of the GnRH antagonist can lower endogenous E_2 levels. Typically, no further decrease in gonadotropin dose is recommended. Rather, most clinicians add back FSH/LH drugs at time of antagonist start.
5. Once follicular size reaches 18–22 mm, administer hCG, typically 5000–10,000 U SC or IM.
6. Oocyte retrieval 34–35 hrs after hCG

Oocyte Retrieval

- Typically performed 34–35 hrs after hCG
- Performed under IV sedation with the placement of a 5-MHz vaginal transducer with associated needle guide. A 16-gauge, 35-cm aspiration needle is inserted transvaginally into multiple preovulatory follicles with sequential aspiration (low-grade suction <100 mm Hg) of oocytes. The aspirate is then given to the embryologist for evaluation.
- Complications can include intraabdominal bleeding and infection, typically occurring in <1–2% of IVF cases.

ASSISTED REPRODUCTIVE TECHNOLOGIES

EMBRYOLOGY

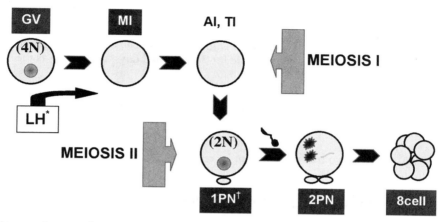

*Arrested at prophase I until luteinizing hormone (LH) surge. †Arrested at metaphase II until fertilization. AI, anaphase I; GV, germinal vesicle; MI, metaphase I; N, nuclei; PN, pronuclei; TI, telophase I.

- Retrieved eggs are identified in the follicular aspirate. Once they are identified, they are removed from the aspirate and placed in culture dishes.
- Standard IVF insemination is performed by culturing the identified eggs for approximately 16 hrs with ≥50,000 sperm/mL. The next morning, the eggs are identified and evaluated for fertilization. The first sign of fertilization is two pronuclei within the cytoplasm.
- ICSI is performed in cases of severe male factor infertility, failed fertilization in a previous cycle, or severe antisperm antibody levels. After identification of the eggs in the follicular aspirate, the eggs are then placed into culture dishes. The cumulus cell complex surrounding the eggs is then removed in a process called *stripping*. Once the eggs are stripped, they are evaluated for maturity. Only metaphase 2 (MII) eggs can be fertilized. All MII eggs are then inseminated by taking one motile, morphologically normal–appearing sperm and injecting it into each mature egg.
- Fertilization rate with standard insemination is approximately 70%. With ICSI fertilization, rates range from 50–70%.

ASSISTED REPRODUCTIVE TECHNOLOGIES

- Embryos are then cultured, typically for 3–5 days, in incubators maintained at body temperature and media specific for human embryo culture. Embryos are typically evaluated on day 3 for their cell number and overall morphology.
- It is most common for embryo transfer to be performed on day 3. In some centers, patients with a large number of embryos of high cell count and grade are placed into extended embryo culture for 2 additional days, referred to as the *blastocyst stage.*
- Extended embryo culture to the blastocyst stage may help to identify embryos with the highest prognosis for pregnancy. Cochrane Review concludes that there is little difference in the major pregnancy outcome parameters between day 2–3 embryo transfer and blastocyst culture (Blake et al., 2002).
- Blastocyst embryo transfer seems to increase the risk of monozygotic twins compared to day 2–3 embryo transfers (Behr et al., 2000).

POSTRETRIEVAL HORMONAL MANAGEMENT
- Due to the use of GnRH-as and antagonists, there is concern about diminished progesterone secretion by the corpus luteum. Accordingly, the vast majority of ART cycles use supplemental progesterone via IM progesterone or vaginally administered progesterone. This is typically continued until 9–12 wks of pregnancy.
- Some centers also replace E_2, which is also concomitantly secreted by the corpus luteum.

EMBRYO TRANSFER
- On either day 3 or day 5, the embryos are typically transferred transcervically into the uterine cavity.
- The number of embryos transferred is ultimately based on the patient's age, prior IVF history, egg quality, embryo quality, and the IVF center's success rates. Typically, patients <35 yrs old have two embryos transferred, whereas those >35 yrs old have three embryos transferred.

ASSISTED REPRODUCTIVE TECHNOLOGIES

- ASRM practice committee guidelines on number of embryos transferred:

Parameter	Number	Notes
<35 yrs old	≤2	1 if 1st IVF, good quality of embryos, and excess number of embryos.
35–37 yrs old	≤2 if favorable prognosis ≤3 for all others	
38–40 yrs old	≤4	With consideration for ≤3 if favorable prognosis.
>40 yrs old	≤5	
≥2 prior failed IVF cycles or those with less favorable prognosis		Additional embryos may be transferred after consultation.
Donor egg cycles		Determine number based on age of donor.
Gamete intrafallopian tube transfer (GIFT)		One more oocyte than embryo may be transferred for each category considering potential for lack of fertilization.

IVF, in vitro fertilization.
Source: Adapted from Guidelines on the number of embryos transferred. The Practice Committee of the Society for Assisted Reproductive Technology and the American Society for Reproductive Medicine. *Fertil Steril* 82[Suppl 1]:S1, 2004.

- Embryo transfer is typically performed under ultrasound guidance. A full bladder helps provide acoustic window and decreases the anterior bend of the cervix in patients with an anteverted uterus. This can ease embryo transfer.
- Patients are typically asked to rest for 12–24 hrs after embryo transfer.

ASSISTED REPRODUCTIVE TECHNOLOGIES

RISKS OF *IN VITRO* FERTILIZATION

- **High-order gestations:** This is by far the greatest risk. Multiple pregnancies ultimately depend on the number of embryos transferred. With the transfer of two high-quality embryos in patients <35 yrs of age, twin pregnancy rates range from 20–40%, and triplet rates range from 1–3%.
- **Ectopic pregnancy:** The uterus at the time of embryo transfer contracts from the cervix to the fundus, and embryos placed in the uterine cavity can be pushed into the fallopian tubes. Ectopic pregnancy rates are 1–2% for patients without tubal disease and as high as 5% for patients with tubal disease.
- **Ovarian hyperstimulation syndrome:** This typically affects 3–5% of IVF cycles and can manifest as increasing abdominal distention, accumulation of ascites, nausea, vomiting, hypercoagulability, electrolyte imbalance, and an increased risk for deep venous thrombosis and stroke. <1% of IVF patients require hospitalization for severe ovarian hyperstimulation syndrome.
- **Bleeding** or **infection** from egg retrieval occurs rarely.

Anomalies

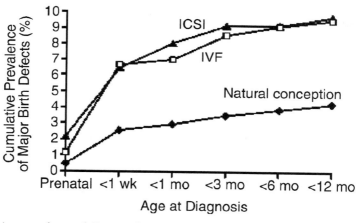

Cumulative prevalence of diagnosed major birth defects (significant differences for musculoskeletal and cardiovascular defects) in singleton infants, according to age at diagnosis (approximately 9% for *in vitro* fertilization [IVF] or IVF/intracytoplasmic sperm injection [ICSI] vs. approximately 4% for non-IVF). (Source: Reproduced with permission from Hansen M, Kurinczuk JJ, et al. The risk of major birth defects after intracytoplasmic sperm injection and in vitro fertilization. *N Engl J Med* 346[10]:725, 2002.)

- A systematic review in 2005 suggests that there is an increased risk of birth defects associated with ART compared with spontaneous conceptions (Hansen et al., 2005).
- Likelihood of low birth weight after IVF or ICSI = 6% (Schieve et al., 2002); nonsignificant difference in gestational carriers
- Likelihood of major defect after IVF or ICSI = 9% vs. 4% for non-IVF (Hansen et al., 2002)

ASSISTED REPRODUCTIVE TECHNOLOGIES

SUCCESS RATES

- Success rates are IVF center–specific and depend on the patient's characteristics, quality of the ovarian stimulation, embryo culture system, and transfer technique. Center-specific pregnancy rates are published by the Centers for Disease Control and Prevention annually and can be found at http://www.cdc.gov/reproductivehealth/art.htm.

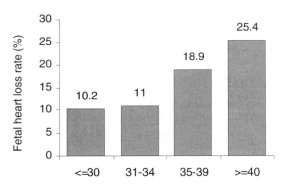

Pregnancy loss by age after documentation of fetal cardiac activity (*in vitro* fertilization, retrospective analysis). (Source: Reproduced with permission from Spandorfer SD, Davis OK, Barmat LI, et al. Relationship between maternal age and aneuploidy in in vitro fertilization pregnancy loss. *Fertil Steril* 81[5]:1265, 2004.)

Terminology

- **Pregnancy rate:** can have many definitions ranging from serum or urine positive for hCG to a live birth
- **Clinical pregnancy rate:** most common reported pregnancy rate from ART centers. This is the percentage of patients with at least one fetus in the uterine cavity with fetal cardiac activity at 7 wks of pregnancy.
- **Live birth rate:** percentage of patients with a live birth from an ART cycle
- **Implantation rate:** This is the chance that each embryo transferred into the uterine cavity will result in a clinical pregnancy (intrauterine pregnancy with

fetal cardiac activity at 7 wks). Calculated by taking the number of clinical pregnancies divided by the number of embryos transferred.

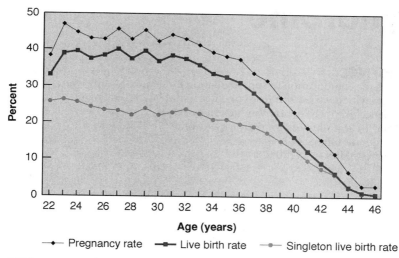

Year 2002 pregnancy, live birth, and singleton live birth rates for assisted reproductive technology cycles using fresh, nondonor eggs. (Source: Reproduced from Centers for Disease Control and Prevention American Society for Reproductive Technology. *2002 Assisted Reproductive Technology Success Rates: National Summary and Fertility Clinic Reports.* Washington, DC: U.S. Department of Health and Human Services, 2004:22.)

23. Ovarian Hyperstimulation Syndrome

INCIDENCE
- Iatrogenic complication of superovulation induction therapy (rarely clomiphene citrate) with a varied spectrum of clinical and laboratory manifestations
- Incidence in superovulation induction cycles:
  - Mild ovarian hyperstimulation syndrome (OHSS) → 33%
  - Moderate OHSS → 3–4%
  - Severe OHSS → 0.1–0.2%
- ↑ Incidence with:
  - Young age
  - More aggressive assisted reproductive technologies
  - Anovulatory women with polycystic ovary syndrome (PCOS)
  - Large numbers of small/medium follicles at time of human chorionic gonadotropin (hCG) administration

OVARIAN HYPERSTIMULATION SYNDROME

CLASSIFICATION

• Clinical, laboratory, and ultrasound findings:

	OHSS Stage		
Grade	Mild	Moderate	Severe
1	Abdominal distention/discomfort.		
2	Features of grade 1 + nausea and vomiting ± diarrhea. Ovaries enlarged to 5–12 cm.		
3		Features of mild OHSS + ultrasound evidence of ascites.	
4			Features of moderate OHSS + clinical evidence of ascites ± hydrothorax or shortness of breath.
5			All of the above + change in blood volume, ↑ blood viscosity due to hemoconcentration, coagulation abnormalities, and diminished renal perfusion and function.

OHSS, ovarian hyperstimulation syndrome.
Source: Data from Golan A, Ron-El R, Herman A, et al. Ovarian hyperstimulation syndrome: an update review. *Obstet Gynecol Surv* 44:430, 1989.

• Symptoms typically start 3–4 days after hCG and peak 7 days after ovulation or follicle aspiration unless patient is pregnant, in which case symptoms persist/worsen.

• Pain is often the first presenting symptom.

OVARIAN HYPERSTIMULATION SYNDROME

PATHOPHYSIOLOGY
- Ovarian enlargement with multiple cysts
- Edema of stroma
- ↑ Capillary permeability (marked arteriolar vasodilation) with acute fluid shift out of intravascular space
  - ↑ Permeability secondary to a *factor* secreted by corpora lutea? *Factors:* Prostaglandins (PGs)? Endothelin-I? Vascular endothelial growth factor? Angiotensin-II?
- Shift of fluid from intravascular space into the abdominal cavity → massive 3rd spacing
- Follicular aspirations may offer partial protection against OHSS.
- Early vs. late form (Papanikolaou et al., 2004):
  - **Early-onset OHSS** is related to exogenous hCG and is associated with a higher risk for preclinical miscarriage; presents 3–7 days after hCG administration.
  - **Late-onset OHSS** is more likely associated with pregnancy and tends to be more severe with a relatively low risk for miscarriage; presents 12–17 days after hCG administration.

HYPERREACTIO LUTEINALIS
- Hyperreactio luteinalis (HL) can mimic OHSS (Foulk et al., 1997).
- HL is the benign hyperplastic luteinization of ovarian theca-interna cells, leading to multicystic ovaries (bilateral) and occasional hyperandrogenism.
- Both may be managed conservatively.
- Comparison features of OHSS and HL:

Ovarian Hyperstimulation Syndrome	Hyperreactio Luteinalis
Ovulation induction	Absence of ovulation induction
1st TM	Anytime during pregnancy (54%, 3rd TM; 16%, 1st TM)
Associated with polycystic ovary syndrome, hypothyroidism	Associated with trophoblastic disease

TM, trimester.

OVARIAN HYPERSTIMULATION SYNDROME

MANAGEMENT

- Conservative management leading to spontaneous resolution with time:
  - 7 days in nonpregnant women
  - 10–20 days in pregnant women
- Have patient drink ≥1 L fluid/day (Gatorade).
- ↓ Physical activity
- Pelvic rest
- Laboratory tests:
  - Electrolytes, creatinine (Cr)
  - Complete blood count (CBC) with platelets (PLTs)
  - Prothrombin time (PT)/partial thromboplastin time (PTT)
- Management scheme:

Classification	Clinical Characteristics/ Biochemical Parameters	Management
A: Mild	Abdominal distention Inconvenience	Accept as inevitable
B: Moderate	A plus: Ascites on sonogram Variable ovarian enlargement	Instruct patient carefully Self-monitoring of body weight Bed rest Abundant fluid intake Frequent follow-up (outpatient basis)
C: Severe	B plus: Massive ascites Hypovolemia	Hospitalization Consider paracentesis IV fluids (crystalloids/plasma expanders/ albumin) Monitoring fluid balance Low-dose heparin prophylaxis Diuretics only when hemodilution achieved Correction of electrolytes
D: Critical	C plus: Hematocrit >55% Impaired renal perfusion Thromboembolism Impending multiorgan failure	C plus: Intensive care unit Continuous monitoring of hemodynamics Perform paracentesis/transvaginal drainage IV heparin/SC heparin Consider termination of pregnancy

Source: Adapted from Beerendonk CC, van Dop PA, Braat DD, et al. Ovarian hyperstimulation syndrome: facts and fallacies. *Obstet Gynecol Surv* 53:439, 1998.

OVARIAN HYPERSTIMULATION SYNDROME

- Hospitalize **if:**
  - **History:** intolerance of food/liquid, severe abdominal pain
  - **Physical examination:**
    - ⇨ Hypotensive blood pressure (BP)
    - ⇨ ↓ Breath sounds
    - ⇨ Tense, distended abdomen
    - ⇨ Peritoneal signs
  - **Blood tests:**
    - ⇨ Hematocrit (Hct) >48% (more than 30% increment over baseline value)
    - ⇨ Na^+ <135 mEq/L
    - ⇨ K^+ >5.0 mEq/L
    - ⇨ Cr >1.2 mg/dL

TREATMENT
Oliguria Management
See algorithm on following page.

OVARIAN HYPERSTIMULATION SYNDROME

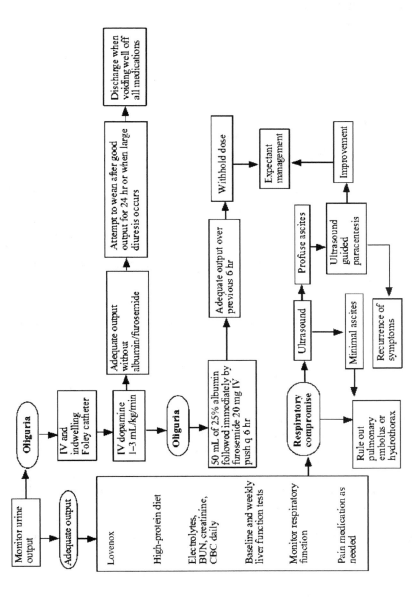

BUN, blood urea nitrogen; CBC, complete blood count. (Source: Adapted from Morris RS, Paulson R. Ovarian hyperstimulation syndrome: classification and management. *Cont Ob/Gyn* Sept: 43, 1994.)

OVARIAN HYPERSTIMULATION SYNDROME

Hospital Management

Admission Orders for Severe Ovarian Hyperstimulation Syndrome

1. Daily weight
2. Strict intake and output (I&O)
3. CBC, PT/PTT, electrolytes, liver function tests (LFTs), and β-human chorionic gonadotropin (β-hCG) on admission and p.r.n.
4. Chest x-ray (CXR) and arterial blood gas (ABG) if short of breath
5. Bed rest with bathroom privileges
6. Enoxaparin (Lovenox) if hemoconcentrated:
   • Prophylaxis: 30 mg SC q12 hrs
   • Treatment: 1 mg/kg SC q12 hrs
7. Regular diet
8. IV fluid dextrose 5% in normal saline solution (D5NS) at 120 mL/hr without added potassium (see below)
9. Continue progesterone for luteal support.
10. Acetaminophen with narcotics as needed; avoid nonsteroidal antiinflammatory drugs (NSAIDs).
11. Paracentesis/transvaginal aspiration for discomfort, shortness of breath (SOB), and/or persistent oliguria
12. If hypovolemic, oliguric (<30 cc/hr), see treatment algorithm on the previous page.

- No pelvic/abdominal examinations secondary to fragility of ovaries (can precipitate ovarian rupture and hemorrhage)
- CXR if SOB ensues
- White blood cell count (WBC) >22,000 is an ominous sign of imminent thromboembolism (Kodama et al., 1995).
- K-exchange resins (i.e., Kayexalate) p.r.n.; no diuretics; electrocardiogram (ECG) p.r.n. for elevated K
- Anticoagulation in severely hemoconcentrated patients
- Transvaginal aspiration of ascites or of follicular structures
- Fluid replacement management (also see treatment algorithm above):
  - **Initial:** 1 L of normal saline (NS) × 1 hr (Lactated Ringer solution [LR] not recommended, as patients with severe OHSS are hyponatremic)
  - **Maintenance:** D5NS at 125–150 mL/hr; assess urinary output (UO) q4 hr
  - **On diuresis:** Restrict oral fluids to 1 L/day and stop IV fluid
- A falling Hct + diuresis is an indication of resolution, not hemorrhage.
- Patient may be given indomethacin, or perhaps captopril or antihistamines.

- Surgery if suspicion of intraperitoneal bleeding (↓ Hct without diuresis) or torsion of ovarian cyst

Thrombosis Prevention in Patients with Severe Ovarian Hyperstimulation Syndrome

- 30 mg Lovenox SC q12 hr (treatment dosage → 1 mg/kg SC q12 hr)
- Thigh-high venous support stockings

Ascites Management

- Consider **indwelling "pig-tail"** catheter for extended drainage.
- Indications for paracentesis:
  - Severe discomfort/pain
  - Pulmonary compromise
  - Evidence of renal compromise unresponsive to fluid management
- Technique:
  1. Empty bladder and identify suprapubic target.
  2. Prep, drape, and inject local anesthetic.
  3. Insert 18–20 gauge Angiocath with 1 $\frac{1}{2}$-in. needle while aspirating until free flow is obtained, then advance catheter and withdraw needle.
  4. Connect Angiocath to evacuated IV bottle and tilt patient forward.

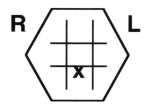

- Alternate management: early intervention with transvaginal aspiration of ascites

OVARIAN HYPERSTIMULATION SYNDROME

COMPLICATIONS

Tension Ascites
- Manifestation of capillary leakage
- Pleural effusions may be associated with tension ascites
- Treatment with paracentesis suggested by some

Thromboembolic Phenomena
- Coagulation abnormalities
- Hemoconcentration $\rightarrow$ arterial thromboemboli

Liver Dysfunction
- Hepatocellular and cholestatic changes

Renal Impairment
- Prerenal failure secondary to $\downarrow$ perfusion from hypovolemia
- Sign of recovery from OHSS = $\uparrow$ urine output
- Renal-dose dopamine after restoration of plasma volume

Acute Respiratory Distress Syndrome
- Due to $\uparrow$ capillary leakage
- Treat with positive end-expiratory pressure respiration

PREVENTION
- Choice of stimulation protocol may help avoid this situation.
- Cancel cycle, withhold hCG.
- Give hCG, aspirate, then cryopreserve all embryos.
  - Aspiration of follicles has a protective effect (decreasing volume of granulosa cells and subsequent vascular endothelial growth factor [VEGF] production for late-onset OHSS but not necessarily for early-onset OHSS)
- Induce ovulation/oocyte maturation with:
  - Minimal effective dose of hCG: 5000 IU and avoid hCG in luteal phase
  - Gonadotropin-releasing hormone (GnRH) agonist (need to support the luteal phase with estradiol, 4 mg/day, and progesterone [micronized progesterone], 200 mg t.i.d.)
    ⇨ Acceptable in cycles without GnRH agonist or in those using GnRH antagonist:
      - ❖ 3 puffs of nafarelin (Synarel) q8 hr, or
      - ❖ 2 injections of 0.5 mg leuprolide SC 8 hrs apart, or
      - ❖ 50 μg intranasal buserelin

OVARIAN HYPERSTIMULATION SYNDROME

- Luteal phase support with progesterone rather than hCG
- Human albumin may prevent severe OHSS in high-risk women (metaanalysis odds ratio, **0.28**; 95% confidence interval [CI], 0.11–0.73); for every **18** women at risk of severe OHSS, albumin infusion **prevents one** more case (Aboulghar et al., 2002).
  - ⇨ 50 g IV albumin just before or immediately after oocyte retrieval

24. Hyperemesis in Pregnancy

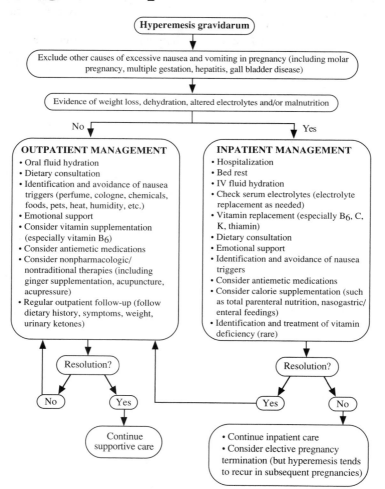

Hyperemesis gravidarum

↓

Exclude other causes of excessive nausea and vomiting in pregnancy (including molar pregnancy, multiple gestation, hepatitis, gall bladder disease)

↓

Evidence of weight loss, dehydration, altered electrolytes and/or malnutrition

No ↓   ↓ Yes

OUTPATIENT MANAGEMENT
- Oral fluid hydration
- Dietary consultation
- Identification and avoidance of nausea triggers (perfume, cologne, chemicals, foods, pets, heat, humidity, etc.)
- Emotional support
- Consider vitamin supplementation (especially vitamin B$_6$)
- Consider antiemetic medications
- Consider nonpharmacologic/nontraditional therapies (including ginger supplementation, acupuncture, acupressure)
- Regular outpatient follow-up (follow dietary history, symptoms, weight, urinary ketones)

INPATIENT MANAGEMENT
- Hospitalization
- Bed rest
- IV fluid hydration
- Check serum electrolytes (electrolyte replacement as needed)
- Vitamin replacement (especially B$_6$, C, K, thiamin)
- Dietary consultation
- Emotional support
- Identification and avoidance of nausea triggers
- Consider antiemetic medications
- Consider calorie supplementation (such as total parenteral nutrition, nasogastric/enteral feedings)
- Identification and treatment of vitamin deficiency (rare)

Resolution?   Resolution?

No   Yes   Yes   No

Continue supportive care

- Continue inpatient care
- Consider elective pregnancy termination (but hyperemesis tends to recur in subsequent pregnancies)

Source: Adapted from Erick M. Hyperemesis gravidarum: a practical management strategy. *OBG Management*, November 2000, 25–35. Reproduced with permission of Dr. Errol Norwitz, Department of Obstetrics, Gynecology and Reproductive Sciences, Yale School of Medicine, New Haven, Connecticut.

Therapy	Route of Administration/Dose	Efficacy	Comments
Antiemetics			
Metoclopramide (Reglan)	PO (10–30 mg q.i.d.) IM/IV (10 mg q4–6 hr)	Effective	Concern over possible teratogenic effects not well founded in humans, often given with hydroxyzine (Atarax), 25–50 mg q4–6 hr.
Ondansetron (Zofran)	PO (4–8 mg q4–8 hr) IV (8 mg q4–8 hr)	Probably effective	A serotonin receptor antagonist, common side effects include mild sedation and headache.
Droperidol (Inapsine)	IV/IM (2.5 mg q3–6 hr) IV continuous infusion (1.0–2.5 mg/hr)	Probably effective	No known teratogenicity.
Phenothiazines/antipsychotics			
Promethazine (Phenergan)	PO/PR/IM (12.5–50.0 mg q4–6 hr)	Effective	No known teratogenicity, may cause extrapyramidal (parkinsonian) side effects, hypertension, sedation.
Prochlorperazine (Compazine)	PO/IV/IM (5–10 mg q4–6 hr) PR (25 mg q12 hr)	Probably effective	No known teratogenicity.
Chlorpromazine (Thorazine)	PO/IM (10–50 mg q6–8 hr)	Probably effective	No known teratogenicity.
Antihistamines			
Doxylamine succinate (Unisom)	PO (12.5–25.0 mg daily)	Probably effective	No known teratogenicity.
Doxylamine succinate 10 mg + pyridoxine 10 mg (Bendectin)	PO (1–2 tablets q6–8 hr)	Effective	Initial concern over teratogenic effects not well founded in humans.

255

HYPEREMESIS IN PREGNANCY

Therapy	Route of Administration/Dose	Efficacy	Comments
Meclizine (Antivert)	PO (25–100 mg daily)	Possibly effective	No known teratogenicity.
Chlorpheniramine (Chlor-Trimeton)	PO (8–12 mg daily)	Possibly effective	No known teratogenicity.
Diphenhydramine (Benadryl)	PO/IM/IV (50–75 mg q4–6 hr)	Possibly effective	No known teratogenicity.
Trimethobenzamide (Tigan)	PO (250 mg t.i.d./q.i.d.) PR/IM (200 mg q6–8 hr)	Possibly effective	No known teratogenicity.

Source: Adapted from Erick M. Hyperemesis gravidarum: a practical management strategy. *OBG Management*, November 2000: 25–35. Reproduced with permission of Dr. Errol Norwitz, Department of Obstetrics, Gynecology, and Reproductive Sciences, Yale School of Medicine, New Haven, Connecticut.

25. Gamete Preservation

FEMALE GAMETE PRESERVATION
Indications
- Cancer (chemotherapy, radiotherapy, radical surgery)
- Collagen vascular disease (chemotherapy, radiotherapy)
- Endometriosis (oophorectomy)
- Hematologic disease (chemotherapy, radiotherapy)

Premature Ovarian Failure/Gonadotoxicity
- Potential sequela of chemotherapy (e.g., cyclophosphamide) or radiotherapy
- Manifested as hypergonadotropic hypogonadism ($\uparrow$ follicle-stimulating hormone [FSH] and luteinizing hormone [LH], $\downarrow$ estradiol) → amenorrhea → ovarian dysfunction and infertility
- Risk of premature ovarian failure (POF) increases with age and cumulative dosage of chemotherapy.
- Gonadotropin-releasing hormone (GnRH) antagonists: No protection from cyclophosphamide in mice, and, in fact, GnRH antagonists depleted primordial follicles in this murine model (Danforth et al., 2003).

Options for Female Gamete Preservation
Oral Contraceptives (Slater et al., 1999)
- **Possible** protective effect on fertility
- Avoid in patients with systemic lupus erythematosus + antiphospholipid antibodies and others with high risk for hypercoagulability.

Gonadotropin-Releasing Hormone Agonists
- Administered to down-regulate hypothalamic-pituitary-ovarian (HPO) axis to $\downarrow$ susceptibility to gonadotoxicity
- Possible mechanism(s):
  - GnRH receptors (ovarian cancer cells) mediate antiproliferative effects (Volker et al., 2002).
  - $\downarrow$ Gonadotropin concentrations
  - $\downarrow$ Ovarian perfusion due to hypoestrogenic milieu
  - Antiapoptotic effect mediated by sphingosine-1-phosphate
  - Germline stem cell preservation
- Study of young women with lymphoma receiving chemotherapy (Blumenfeld et al., 1996):
  - **GnRH agonist + chemotherapy group:** 94% with spontaneous ovulation and menses within 3–8 mos of completing treatment
  - **Chemotherapy-only group:** 61% with POF

GAMETE PRESERVATION

Dosage

University of Michigan (Slater et al., 1999):
> Leuprolide (Lupron Depot), 3.75 mg IM, given 10 days before cyclophosphamide (when this is not done before 1st pulse, start Lupron between 1st and 2nd pulses; give for 6 mos when considering change from cyclophosphamide to azathioprine); possible estrogen supplement after 1–2 mos

Brigham & Women's (Slater et al., 1999):
> Lupron Depot, 11.25 mg IM, every 3 mos × 2, with 1st dose given 3–4 wks before chemotherapy
>
> Lupron Depot, 7.5 mg IM, 1 mo before and on day of pulse chemotherapy (may give Lupron Depot closer to 1st chemotherapy dose if necessary)
>
> Recommend pretreatment bone mineral density (dual-energy x-ray absorptiometry [DXA])
>
> Repeat DXA if patient is on GnRH agonist >6 mos

In Vitro Fertilization Cycle to Cryopreserve Embryos before Potentially Gonadotoxic Treatment

- Viable option for reproductive-aged woman and partner
- May delay treatment for disease to complete ovulation/stimulation protocol
- Not acceptable for single woman who declines use of donor sperm
- Not acceptable for pediatric patients

Oocyte Cryopreservation

- After thaw and *in vitro* fertilization (IVF)/intracytoplasmic sperm injection (ICSI), pregnancies and live births reported (Falcone et al., 2004), but fecundability not high enough for routine clinical use.
- Consider for single, adult women, provided that they are counseled regarding:
  - Low pregnancy rates
  - Time needed for ovulation stimulation
  - Institutional review board (IRB) approval recommended

Ovarian Tissue Cryopreservation and Transplantation

- Area of extensive research with great potential
- Future applications include patients with cancer and those who decline donor oocytes.
- Concern for reintroduction of cancerous cells
- Advancements are being made (Oktay et al., 2004).
- One study reported a liveborn after orthotopic autotransplantation of cryopreserved ovarian tissue. This may be the first such liveborn (Donnez et al., 2004).

258

MALE GAMETE PRESERVATION

Indications

- Chemotherapy
- Radiotherapy
- Retroperitoneal surgery
- Postmortem

Options

Cryopreservation of Sperm/Testicular Tissue

- Avoids need for repeat biopsies/aspiration in azoospermic men who have undergone testicular sperm extraction or percutaneous epididymal sperm aspiration
- The patient may father his own child via IVF/ICSI.
- Required for donor-insemination programs as cryopreservation allows for infectious disease screening (i.e., human immunodeficiency virus [HIV], hepatitis B) (Donnelly et al., 2001).

Cryopreservation of Embryos

- Viable option for reproductive-aged male and partner
- May delay treatment of disease to perform complete cycle of IVF.

26. Luteal Phase Deficiency

DEFINITION
- Classic definition: >2-day lag in endometrial histologic development (Noyes criteria [Noyes et al., 1950] although recently updated as shown in figure below [Murray et al., 2004]) and day of cycle. If found in **two consecutive** cycles, then considered a possible cause of infertility.

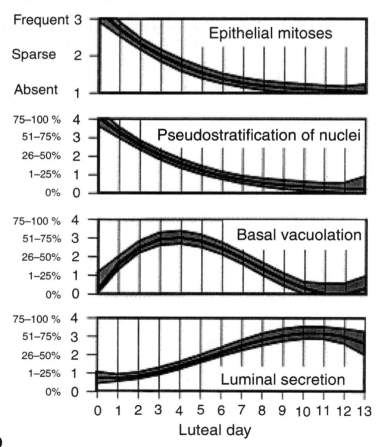

LUTEAL PHASE DEFICIENCY

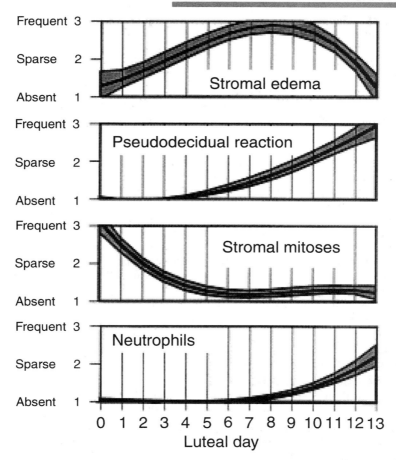

Source: Adapted from Murray MJ, Meyer WR, et al. A critical analysis of the accuracy, reproducibility, and clinical utility of histologic endometrial dating in fertile women. *Fertil Steril* 81(5):1333, 2004.

- However, it is no longer recommended to obtain endometrial biopsies, because histologic endometrial dating is neither accurate nor precise (Murray et al., 2004; Coutifaris et al., 2004).

261

LUTEAL PHASE DEFICIENCY

INCIDENCE
- 30% of isolated cycles in fertile women; 30–40% of infertile women

ETIOLOGY
- Plausible etiologies:
  - ↓ Hormone production by corpus luteum
  - ↓ Follicle-stimulating hormone (FSH) in follicular phase (FSH stimulates granulosa cell proliferation and luteinizing hormone [LH] receptors on granulosa cells)
  - Abnormal patterns of LH secretion
  - ↓ Levels of LH and FSH at the time of ovulatory surge
  - ↓ Response of the endometrium to pregnancy
  - Hyperprolactinemia leading to abnormal gonadotropin-releasing hormone (GnRH) pulsatility
- Consider search for luteal phase deficiency (LPD) if:
  - Normal cycles and unexplained infertility
  - >35 yrs old
  - Short luteal phases (<**13 days** from positive LH peak to menses)
  - History of recurrent losses (28% associated with LPD) (Vanrell and Balasch, 1986)
- LPD occurs in approximately 1/3 of rhesus monkeys after aspiration of preovulatory follicles (Kreitmann et al., 1981).

DIAGNOSIS
- No definitive diagnostic approach presently exists.

Luteal Phase Duration
- Short luteal phase duration (<13 days) as defined by the interval from midcycle LH surge to the onset of menses may define LPD.

Mid-Luteal Phase Progesterone Level and Endometrial Biopsy?

Progesterone Level
- Insufficient evidence, because the level is subject to variation associated with pulsatile LH secretion and poor correlation with histologic stage of endometrium (i.e., endometrial inadequacy can be found in the presence of normal progesterone [P_4] levels)
  - Pulsatile, mid-luteal P_4 is higher in the a.m. (Syrop and Hammond, 1987).
  - Historically, a P_4 level <10 ng/mL (32 nmol/L) or the sum of three serum P_4 levels that is <30 ng/mL (Jordan et al., 1994) 7 days before menses → LPD.

- Argument for measuring P_4 8 days after a positive LH-kit change: Mid–luteal phase P_4 <9.4 ng/mL is associated with a lower pregnancy rate (Hull et al., 1982).
- Argument for mid-luteal P_4 supplementation: LPD successfully treated if P_4 <6.6 ng/mL (receiver operator curve) (Daya et al., 1988)

Endometrial Biopsy
- Timed endometrial biopsy with histologic dating provides no clinically useful information as a subfertility screening test:
  - Out-of-phase biopsy results poorly discriminated between women from fertile and subfertile couples (in either mid-luteal or late luteal phase) (Coutifaris et al., 2004).
  - Out-of-phase biopsy found in approximately 20–30% of normal cycles
  - Randomized, observational study concluded that there is poor accuracy and reproducibility in histologic endometrial dating (Murray et al., 2004).
  - Historically performed 1–2 days before menses, with dating reference being the **subsequent** menses.

TREATMENT
- Treat after checking prolactin (PRL) and thyroid-stimulating hormone (TSH).
- Aromatase inhibitor: letrozole (Femara) 5 mg days 3–7 (or 20 mg single dose on day 3 [Mitwally and Casper, 2005]), ultrasound day 14, human chorionic gonadotropin (hCG) booster and intrauterine insemination depending on semen analysis
- Clomiphene citrate (CC):
  - 50 mg q.d. × 5 days beginning on day 3, 4, or 5 of cycle
  - Drawbacks:
    - ⇨ 10% chance of multiple gestation
    - ⇨ Occasional hot flashes
    - ⇨ Occasional severe mood changes
    - ⇨ Rare visual changes (*palinopsia* = prolonged afterimages or shimmering of the peripheral field) that may be irreversible (Purvin, 1995)
    - ⇨ Potential for inducing LPD (Manners, 1990), although this may just reflect underlying anovulation (Hecht et al., 1990)
- FSH: risk of ovarian hyperstimulation → multiple births
- Progesterone:
  - 25-mg P_4 suppositories b.i.d., Crinone 8% every evening, or Prometrium, 100 mg b.i.d. per vagina starting 3 days after ovulation (i.e., after 3 days of temperature rise >97.8°F); treatment is maintained until menses, or if pregnant, continue until 12th wk, although literature support is weak for use past 9 wks (Csapo and Pulkkinen, 1978).

LUTEAL PHASE DEFICIENCY

- Drawback: can prolong the luteal phase and thus delay menses (causes patient frustration!)
- No difference in outcome between CC vs. P_4 treatment of LPD (Huang, 1986; Murray et al., 1989)

LUTEAL PHASE SUPPORT IN *IN VITRO* FERTILIZATION CYCLES

- Need may reflect:
  - GnRH agonist down-regulation
  - Removal of granulosa cells with oocyte retrieval/poor corpus luteum function

Regimens

- hCG: 2500 IU IM 4 days after embryo transfer, then every 4 days
- P_4: (treat through luteal-placental shift)
  - Oral: micronized 300–800 mg/day
  - Vaginal: micronized P_4, 200 mg t.i.d.; suppositories, 10–600 mg/day; Crinone, 90 mg/day
  - IM: P_4 in oil, 50–100 mg/day; 17α-hydroxyprogesterone caproate, 341 mg q3d
- Recent metaanalysis: IM hCG and IM P_4 better than no treatment; IM P_4 better than oral and vaginal P_4 (Pritts, 2002)
- The addition of oral **estrogen** (estradiol, 2–6 mg PO/day) to luteal support regimens may improve the implantation rate, but it has not been shown to improve the clinical pregnancy rate (Pritts, 2002)
- hCG booster is associated with ↑ incidence of ovarian hyperstimulation syndrome.

27. Hyperprolactinemia and Galactorrhea

DEFINITION
- Consistently elevated fasting serum prolactin (PRL >20 ng/mL) in the absence of pregnancy or postpartum lactation; nonpuerperal lactation

PROLACTIN
- Little PRL = polypeptide hormone of 198 amino acids, but there are several different circulating forms:

Name	Molecular Weight	Biologically Active	Immunologically Active
Little PRL	22 kd	Yes	Yes
Glycosylated little PRL	25 kd	Yes, but decreased	No
Big PRL	50 kd	No	Yes
Big-big PRL	>100 kd	No	Yes

PRL, prolactin.

- Big and big-big forms have lower receptor-binding properties; normal fertility can be present with hyperprolactinemia due primarily to big-big PRL; however, circulating big PRL can be converted to little PRL by disulfide bond reduction.
- Synthesized and stored in the pituitary gland in lactotrophs (also synthesized in decidua and endometrium, although not under dopaminergic control)
- Mean levels of 8 ng/dL in adult women; $t_{1/2}$ = 20 mins
- Cleared by the liver and kidney (hence ↑ PRL with renal failure)
- Functions:
  - Mammogenic → stimulates growth of the mammary tissue
  - Lactogenic → stimulates mammary tissue to produce and secrete milk

PHYSIOLOGY
- Synthesis and release controlled by central nervous system (CNS) neurotransmitters (usually inhibitory)
- Dopamine (DA; PRL-inhibiting factor) and cannabinoids inhibit secretion through D_2 DA receptors (DA-Rs) on lactotrophs (Pagotto et al., 2001).
- PRL-releasing peptide (PrRP), thyrotropin-releasing factor, and estrogen stimulate release (Rubinek et al., 2001).

HYPERPROLACTINEMIA AND GALACTORRHEA

- Follicle-stimulating hormone (FSH) may be suppressed by ↑ PRL through gonadotropin-releasing hormone (GnRH) suppression.
- Episodic secretion varying throughout the day and cycle (↑ PRL at time of luteinizing hormone [LH] surge) (Djahanbakhch et al., 1984)
- No clinically relevant changes over the menstrual cycle, although there is a significant albeit subtle midcycle peak in PRL (Fujimoto et al., 1990).
- Hypertrophy and hyperplasia of lactotrophs in pregnancy in response to ↑ estrogen
- PRL:
  - Steadily ↑ during pregnancy, reaching 200 ng/mL in the 3rd trimester (TM)
  - Return to normal in nonlactating women 2–3 wks postpartum
  - Return to normal in lactating women 6 mos postpartum
  - ↑ With breast stimulation, exercise, sleep, stress

PREVALENCE OF INCREASED PROLACTIN WITH THE FOLLOWING SIGNS AND SYMPTOMS

Sign/Symptom	↑ Prolactin (%)
Anovulation	15
Amenorrhea	15
Galactorrhea	30
Amenorrhea + galactorrhea	75
Infertility	34

Source: Adapted from Molitch ME, Reichlin S. Hyperprolactinemic disorders. *Dis Mon* 28(9):1, 1982.

- ↑ PRL induces a dose-dependent ↑ DA secretion, which in turn inhibits GnRH pulsatile release through the D_1 receptor on GnRH neurons and by the activation of the β-endorphin neuronal system that further inhibits GnRH release (Seki et al., 1986).
- Autopsy: pituitary adenomas in 27% of women (Burrow et al., 1981) (**PRL-secreting** incidence in autopsies: 11%)

ETIOLOGY
Pituitary Causes
Prolactinoma (Most Common)
- Even with normal values or only mildly elevated PRL, patient may have a large tumor.
- Arise most commonly from the lateral wings of the anterior pituitary

HYPERPROLACTINEMIA AND GALACTORRHEA

- Islands of pituitary lactotrophs may be released from the normal tonic inhibitory effect of DA through spontaneous or estradiol (E_2)-dependent generation of arteriolar shunts (Elias and Weiner, 1984).
- Found in 10% of general population (most asymptomatic)
- **Found in 50% of women with hyperprolactinemia**
- Incidence increases with (a) increasing PRL levels and (b) severity of symptoms.
- Microadenoma <1 cm
  - Prevalence of up to 27% in autopsy series (Burrow et al., 1981)
  - Enlargement uncommon (≤5%) (Schlechte et al., 1989)
  - Most regress spontaneously.
- Macroadenoma >1 cm and usually PRL >200 ng/mL
  - Prevalence unknown
- The risk of diminished secretion of other pituitary hormones due to the presence of a prolactinoma is based on their proximity to the prolactinoma mass and their overall cell number: mnemonic for the adenohypophyseal hormones with the greatest to least propensity to be affected → **GnTAG** (% relates to the number of cells):
  - Gonadotropins (Gns) (5%, close to lactotrophs), thyroid-stimulating hormone (TSH) (5%), adrenocorticotropic hormone (ACTH) (20%), growth hormone (GH) (50%), antidiuretic hormone (ADH) (rare, posterior pituitary)

Acromegaly
- GH-secreting pituitary adenoma
- Associated symptoms: macrognathia, spread teeth, sweaty palms, carpal tunnel syndrome
- Affected patients experience symptoms of the disease ~7 yrs before diagnosis.
- GH can bind to PRL receptors (but PRL does not bind to GH receptors).
- ~20% of GH-secreting pituitary adenomas secrete PRL.
- Check serum insulin-like growth factor-I (IGF-I) (need age-adjusted and sex-adjusted IGF-I levels) as GH-secreting pituitary adenomas may not be visible on magnetic resonance imaging (MRI).
- Diagnosis: Elevated basal fasting GH and IGF-I; 1-hr glucose (100 mg) challenge test does not lead to GH levels <2 ng/mL in patients with acromegaly.
- Currently, surgery is the 1st choice for acromegaly.

Cushing Disease
- Diagnosis: elevated 24-hr urinary free cortisol excretion and abnormal cortisol suppressibility to low-dose dexamethasone
- Adenoma secretes ACTH. ↑ Supraclavicular/posterior dorsal fat.
- Patients present with hirsutism, coarse facial features, arthritis, and ↑supraclavicular/posterior dorsal fat
- 10% secrete PRL.

HYPERPROLACTINEMIA AND GALACTORRHEA

Other Pituitary Tumors
- Clinically nonfunctioning pituitary tumor (most are classified as gonadotrophic tumors; PRL usually ↓ with DA-agonist treatment), lymphocytic hypophysitis, craniopharyngioma, Rathke's cleft cyst, TSH-pituitary adenoma (rarest)

Lactotroph Hyperplasia
- 8% of pituitary glands at autopsy
- Can only be distinguished from microadenoma by surgery
- Follistatin is a specific marker.

Empty Sella Syndrome
- Congenital or acquired defect in the sella diaphragm
- Intrasellar extension of the subarachnoid space results in compression of the pituitary gland and an enlarged sella turcica.
- 5–10% have hyperprolactinemia (usually <100 ng/mL).
- Diagnose with MRI.
- Benign course, although headaches (mostly localized anteriorly) are a frequent symptom (Catarci et al., 1994).

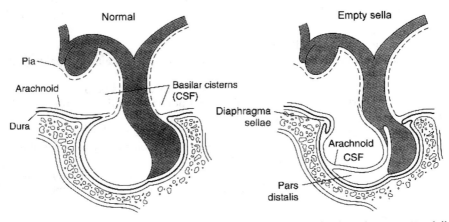

CSF, cerebrospinal fluid. (Source: Reproduced with permission from Jordan RM, Kendall JW, Kerber CW. The primary empty sella syndrome: analysis of the clinical characteristics, radiographic features, pituitary function and cerebrospinal fluid adenohypophysial hormone concentrations. *Am J Med* 62[4]:569, 1977.)

Hypothalamic Disease
- Alters normal portal circulation of DA

HYPERPROLACTINEMIA AND GALACTORRHEA

- Craniopharyngioma (most common)
- Infiltration of hypothalamus by sarcoidosis, histiocytosis, leukemia, carcinoma

Pharmacologic Agents

- Interfere with DA production, action, uptake, or receptor binding
- PRL levels range from 25–100 ng/mL.
- Return to normal level within days after the cessation of the offending drug (Rivera et al., 1976)
- Examples:
  - Neuroleptics (phenothiazines, haloperidol)
  - Antidepressants (selective serotonin reuptake inhibitors, not tricyclics)
  - Opiates
  - Antihypertensives (α-methyldopa, reserpine, verapamil)
  - Metoclopramide (a DA-R blocker)
  - H-2 blockers (intravenous cimetidine)

Hypothyroidism

- Found in 3–5% of patients with hyperprolactinemia; 20–30% of patients with primary hypothyroidism have ↑PRL.
- Galactorrhea secondary to ↑ thyroid-releasing hormone (TRH) → ↑ PRL
- Primary hypothyroidism: ↓ thyroxine (T_4) → ↑ TRH → pituitary → ↑ TSH and ↑ PRL
- Secondary hypothyroidism (from a pituitary tumor): normal TSH! Therefore, need to check T_4.

Chronic Renal Disease

- ↓ PRL clearance and ↑ production rate

Chronic Breast Nerve Stimulation

- Status post–thoracic surgery, herpes zoster, chest trauma

Stress

Idiopathic Hyperprolactinemia

- PRL levels later return to normal in $1/3$.
- Unchanged PRL levels in nearly $1/2$
- 10% have radiographic evidence of a pituitary tumor during a 6-yr follow-up (Sluijmer and Lappohn, 1992).

DIAGNOSTIC TECHNIQUES

Magnetic Resonance Imaging with Gadolinium Enhancement

- Preferred technique with resolution to 1 mm
- Accurate soft-tissue imagery without radiation exposure

HYPERPROLACTINEMIA AND GALACTORRHEA

DIAGNOSTIC EVALUATION

Fasting a.m. laboratory tests: **PRL, IGF-I, T$_4$, TSH**
IGF-I obtained because 25% of acromegalics secrete ↑ PRL.
T$_4$ obtained to rule out *other* pituitary tumor leading to low-normal TSH and low T$_4$.

Cortisol, LH, FSH, α-subunit, if hyperprolactinemia and no response to medication, especially in cases with hypertension

Routine breast examination does not acutely alter serum PRL levels in normal women (Hammond et al., 1996).

If PRL values are <200 ng/mL, and a macroadenoma (>10 mm) is seen on MRI, it is most likely **not** a prolactinoma (probably gonadotrope tumor or nonsecretory).

MANAGEMENT

- Microadenoma or functional hyperprolactinemia: risk of progression for PRL-secreting tumors to macroadenomas is <5% (Weiss et al., 1983).
- Macroadenomas should be treated no matter the severity of symptoms.
- Without treatment of microadenomas, there is a 24% chance of PRL normalization within 5 yrs, and 95% do not grow (Schlechte et al., 1989).
- Management scheme:

Low E$_2$ (<40 pg/mL)
Estrogen treatment or oral contraceptives (OCs) (no ↑ size of microadenoma or ↑ [serum PRL]) to prevent osteopenia/osteoporosis
Yearly PRL levels

Normal E$_2$
Normal cycles
Yearly PRL levels

Oligomenorrhea or amenorrhea and E$_2$ >40 pg/mL
Progestin withdrawal or OCs
Yearly PRL levels

TREATMENT ENDPOINTS (EFFECTS OF MEDICAL THERAPY)

- Bromocriptine (Parlodel) or cabergoline is used to achieve desired fertility (80% restored), relieve intolerable galactorrhea (60% eradicated), and reduce mass effect (reduced tumor size in 80–90%).

HYPERPROLACTINEMIA AND GALACTORRHEA

DRUGS

- **Bromocriptine** or **cabergoline** (DA-R agonists):
  - Impair PRL synthesis and release
  - DA agonists do not restore bone mass to clinically meaningful degree (Colao et al., 2000).
  - Discontinue once pregnancy is achieved and restart if symptoms develop (no evidence of teratogenicity).
  - Discontinue after 2 yrs of therapy for galactorrhea to assess for remission (11% after 1 yr, 22% after 2 yrs) (Ciccarelli and Camanni, 1996).
  - Measure PRL 4–6 wks later.
  - Long-term treatment usually necessary for large tumors:
  - Does not lead to pituitary insufficiency (including diabetes insipidus [DI]) like surgical or radiation treatment
  - Response occurs in 6 wks in 2/3 and can take up to 6 mos in 1/3.
  - **Bromocriptine: 1.25 mg b.i.d.–t.i.d.**
    - ⇨ Side effects: syncope, mood changes, nausea and vomiting (N/V), nasal congestion; efforts to minimize include:
      - ❖ Begin with 1.25 mg q.h.s. only, then gradually increase dose, maximum of 10 mg/day; repeat **serum PRL after 1 mo of treatment.**
      - ❖ **No need to repeat MRI if *micro*adenoma and ↓ PRL; if *macro*adenoma, regardless of PRL, repeat MRI after 3 mos of treatment.**
      - ❖ Take medicine in the middle of a bulk meal.
      - ❖ 2.5 mg **per vagina** q.d. (fewer side effects) (Jasonni et al., 1991)
    - ⇨ Depot form (q month injection) not yet available
    - ⇨ Follow PRL every 6–12 mos once stabilized—no need to repeat MRI scans; visual field testing is more sensitive than MRI for detecting tumor shrinkage.
  - **Cabergoline:**
    - ⇨ Start at 0.25 mg 2× a week, ↑ to **0.5 mg once a week;** maximum: 1 mg 2× a week
    - ⇨ More specific D_2 agonist; approximately 1/2 of those who do not respond to bromocriptine respond to cabergoline (Verhelst et al., 1999).
    - ⇨ Far fewer side effects than bromocriptine but costly (0.5 mg, 8 tabs = $218 vs. Parlodel, 2.5 mg, 30 tabs = $65)
    - ⇨ Higher rate of restoration of ovulation than bromocriptine with similar rate of tumor size reduction and better tolerance
- Follow-up after cabergoline withdrawal (Colao et al., 2003):
  - 2–5 yrs after normalization of hyperprolactinemia:
    - ⇨ ↑ PRL in 24% of nontumoral hyperprolactinemia
    - ⇨ ↑ PRL in 31% with microadenomas
    - ⇨ ↑ PRL in 36% with macroadenomas
    - ⇨ 22% showed gonadal dysfunction.

HYPERPROLACTINEMIA AND GALACTORRHEA

⇨ 0% renewed tumor growth
⇨ Rate for recurrence of hyperprolactinemia was **19% for each mm increment** in the maximal tumor diameter.
⇨ Taper cabergoline from 0.25 mg twice a week to 0.25 mg once a week and then to 0.25 mg every other week before discontinuation.

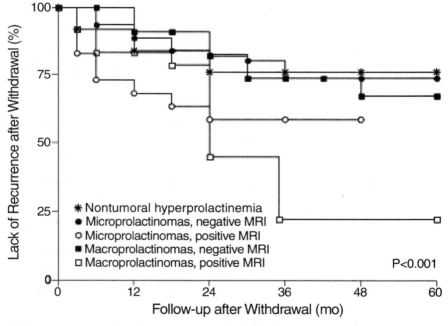

MRI, magnetic resonance imaging. (Source: Adapted from Colao A, Di Sarno A, Cappabianca P, et al. Withdrawal of long-term cabergoline therapy for tumoral and nontumoral hyperprolactinemia. *N Engl J Med* 349[21]:2023, 2003.)

Pregnancy and Prolactinomas

• 70% increase in pituitary size during pregnancy
• Risk of symptomatic tumor enlargement during pregnancy (Molitch, 1985):

Microadenoma: 1.6%
Macroadenoma: 15.5%; check visual-field testing, a.m. cortisol, and TSH every trimester.

HYPERPROLACTINEMIA AND GALACTORRHEA

Operative Approach

Transsphenoidal Microsurgical Resection

- Mortality: <0.5%
- Pituitary insufficiency rate of 19%
- Temporary DI, 10–40%; permanent DI, <2%
- 3.9% glucocorticoid replacement therapy (Feigenbaum et al., 1996)
- 3% chronic sinusitis; 2% septal defect (i.e., epistaxis) (Feigenbaum et al., 1996)
- Initial cure rate (Amar et al., 2002):
  - Microadenoma: 65–91%
  - Macroadenoma: 20–40%
- Effect on reproductive function (those actively attempting postoperatively):
  - 6 mos: 82% pregnancy rate
  - 12 mos: 88% pregnancy rate
- Better prognosis: PRL <100 ng/mL
- Poor prognosis: PRL >200 ng/mL, >26 yrs old, amenorrhea >6 mos
- Cure rates based on pre- and postoperative PRL levels (Feigenbaum et al., 1996):
  - Preoperative levels <100 ng/mL: 69% cure rate
  - Preoperative levels <200 ng/mL: 60% cure rate
  - Immediate postoperative levels <5 ng/mL: 84% cure rate
  - Immediate postoperative levels <20 ng/mL: 74% cure rate
- Recommended after failure of medical treatment (i.e., cabergoline) or if patient is intolerant of side effects
- Transsphenoidal approach provides a decompression of the bony confines of the sella turcica, so that recurrence of the tumor tends to follow the path of least resistance into the sphenoid sinus rather than the intracranial compartment.

Radiation Therapy

- Cobalt, proton beam, heavy particle therapy, or brachytherapy
- Inconsistent results and takes years to ↓ tumor
- Delay in symptom resolution
- Only used in adjunctive management with surgery for large tumors

Other Possible Therapies

- **Gamma knife:** inconclusive data but may be preferred over conventional radiation treatment for patients not responding to DA with residual tumor after surgery

HYPERPROLACTINEMIA AND GALACTORRHEA

NOTES

- Oral contraceptives are safe in women with hyperprolactinemia, but they do not normalize bone density (they can prevent progressive bone loss) (Corenblum and Donovan, 1993).
- Prospective data suggest that higher PRL levels are associated with an ↑ risk of breast cancer in postmenopausal women (Hankinson et al., 1999).
- Osteoporosis: ↓ bone mineral density in women with hyperprolactinemia; although bone density may ↑ when prolactin levels are normalized, it typically remains subnormal, continuing the risk of vertebral and hip fractures.
- Hirsutism: PRL receptors have been found on the human adrenal gland, thereby influencing the secretion of androgens (Glasow et al., 1996).

A. Clinically Nonfunctional Pituitary Mass

- Hormonal assessment to rule out:
  - Pituitary hormone excess from clinically silent adenoma
  - Pituitary hormone deficiency attributable to a pituitary tumor/infiltrative disease with mass effects

Axis	Hypersecretion Assessment	Reserve Assessment
Somatotropic	100 mg oral glucose tolerance test suppression testing	GH level does not decrease to <2 ng/mL if there is a GH-producing adenoma.
PRL	a.m. PRL (normal range, 1.4–24.2 ng/mL)	TRH stimulation test → PRL should ↑ 2× 15–30 mins after TRH.
Gonadotropic	LH, FSH, E_2, free α-subunit	E_2 should be >30 pg/mL; gonadotropin-releasing hormone agonist (100 μg) → LH, FSH.
Corticotropic	Low-dose dexamethasone test (normal if cortisol <1.8 μg/dL)	Metyrapone test (normal if 11-deoxycortisol >10 μg/L).
Thyrotropic	Free T_4, free T_3, TSH	Free T_4, free T_3, TSH; TRH stimulation test.

E_2, estradiol; FSH, follicle-stimulating hormone; GH, growth hormone; LH, luteinizing hormone; PRL, prolactin; T_3, triiodothyronine; T_4, thyroxine; TRH, thyroid-releasing hormone; TSH, thyroid-stimulating hormone.

28. Hypothyroidism

PREVALENCE
- ↑ Thyroid-stimulating hormone (TSH) is found in >7% of all adult women (21% if >74 yrs old).

THYROID FUNCTION
- Most of the released hormone is thyroxine (T_4), which is then peripherally converted to triiodothyronine (T_3).
- T_3 is more biologically active than T_4.

SIGNS AND SYMPTOMS
- Fatigue
- Menstrual cramps
- Weakness
- Myalgia
- Weight gain
- Constipation
- Coarse or dry hair
- Depression
- Dry or rough skin
- Irritability
- Hair loss
- Memory loss
- Cold intolerance
- Abnormal menses
- Deepened voice
- ↓ Libido

- Primary thyroid failure → menometrorrhagia; hyperthyroidism → oligomenorrhea
- Pituitary failure → amenorrhea and loss of pubic hair

DEFINITIONS
- Subclinical hypothyroidism: asymptomatic; normal T_4,T_3 but ↑ TSH ± thyroid antibodies (Abs); incidence, 4–10% of the general population
- Progression to overt hypothyroidism is dependent on the magnitude of TSH and antithyroid Ab titers.
- **Antithyroperoxidase Abs** (APA) = antimicrosomal Abs (AMA)
- Antithyroglobulin Abs (Vanderpump et al., 1995) (<1:1600 titer → no progression seen)

	Odds Ratio to Develop Overt Hypothyroidism over 20 Yrs
↑ TSH, no Abs	8
Normal TSH, ↑ Abs	8
↑ TSH, ↑ Abs	38

Abs, antibodies; TSH, thyroid-stimulating hormone.
Source: Adapted from Vanderpump MP, Tunbridge WM, French JM, et al. The incidence of thyroid disorders in the community: a twenty-year follow-up of the Whickham Survey. *Clin Endocrinol (Oxf)* 43(1):55, 1995.

FERTILITY AND PREGNANCY (Lincoln et al., 1999)
- Screening for hypothyroidism useful in women with ovulatory dysfunction
- Prepubertal hypothyroidism → short stature, delay in sexual maturity
- Infertility from anovulation and menorrhagia from estradiol (E_2)-withdrawal bleed
- APA-positive patients are at an ↑ risk of miscarriage: 50% vs. 23% for those women negative for thyroid antibodies (Poppe et al., 2003); other studies show no such relationship; benefit of thyroid hormone supplement not studied as yet.
- During pregnancy, T_4 needs rise approximately 45% (secondary to [a] ↑ thyroxine-binding globulin and [b] ↓ free thyroid hormone concentrations as pregnancy progresses)

As soon as pregnancy is confirmed (Toft, 2004):
  ↑ Levothyroxine (LT4) 25–50 μg daily
  Check TSH in 4 wks

SCREENING
- Check TSH at age 35 yrs and then every 5 yrs; yearly for fertility patients.
- Non–fertility patient: TSH >10 mIU/L, progression likely; start LT4 (Surks, 2005)
- Non–fertility patient: TSH >5 mIU/L, check Abs
  - Positive Abs → progression likely, start LT4
  - Negative Abs → lower rates of progression, but still may have 2–3× ↑ risk of atherosclerosis (Hak et al., 2000), start LT4
- Fertility patient: TSH >5 mIU/L → start LT4

TREATMENT (Cooper, 2001)
- 50–75 μg/day initially; recheck 4 wks, ↑ by 25 μg p.r.n.
- Once stable (TSH 0.45–4.50 mIU/L), the TSH can be monitored annually.

29. Recurrent Pregnancy Loss

INCIDENCE

- Fetal viability is only achieved in 30% of all human conceptions, 50% of which are lost before the first missed menses (Edmonds et al., 1982).
- 15–20% of clinically diagnosed pregnancies are lost in the 1st or early 2nd trimester (TM) (Warburton and Fraser, 1964; Alberman, 1988).
- Risk of loss:
  - 12% after one successful pregnancy
  - 24% after two consecutive losses
  - 30% after three consecutive losses
  - 40% after four consecutive losses
- Risk of a 4th loss after three prior losses:
  - If no prior live birth → 40–45%
  - If ≥1 prior live birth → 30%
- ↑ Rate of pregnancy loss with advanced maternal age (most commonly, isolated nondisjunction)
- 80% of spontaneous abortions (SABs) occur within first 12 wks of pregnancy, and 60% of these are due to chromosome abnormalities.
- Recurrent pregnancy loss (RPL) is a risk factor for ectopic pregnancies (2.5%), complete molar gestations (5 in 2500), and neural tube defects (Adam, 1995).
- Prognostic value of transvaginal ultrasound observation of embryonic heart activity:

Maternal Age (Yrs)	Risk of Loss (%)
≤35	<5
36–39	10
≥40	29
History of recurrent pregnancy loss	15–25

Source: Adapted from van Leeuwen I, Branch DW, et al. First-trimester ultrasonography findings in women with a history of recurrent pregnancy loss. *Am J Obstet Gynecol* 168(1 Pt 1):111, 1993; Laufer MR, Ecker JL, et al. Pregnancy outcome following ultrasound-detected fetal cardiac activity in women with a history of multiple spontaneous abortions. *J Soc Gynecol Investig* 1(2):138, 1994; and Deaton JL, Honore GM, et al. Early transvaginal ultrasound following an accurately dated pregnancy: the importance of finding a yolk sac or fetal heart motion. *Hum Reprod* 12(12):2820, 1997.

RECURRENT PREGNANCY LOSS

DEFINITIONS

- RPL (≥2 consecutive or ≥3 spontaneous losses ≤20 wks) occurs in **approximately 1–4%** (Salat-Baroux, 1988).
- **Abortion:** pregnancy loss before 20 wks' gestation or a fetal weight of <500 g
- **Primary RPL:** refers to a woman who has never carried a pregnancy to viability
- **Secondary RPL:** refers to a history of ≥1 viable term pregnancy before a series of losses
- **Early pregnancy loss:** refers to a loss <12 wks' estimated gestational age (EGA)
- **Late pregnancy loss:** refers to a loss between 12 and 20 wks' EGA

ETIOLOGY

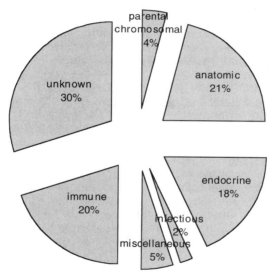

Etiologies of recurrent pregnancy loss.

- In approximately 30% of couples with RPL, there is no identifiable cause after sufficient workup (Boue et al., 1985).

Genetic Factors

Parental Chromosome Abnormality

- Approximately 4% in couples with RPL (vs. 0.2% in normal population)
- The maternal to paternal ratio is 3 to 1.
- One aneuploid SAB ↑ the risk of a subsequent loss to aneuploidy (Golbus, 1981).

RECURRENT PREGNANCY LOSS

- 4% probability that either parent is a carrier of a balanced translocation if there are ≥2 SABs or one SAB + a malformed fetus.
- Majority of abnormalities are balanced translocations (no DNA is lost and phenotype of the parent is normal), resulting in an unbalanced translocation in the fetus.
- Approximately 60% of balanced translocations are **reciprocal**, and 40% are **Robertsonian:**
  - **Reciprocal translocation:** even exchange of chromatin between two nonhomologous chromosomes; *risk of a malformed, chromosomally abnormal liveborn varies depending on the size, specific translocation, and breakpoint: approximately 10–15%.*
  - **Robertsonian translocation:** involves group D (13–15) and G (21 and 22) chromosomes (i.e., 14/21 translocation = long arms join up, but some short-arm material may be lost; breakage occurs close to the centromere; there are 45 chromosomes present (one normal 14 and 21, along with the balanced 14/21); *risk of an abnormal live birth ~10% if the mother is the carrier of a 21 translocation and 1% if the father carries the translocation.*

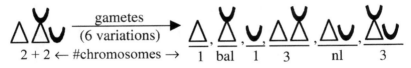

Robertsonian transfer. Robertsonian translocation: 1/3 of gametes are normal (including balanced). Reciprocal translocation: 1/2 of gametes are normal (including balanced). bal, balanced; nl, normal.

  ⇨ Robertsonian translocation of homologous chromosomes (incidence of 1 in 2500 with RPL) necessitates donor gametes for the affected partner.
  - *De novo* translocations (Warburton, 1991):
    ⇨ Reciprocal translocation: 1 in 2000
    ⇨ Robertsonian translocation: 1 in 9000

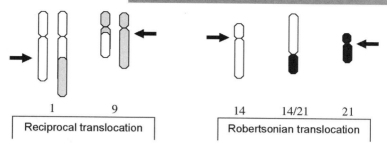

1 9	14 14/21 21
Reciprocal translocation	Robertsonian translocation

Source: Reproduced with permission from PROLOG. *Reproductive Endocrinology and Infertility*, 4th ed. Washington, DC: American College of Obstetricians and Gynecologists, 2000:23.

- Parental chromosomal testing may or may not demonstrate abnormality; there may be single gene defects that are not manifested by abnormalities; if an abnormal chromosome pattern is defined, there is nothing that can be done to lessen the chance for another loss (may offer controlled ovarian hyperstimulation with follicle-stimulating hormone [FSH]), although preimplantation genetic diagnosis may offer a remedy; the parents should be referred to genetic counseling/prenatal diagnosis.

- Turner mosaics are more susceptible to spontaneous miscarriages (Tarani et al., 1998):
  - Out of 160 pregnancies:
    ⇨ 29%: spontaneous loss
    ⇨ 20%: malformed babies (Turner syndrome [TS], trisomy 21, and so forth)
    ⇨ 7%: perinatal death

Fetal Chromosomal Abnormality

- Approximately 60–75% of SABs (Fritz et al., 2001)
- Karyotyping of the conceptus may reveal need for parental karyotype testing.
- The karyotype of a 2nd successive spontaneous loss was abnormal in approximately 50–70% when aneuploidy was found in the 1st abortus, but in only 20% of cases in which the 1st abortus was chromosomally normal (Daniely et al., 1998; Hassold, 1980).
- It is generally held that fetal chromosomal abnormalities play a prominent role in affecting single pregnancy losses but not recurrent losses; in fact, as the number of losses increases, the chance of a fetal chromosomal aberration decreases (Ogasawara et al., 2000; Christiansen et al., 2002).

RECURRENT PREGNANCY LOSS

- A woman who loses a chromosomally abnormal fetus has a greater chance of a live birth than the woman losing a euploid embryo.

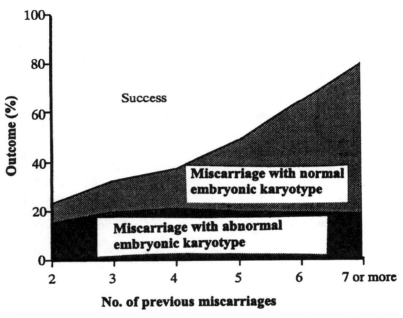

Source: Reproduced with permission from Ogasawara M, Aoki K, et al. Embryonic karyotype of abortuses in relation to the number of previous miscarriages. *Fertil Steril* 73(2):300, 2000.

- As a group, the trisomies are the most common anomaly, and of these, trisomy 16 is the *most common trisomy* found in abortuses, although the *single most common aneuploidy* for 1st TM losses is 45,XO.

RECURRENT PREGNANCY LOSS

Anatomic Factors

Congenital Uterine Anomalies

- Incidence of uterine malformations:

	Fertile (%)	Recurrent Pregnancy Loss (%)	Subfertile (%)
Total	3.8^w	6.3^x	2.4^w
Bicornuate	0.4^y	1.9^z	0.5^y
Septate	1.5	2.0	0.6
Arcuate	1.6	1.0	1.1

Note: Statistical significance by **row**: $w/x = P <.05$; $y/z = P <.01$.
Source: Adapted from Raga F, Bauset C, et al. Reproductive impact of congenital Mullerian anomalies. *Hum Reprod* 12(10):2277, 1997.

- Reproductive performance of different uterine malformations:

	Spontaneous Abortion (%)	Preterm Delivery (%)	Live Birth (%)
Didelphys	20.0	53.3^{b,c}	40.0^f
Unicornuate	37.5^b	25.0^b	43.7^f
Bicornuate	25.0	25.0^b	62.5^e
Septate	25.5	14.5^{b,d}	62.0^e
Arcuate	12.7^a	4.5^a	82.7^e

Note: Statistical significance by **column**: $a/b = P <.05$; $c/d = P <.01$; $e/f = P <.001$.
Source: Adapted from Raga F, Bauset C, et al. Reproductive impact of congenital Mullerian anomalies. *Hum Reprod* 12(10):2277, 1997.

- A more recent study suggested that a bicornuate uterus is not generally associated with RPL (Proctor and Haney, 2003).
- Incomplete caudal to cephalad septum reabsorption, type V (**septate**) anomaly, is associated with a 60% rate of RPL (Buttram, 1983).
- Note: The vascular density in uterine septa removed at the time of metroplasty is similar to that of the normal uterine wall (Dabirashrafi et al., 1995).
- Pregnancy loss is more common among women with diethylstilbestrol (DES) exposure (Kaufman et al., 2000).

Acquired Uterine Anomalies

- Intrauterine synechiae (also known as *Asherman syndrome*) from vigorous uterine curettage have been found to occur in 5% of women with RPL.
- Submucosal leiomyomas may cause an unfavorable implantation site by interfering with vascularization or by reducing the intrauterine cavity size; likewise, subserosal and myometrial fibroids may cause reproduction failure if they distort the uterine cavity.
- Miscarriage rates are reduced after removal of large intramural fibroids (>5 cm) (Bajekal and Li, 2000).

283

RECURRENT PREGNANCY LOSS

- Uterine polyps may act like a foreign body and disrupt pregnancy.

Diagnosis

- Hysterosalpingogram/hysteroscopy/hysterosonography/laparoscopy/magnetic resonance imaging (MRI)
- Imaging for septate uterus (Pellerito et al., 1992):
  - *Transvaginal sonography* (TVS) has a sensitivity of 100% and specificity of 80%.
  - *MRI* has a sensitivity and specificity of 100%.

Treatment

- **Primary method of treatment in all cases is corrective surgery.** In the case of congenital anomalies, unification procedures such as the Strassman procedure are rarely undertaken. Septum resection is warranted. In the case of Asherman syndrome, hysteroscopy to lyse adhesions is advisable. Hysteroscopic myomectomy, when feasible, is recommended for submucosal fibroids.

Endocrinologic Factors

Luteal Phase Deficiency

- The insufficient level of progesterone, presumably from a deficient corpus luteum in the 2nd half of the menstrual cycle, is hypothesized to prevent implantation of conceptus or impair maintenance of pregnancy; luteal phase deficiency (LPD) is more clearly associated with RPL than subfertility; histologic differences between fertile and infertile women are not significant (Coutifaris et al., 2004); diagnose LPD if duration of luteal phase is <13 days (from positive luteinizing hormone [LH] kit to start of menses).
  - Normal women have endometrial histology suggestive of LPD in up to 50% of single menstrual cycles and 25% of sequential cycles (Davis et al., 1989).
  - Suggested treatment options include aromatase inhibitor, clomiphene citrate, recombinant human follicle-stimulating hormone (rhFSH), human chorionic gonadotropin (hCG), and progesterone supplementation (beginning 3 days after positive ovulation prediction kit [OPK] until 10 wks' EGA).
  - **Hyperprolactinemia** has been shown to induce an LPD (possibly by ↓ progesterone from luteal cells); diagnose by prolactin (PRL) level and treat with **bromocriptine or cabergoline.**

Polycystic Ovary Syndrome

- Sonographic evidence of polycystic-appearing ovaries (PCAOs) in women with RPL does not predict worse pregnancy outcome than in women with RPL without PCOS (Rai et al., 2000).
- Data from small retrospective studies with poor control groups suggest that metformin may ↓ RPL in PCOS patients (Glueck, 2001; Jakubowicz et al., 2002) (see Chapter 18, Polycystic Ovary Syndrome).

RECURRENT PREGNANCY LOSS

Insulin

- ↑ Prevalence of **insulin resistance** in women with RPL (Craig et al., 2002):
  - 27.0% vs. 9.5%; odds ratio (OR), 3.55; 95% confidence interval (CI), 1.40–9.01
- Poorly controlled diabetes has been associated with ↑ rate of pregnancy loss; intervention with appropriate **insulin therapy** has been shown to reduce this risk (Dorman et al., 1999).

Thyroid

- **Hyper-** and **hypothyroidism** have been associated with ↑ pregnancy loss; no direct causal relationship specifically known toward RPL.
- **Antithyroperoxidase antibodies** (APA)–positive patients are at an ↑ risk of miscarriage: 50% vs. 23% for those women negative for thyroid Abs (Poppe et al., 2003); other studies show no such relationship; benefit of thyroid hormone supplement not studied as yet.

Obesity

- Obesity (body mass index >30 kg/m^2) is associated with ↑ risk of 1st TM and recurrent miscarriage (Lashen et al., 2004).
  - Early miscarriage OR 1.2; 95% CI, 1.01–1.46
  - RPL OR, 3.5; 95% CI, 1.03–12.01

Microbiologic Factors

- Several infectious agents have been implicated as etiologic factors in sporadic pregnancy loss, but no infectious agent has been clearly proven to cause RPL.
- Studies of women with RPL show an increased colonization with *Ureaplasma urealyticum* in the endometrium (Kundsin et al., 1981).
- Other commonly linked infections include *Toxoplasma gondii*, rubella, herpes simplex virus (HSV), measles, cytomegalovirus (CMV), coxsackievirus, *Listeria monocytogenes*, and *Mycoplasma hominis*, although none has been convincingly associated with RPL.
- Bottom line: more cost effective and time efficient to empirically treat each partner with azithromycin (1 g × 1 dose) or doxycycline (100 mg b.i.d. × 10 days) than to pursue multiple and repeated cultures.
- Reasonable to omit infectious testing or treatment

Inherited Thrombophilia   (Seligson and Lebetsky, 2001)

Who should be tested?
Unexplained fetal death >10 wks' EGA
Patient with a history of venous thromboembolism (VTE)
Family history suggestive of thrombophilia disorder
Consider if ≥ three 1st-TM losses.

RECURRENT PREGNANCY LOSS

- Factor V Leiden (FVL) and **prothrombin G20210A (ProG)** mutation, found in approximately 9% (1% of these are homozygous for the FVL mutation) and 3%, respectively, of white women in the United States; these mutations are associated with approximately 25% of isolated thrombotic events and approximately 50% of familial thrombosis.
- Although all who carry the FVL mutation show phenotypic resistance to activated protein C (PC), approximately 15% of all cases of activated PC resistance are not due to being a carrier of the FVL mutation.
- In the subgroup of case patients with three or more pregnancy losses and no successful pregnancies, prevalence of the FVL mutation was 9% (OR, 2.6 [CI, 1.0, 6.7]; P = .048) (Ridker et al., 1998).
- Other less common thrombophilias include autosomal-dominant deficiencies of the anticoagulants **PC, protein S (PS**; bad if <60%, then test antigenic levels of PS), **antithrombin III deficiency (ATdef)**, or **hyperhomocystinemia.**
  - Oral contraceptives (OCs) ↑ PC and PS but ↓ ATIII.
  - Smoking ↓ PC and PS.
  - Origin of nomenclature:
    ⇒ PC = presence in *peak* C in the electrophoretic procedure used in its isolation
    ⇒ PS = isolation originally occurred in *Seattle.*
- Relative risk of abortion and stillbirth per pregnancy for deficient women (ATdef, PC, PS) as compared to nondeficient women was 2.0 (95% CI, 1.2, 3.3) (Sanson et al., 1996).
- Methylene *tetra*hydro*f*olate *r*eductase (MTHFR) mutations and low vitamin B_6 or B_{12} may lead to **hyperhomocystinemia:**
  - Mild: 16–24 µmol/L
  - Moderate: 25–100 µmol/L
  - Severe: >100 µmol/L

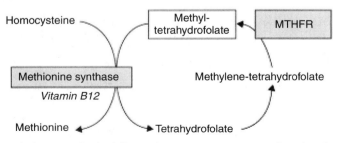

MTHFR, methylene tetrahydrofolate reductase. (Source: Reproduced with permission from Quere I, Perneger TV, Zittoun J, et al. Red blood cell methylfolate and plasma homocysteine as risk factors for venous thromboembolism: a matched case-control study. *Lancet* 359[9308]:747, 2002.)

RECURRENT PREGNANCY LOSS

⇨ Supplementation (see Treatment section for recommended doses) with vitamin B_6, B_{12}, and folate can often reduce homocysteine levels to normal, but this therapy has not yet been shown to result in a ↓ risk of thrombosis (Makris, 2000).

⇨ Compound heterozygotes for FVL and MTHFR alleles may experience worse outcomes.

• Lifetime risk of DVT compared to those without defect:

Defect	Prevalence in General Population (%)	Estimated ↑ Risk of Thrombosis (×-Fold Increase)	Risk of Deep Venous Thrombosis in Pregnancy (%)
Antithrombin III deficiency	0.02	10–20×	50
Protein C deficiency	0.2–0.4	10×	<1.0
Protein S deficiency	0.03–.013	10×	<1.0
Factor V Leiden	1–15	5×	0.2
Hyperhomocystinemia	5	3×	?
Prothrombin G20210A	2–5	3×	0.5

Source: Adapted from Martinelli I, Mannucci PM, et al. Different risks of thrombosis in four coagulation defects associated with inherited thrombophilia: a study of 150 families. *Blood* 92(7):2353, 1998.

• Risk of pregnancy loss (early + late pregnancy losses):

Defect	Prevalence in Control Subjects (%)	Prevalence in Women with Pregnancy Loss[a] (%)	Risk of Pregnancy Loss (Odds Ratio)
Factor V Leiden	9	8–32	2–5
Prothrombin G20210A	3	4–13	2–9
Antithrombin III deficiency	0–1.4	0–2	2–5
Protein C deficiency	0–2.5	6	2–3
Protein S deficiency	0–0.2	5–8	3–40
Hyperhomocystinemia	5–16	17–27	3–7

[a]Defined as first or recurrent early and/or late pregnancy loss.
Source: Adapted from Martinelli et al., 1998; Brenner et al., 1999; Ridker et al., 1998; Foka et al., 2000; Preston et al., 1996; Rai et al., 2001; Many et al., 2002; Sanson et al., 1996.

• Treatment is uncertain (see Treatment section at the end of chapter).

RECURRENT PREGNANCY LOSS

Immunologic Factors (20%)

Endometriosis

- Although few clinical data support a direct association of endometriosis with RPL (Vercammen and D'Hooghe, 2000; Balasch, 1988), several underlying pathophysiological features are common to the two conditions (Somigliana et al., 1999).

Autoimmunity (Self-Antigens) or Acquired Thrombophilia

- **Antiphospholipid-Ab syndrome** (APS or Hughes syndrome) believed to be a cause in approximately 5% of women with RPL; fetal loss more commonly occurs >10 wks of gestation (Simpson et al., 1998). It is characterized by
  - ↑ Antiphospholipid antibodies (Abs) (**anticardiolipin immunoglobulins IgG or IgM** [Katsuragawa et al., 1997]) or **lupus anticoagulant** with one or more clinical features:
    ⇨ RPL, thrombosis, autoimmune thrombocytopenia
  - APS actually comprises two syndromes:
    ⇨ Not associated with another illness (*primary APS*)
    ⇨ Additional burden of systemic lupus erythematosus or other rheumatic disease (*secondary APS*)
  - 1/3 of patients with lupus have antiphospholipid Abs.
  - Mechanism: uteroplacental thrombosis and vasoconstriction secondary to immunoglobulin binding to platelets and vascular endothelial membrane phospholipids
    ⇨ Note: True blood flow through placental vasculature does not occur until 9 to 10 wks' EGA (Jaffe et al., 1997).

- Diagnosis:
  ⇨ APS if **one** from A and **one** from B:

A: Clinical criteria

1. ≥1 Clinical episode of arterial, venous, or small-vessel **thrombosis**
2. **Pregnancy morbidity:**
   (a) ≥1 SAB morphologically normal fetus ≥10 wks' EGA, **or**
   (b) ≥1 Premature birth morphologically normal neonate ≥34 wks because of severe preeclampsia or severe placental insufficiency, **or**
   (c) ≥3 SABs <10 wks' EGA (without maternal anatomic or hormonal abnormalities; no maternal/paternal chromosomal causes)

B: Laboratory criteria

1. Medium-high maternal antiphospholipid antibody levels,[a] on ≥2 occasions ≥6 wks apart
2. Lupus anticoagulant, on ≥2 occasions ≥6 wks apart:

   (a) Dilute RVVT[a] (Russell's viper venom time) = prolonged phospholipid-dependent coagulation

   (b) Exclusion of other coagulopathies

EGA, estimated gestational age; SAB, spontaneous abortion.
[a]Abnormal values for antiphospholipid antibodies and lupus anticoagulant: See table below.
Source: Adpated from Wilson WA, Gharavi AE, et al. International consensus statement on preliminary classification criteria for definite antiphospholipid syndrome: report of an international workshop. *Arthritis Rheum* 42(7):1309, 1999.

Anticardiolipin[a]
>20 GPL or MPL units
Dilute Russell's viper venom time (lupus anticoagulant)[b]
≥1.2

---

[a]Immunoglobulin (Ig) G or IgM.
[b]Russell's viper venom time: venom has thromboplastin activity that activates factor X and bypasses the extrinsic pathway (factor VIII); more specific way to document deficiency in intrinsic pathway is usually assessed by partial thromboplastin time (>1.5 of normal).

- Treatment:
  ⇨ **Low-dose aspirin (81 mg/day) + low-molecular-weight heparin (LMWH; once + βhCG):** approximately 70–75% reported successful pregnancy outcome if treated compared with <50% for untreated (Kutteh, 1996). The combination (acetylsalicylic acid [ASA] + heparin) ↓ pregnancy loss by 54% compared with ASA alone (relative risk [RR], 0.46, 0.29–0.71) (Empson et al., 2002).

RECURRENT PREGNANCY LOSS

⇨ **LMWH may be an effective alternative to unfractionated heparin** (Rai et al., 1997; Greer, 2002); initiate at positive pregnancy test, should stop at 36 wks and potentially convert to unfractionated heparin to reduce risk of epidural hematoma.

Enoxaparin (Lovenox), 40 mg SC q.d. (Rai et al., 1997); adjust doses by weight (1 mg/kg/day) if obese (therapeutic dose: 1 mg/kg/day SC; full dose: q12 hrs)

Dalteparin (Fragmin), 5000 IU SC q.d.; adjust doses by weight (200 IU/kg/day) if obese (therapeutic dose: 100 IU/kg SC divided q12hrs)

⇨ **Therapeutic unfractionated heparin** levels recommended if history of thrombosis (may use prophylactic unfractionated heparin, 5000 U b.i.d., if no history of thrombosis)

⇨ **Risk of thrombosis presumably highest first 6 wks postpartum**

⇨ Initiating heparin before conception is potentially dangerous because of the risk of hemorrhage at the time of ovulation.

⇨ Need close maternal and fetal surveillance secondary to high risk for complications (i.e., preeclampsia, fetal distress, intrauterine growth restriction [IUGR], preterm labor [PTL], and so forth)

⇨ Low-dose aspirin vs. placebo prospective study now under way

⇨ If surgery planned while on LMWH, stop 18–24 hrs before procedure and restart 12 hrs postprocedure. If emergent, can reverse with **protamine sulfate; slow infusion, no need to reverse if >18 hrs from last dose.** For enoxaparin, use *mg/mg*, for dalteparin, *50 mg/5000 IU*.

Alloimmunity

- Controversy on how to diagnose and treat
- Refers to all causes of recurrent abortion related to an abnormal maternal immune response to antigens on placental or fetal tissues (i.e., T-helper [Th] 1 immunity)
- Th1 immunodystrophism: a dichotomous **Th1** (↑) and **Th2** (↓) cytokine profile directed toward trophoblasts (Hill et al., 1995); although an aberrant cytokine profile by peripheral blood mononuclear cells was not seen in RPL patients by one more recent report (Bates and Hill, 2002).
- Aberrant cytokine profile not detected in peripheral serum
- Treatment: immunosuppressive doses of progesterone vaginal suppositories (100 mg b.i.d., beginning 3 days after ovulation)
- It has been proposed that maternal production of blocking factors may prevent maternal rejection of fetus, and RPL mothers do not make this blocking factor (Sargent et al., 1988):
  - Treatment: Immunotherapy to stimulate maternal immune tolerance of fetal material is **not effective** (Ober et al., 1999).
  - Furthermore, agammaglobulinemic women are not at ↑ risk for fetal loss.

RECURRENT PREGNANCY LOSS

Ovarian Reserve Factors
- Prevalence of elevated FSH in women with RPL is the same as for an infertility population (Hofmann et al., 2000).
- Women with **unexplained** RPL have a greater incidence of ↑ day 3 serum FSH than women with a known cause of RPL (Trout and Seifer, 2000).

	Day 3 Follicle-Stimulating Hormone ≥10 mIU/mL (%)
57 Women with ≥3 spontaneous abortions	
36 Unexplained RPL	31
21 Explained RPL	5

RPL, recurrent pregnancy loss.

Environmental Factors
- Exposure to nonsteroidal antiinflammatory drugs and risk of miscarriage (note: small numbers):

	Nonsteroidal Antiinflammatory Drugs
Hazard ratio (95% confidence interval)	**1.8** (1.0–3.2)
At conception	**5.6** (2.3–13.7)
>1 wk	**8.1** (2.8–23.4)

Source: Adapted from Li DK, Liu L, et al. Exposure to non-steroidal anti-inflammatory drugs during pregnancy and risk of miscarriage: population based cohort study. *BMJ* 327(7411):368, 2003.

- **Folate ≤2.2 ng/mL** (≤4.9 nmol/L) associated with ↑ SAB; OR. 1.47; CI, 1.01–2.14 (George et al., 2002)

RECURRENT PREGNANCY LOSS

- Smoking, alcohol (**>2 oz/wk**), and heavy coffee (caffeine) consumption are associated with a slight, but statistically significant, ↑ in absolute risk of recurrent abortion.

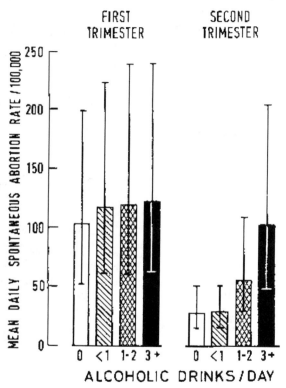

Life-table analysis showed that the age-adjusted relative risks of 2nd TM losses were 1.03 (not significant), 1.98 (*P* <.01), and 3.53 (*P* <.01) for women taking <1, 1–2, and >3 drinks daily, compared with nondrinkers. (Reproduced with permission from Harlap S, Shiono PH. Alcohol, smoking, and incidence of spontaneous abortions in the first and second trimester. *Lancet* 2[8187]:173, 1980.)

RECURRENT PREGNANCY LOSS

- The ingestion of caffeine may ↑ risk of an SAB among nonsmoking women carrying fetuses with normal karyotypes (Cnattingius et al., 2000).
- The half-life of caffeine is halved in smokers and doubled in women taking OCs.

Caffeine/Day (mg)	Spontaneous Abortion Relative Risk (Confidence Interval)
100–299	1.3 (0.9–1.8)
300–499	1.4 (0.9–2.0)
≥500	2.2 (2.3–3.8)

Quantity	Caffeine (mg)
150 mL coffee	If brewed, 115
	If boiled, 90
	If instant, 60
150 mL tea	If tea bag, 39
	If herbal tea, 0
150 mL soft drink	15
(soda can = 355 mL)	(~36)
1 g chocolate bar	0.3

Note: 150 mL = 5.2 oz.

- Exposure to anesthetic gases, tetrachloroethylene (used in dry cleaning), lead, and mercury is linked to abortion.
- Isotretinoin (Accutane) definitely associated with ↑ incidence of SAB.

Dyssynchronous Fertilization
- ↑ SAB due to chromosomal anomalies noted when intercourse occurs remote from ovulation (Boue and Boue, 1973).

HLA Antigens
- Reproductive failure may result from aberrant expression of HLA antigens during any stage of pregnancy (Choudhury and Knapp, 2001).

RECURRENT PREGNANCY LOSS

DIAGNOSIS
- Possible karyotype of conceptus to help decide if parental karyotyping is worthwhile
- Evaluation begun after 2nd consecutive loss, because the risk of RPL after two successive abortions (30%) is similar to the risk of recurrence among women with ≥ three consecutive abortions (33%).

History
- Maternal age
- Current medical illnesses and medications
- Pattern, TM, and characteristics of prior pregnancy losses
- Exposure to environmental toxins, occupation, recent travel
- Gynecologic and/or obstetric infections
- Previous diagnostic tests
- Family history
  - Cycle regularity
  - Spontaneous pregnancy losses
  - Maternal use of DES
  - Genetic syndromes
  - Thrombotic complications

Physical Examination
- General physical and gynecologic examination

Diagnostic Tests

Note: There is no consensus regarding testing for inherited thrombophilias in patients with RPL <10 wks.
Nocturnal gonadotropin-releasing hormone (GnRH) pulses begin 4 wks postpartum. Therefore, wait at least 1 mo after pregnancy loss before obtaining hormonal serum tests (Liu et al., 1983).

Genetic
• Parental and conceptus karyotypes
  ▪ Genetic counseling p.r.n.

Anatomic
• Sonohysterogram or hysteroscopy
  ▪ Intrauterine cavity assessment
  ▪ MRI p.r.n.

Endocrine
• Luteal phase duration (positive kit until 1st day of menses):
  ▪ <13 days → LPD
• Day 3 FSH: ovarian reserve test
• Thyroid-stimulating hormone (TSH) (TPO-Ab debated)
• PRL
• Fasting glucose-insulin ratio (if menses irregular, clinical signs and symptoms of PCOS)
  ▪ Obtain 2 hr-glucose tolerance test (GTT) if (a) glucose–insulin ratio <4.5 or (b) obese PCOS patient

Thrombophilia. (Obtain if >10-wk loss, history of VTE, family history of thrombotic disorder, ≥ three 1st-TM losses)
• Factor V Leiden and prothrombin G20210A mutations
• Homocysteine
• Activated protein C resistance (APCR), AT III, PC, PS

Immunologic. (Note: Low or unsustained, moderately positive values are clinically meaningless.)
• Russell's viper venom time (RVVT) (lupus anticoagulant)
• aCL (anticardiolipin Abs, immunoglobulin [Ig] G or IgM)

RECURRENT PREGNANCY LOSS

TREATMENT
- Thrombophilias and history of RPL:

Defect	Treatment
Factor V Leiden, prothrombin G20210A, antithrombin III, activated protein C resistance	ASA + LMWH
Protein C, protein S	ASA + LMWH if history of venous thromboembolism without risk factor
↑ Homocysteine	ASA + B_6 (10 mg/day), B_{12} (0.4 mg/day), folate (1 mg/day)

ASA, acetylsalicylic acid; LMWH, low-molecular-weight heparin.

- Thrombophilic disorders and fetal loss: a metaanalysis

Early Loss	Late Loss	Disorder	1st Trimester RPL	Non-RPL
SS	SS	Factor V Leiden	2.01 (1.13–3.58)	1.73 (1.18–2.54)
SS	SS	Prothrombin	2.05 (1.18–3.54)	2.30 (1.09–4.87)
SS	SS	Protein S deficiency	14.72 (0.99–218.01)	7.39 (1.28–42.93)
SS		Activated protein C resistance	3.48 (1.58–7.69)	NS
		Protein C deficiency	NS	NS
		Antithrombin III deficiency	NS	NS
		Homomethylene tetrahydrofolate reductase	NS	NS

NS, not significant; RPL, recurrent pregnancy loss; SS, statistically significant.
Source: Adapted from Rey E, Kahn SR, et al. Thrombophilic disorders and fetal loss: a meta-analysis. *Lancet* 361(9361):901, 2003.

- 81 mg aspirin/day improved outcome in unexplained RPL with 2nd TM losses (Rai et al., 2000).
- Other treatment as previously discussed in pertinent sections above (e.g., metformin for PCOS)
- Patients with RPL are anxious and desperate to have "take-home baby." Support and counseling are important.
- Remember, 60–70% of women with unexplained RPL have a successful next pregnancy (Jeng, 1995).
- Oocyte donation has been efficacious in treating RPL (Remohi et al., 1996).
- *In vitro* fertilization (IVF) with preimplantation genetic diagnosis may eventually prove to benefit RPL patients.

RECURRENT PREGNANCY LOSS

- Future pregnancy outcome:

RPL (No.)	RPL Rate with Subsequent Pregnancy (%)
2	24
3	30
4	40
5	44
6	53

RPL, recurrent pregnancy loss.

- Prognosis for viable birth (derived from >1000 cases at Brigham and Women's Hospital):

Status	Intervention	Viable Births (%)
Genetic factors	Timed intercourse and supportive care	20–90
Anatomic factors	Surgery and supportive care	60–90
Endocrine factors		
Luteal phase deficiency	Progesterone ± ovulation induction and supportive care	80–90
Hypothyroidism	Thyroid replacement and supportive care	80–90
Hyperprolactinemia	Dopamine agonist	80–90
Infections	Antibiotics and supportive care	70–90
Antiphospholipid syndrome	Acetylsalicylic acid, heparin, and supportive care	70–90
Unknown factors	Timed intercourse and supportive care	60–90

Source: Adapted from Hill JA. *Recurrent Pregnancy Loss: Male and Female Factor, Etiology and Treatment*. Frontiers in Reproductive Endocrinology. Washington, DC: Serono Symposia USA, Inc., 2001.

30. Management of Early Pregnancy Failure

- Early pregnancy failure (EPF): broader term describing 1st trimester pregnancy failures; preferred term by many
- Incidence of pregnancy loss:
  - 15–20% of all clinically diagnosed pregnancies
  - Mortality for spontaneous abortions: approximately 0.4 in 100,000 (Creinin et al., 2001)

DEFINITIONS

Anembryonic pregnancy: gestational sac >17 mm in diameter without an embryo

Blighted ovum: literally "bad egg"; often used to mean *anembryonic pregnancy* but not currently the preferred terminology

Embryonic demise: demise of an embryo between 4 and 15 mm in length; lack of cardiac activity documented by ultrasound

Fetal demise: demise of a fetus >15 mm in crown–rump length; lack of cardiac activity documented by ultrasound

Incomplete abortion: passage of some but not all fetal or placental tissue <20 wks' gestation

Inevitable abortion: uterine bleeding at gestational age <20 wks, with cervical dilation but without passage of any fetal or placental tissue

Threatened abortion: uterine bleeding at <20 wks' gestation, without cervical dilation or effacement

Missed abortion: historic terminology describing a nonviable pregnancy (<20 wks' gestation) that has been retained in the uterus without spontaneous passage for at least 8 wks (terminology evolved before availability of ultrasound [USN]; **based on size less than expected by date and no fetal heart tones** via fetoscope)

TREATMENT OPTIONS
Surgical Options

- Historically, surgical intervention was standard management and is the most frequently used.
  - **Sharp curettage:** Higher complication rate with sharp curettage as compared to suction curettage; should be avoided (Foma and Gulmezoglu, 2003)
  - Electric suction curettage

MANAGEMENT OF EARLY PREGNANCY FAILURE

- **Manual vacuum aspiration** (see figure in Office Manual Vacuum Aspiration section): Handheld suction device that generates suction pressure equivalent to electric suction devices until the syringe is almost full
- **Anesthesia options:** general, regional, or local (paracervical block)
- **Surgical setting:** Operating room or office
- **Complications (1st trimester evacuations):** 0–10% postprocedural infection; 2–3% incomplete evacuation; up to 15% intrauterine adhesions (many are mild adhesions); <1% hemorrhage, uterine perforation, or cervical laceration (Creinin et al., 2001; Friedler et al., 1993)

Expectant Management

- Two studies have suggested that surgical intervention may result in fewer complications (bleeding, infection) if the gestational sac >10 mm (Hurd et al., 1997), but these studies were small and not randomized (Jurkovic et al., 1998).
- Complete expulsion occurs in 25–80% and may be related to the amount of tissue (Nielsen and Hahlin, 1995; Chipchase and James, 1997).
- Complications: 1–3% infection, 3% hemorrhage

Medical Management (Note: The following applies to nonviable pregnancies only.)

- **Vaginal misoprostol** appears to have higher efficacy than oral administration.
- Use of misoprostol is an off-label indication.
- Probably faster than expectant management but not as fast as surgical
- No clear consensus on best regimen: misoprostol alone vs. mifepristone and misoprostol
  - Multiple trials using different regimens are published based on completion at 14–21 days.
  - Definition of success differed in many studies (from absence of gestational sac to retained products).
  - Efficacy differs by dose and route of administration (see table below).

Regimen	Success (%)	Comments
Misoprostol, 400–600 mg PO	42–95	Side effects include nausea, vomiting, and diarrhea.
Misoprostol, 400–800 mg per vagina	75–85	Vaginal administration has fewer side effects and, in randomized trials, had greater efficacy than oral routes.
Mifepristone + misoprostol	52–95	Mifepristone has not been consistently shown to increase efficacy.

Source: Adapted from Creinin MD, Schwartz JL, et al. Early pregnancy failure—current management concepts. *Obstet Gynecol Surv* 56(2):105, 2001.

MANAGEMENT OF EARLY PREGNANCY FAILURE

- Reasonable regimen (Bagratee et al, 2004):
  - Document intrauterine pregnancy (IUP)
  - Exclusion criteria:
    - ⇨ Prostaglandin allergy
    - ⇨ Cardiac, respiratory, hepatic, renal, or adrenal disease
    - ⇨ Hypertension (HTN), coagulopathy, deep venous thrombosis (DVT), diabetes

Day 0:
Misoprostol, 3 × 200 μg per vagina × 15 mins in recumbent position.
Doxycycline, 100 mg PO b.i.d. × 5 days (metaanalysis of randomized controlled trials of periabortal antibiotics → ↓ 42% risk of infection [Sawaya et al., 1996]).

Day 1: Ultrasound
Repeat misoprostol (600 μg) if incomplete and return on day 2.
If complete, return in 14 days for hCG.

Day 2: Ultrasound
Return on day 7 if incomplete.
If complete, return in 14 days for hCG.

Day 7: Ultrasound
Evacuation of retained products of conception if incomplete.

hCG, human chorionic gonadotropin.

- Pain medications such as Tylenol No. 3 and nonsteroidal antiinflammatory drugs (NSAIDs).
- <42 days from last menstrual period (LMP) → 96% effective; 42–56 days → 86%

Outcome Measures	Misoprostol	Placebo
Overall success	88.5%	44.2%[a]
For early pregnancy failure	86.7%	28.9%[a]
For incomplete miscarriage	100.0%	85.7%
Cumulative success rate over time:		
Day 1	32.7%	5.8%[a]
Day 2	73.1%	13.5%[a]
Day 7	88.5%	44.2%[a]

[a]Statistically significant.
Source: Adapted from Bagratee JS, Khullar V, et al. A randomized controlled trial comparing medical and expectant management of first trimester miscarriage. *Hum Reprod* 19(2):266, 2004.

MANAGEMENT OF EARLY PREGNANCY FAILURE

Office Manual Vacuum Aspiration

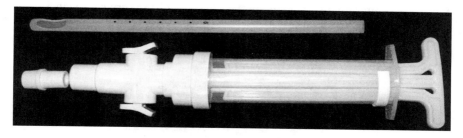

- Conduct a medical history, physical examination, and any indicated laboratory tests.
- Oral pain medications, such as 800 mg of ibuprofen
- Bimanual examination to determine the size and position of the uterus
- Place the speculum and cleanse the cervix with an antiseptic.
- If dilatation is needed, administer a paracervical block and apply a tenaculum.
- Dilate the cervix as needed and then gently insert the cannula.
  - Cannula size = gestational age
  - Size of Pratt dilator needed = 3 × cannula size + 1
- Place the cannula through the cervix to just past the internal os, then attach the prepared aspirator to the cannula.
- Release the pinch valve to transfer the vacuum pressure into the uterus.
- Evacuate the uterine contents by rotating and moving the cannula gently back and forth within the uterine cavity.
- Check for signs of completion, including
  - Red or pink foam passing through the cannula
  - Gritty sensation
  - Contraction of the uterus
  - Products of conception are visible
  - ↑ In cramping
- If patient is Rh negative, administer Rh immune globulin.

How to Administer a Paracervical Block (Modification of Glick Technique)

- Use 10–20 cc of 0.5–1.0% lidocaine.
  - Maximum dose for 60-kg woman:
    - ⇨ Without epinephrine = 270 mg
    - ⇨ With epinephrine = 420 mg
- 23-Gauge 1.5-in. needle or a spinal needle facilitates placement.

MANAGEMENT OF EARLY PREGNANCY FAILURE

- Inject 1–2 cc at tenaculum site (usually at 12 or 6 o'clock).
- Place tenaculum.
- Inject lidocaine at junction between the vaginal wall and cervix (5 o'clock on one side and 7 o'clock on the other)

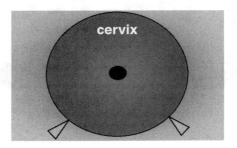

- Always aspirate to avoid intravascular injection (do not inject if blood aspirate).
- Lack of resistance means that you are not in the uterus, but excessive resistance means that you are too close to the internal os.
- Inject to a depth of 1.0–1.5 in.

31. Premature Ovarian Failure

DEFINITION (Rebar and Connolly, 1990)

<40 yrs old
Follicle-stimulating hormone (FSH) > 40 mIU/mL × 2 at least 1 mo apart
Amenorrhea ≥4 mos

- Premature ovarian failure (POF) = hypergonadotropic amenorrhea
- Oocyte physiology: The acme in number of oocytes is reached by 20 wks of gestation when the number reaches 6 million. By birth, this number is down to 2 million, and approximately 400,000 follicles are present at the onset of puberty. Through the process of apoptosis, no responsive oocytes are found by the time of menopause. The timing of ovarian failure is determined by both the original oocyte quantity and the rate of apoptosis.
- The above dogma has recently been challenged by data indicating the presence of **germ stem cells** in rodent ovaries (Johnson et al., 2004).

INCIDENCE (Coulam et al., 1986; Luborsky et al., 2003)
- **1.1%**
  - 0.1% by age 30 yrs
  - 1.1% by age 40 yrs
  - 10–28% of those with primary amenorrhea
  - 4–18% of those with secondary amenorrhea
- Autoimmune polyglandular syndrome comorbidity:
  - 15% rate of POF with type I (hyperparathyroidism, chronic mucocutaneous candidiasis, Addison's disease)
  - 5% rate of POF with type II (Addison's disease, autoimmune thyroid disease, diabetes)

PREMATURE OVARIAN FAILURE

CHARACTERISTICS

	Primary Amenorrhea	Secondary Amenorrhea
Karyotypic abnormalities	56%	13%
Y-chromosome present	10%	None
Symptoms of estradiol deficiency	22%	85%
Progesterone withdrawal bleed	22%	51%
Ovulation after diagnosis	None	24%
Pregnancy after diagnosis	None	8%

Source: Adapted from Rebar RW, Connolly HV. Clinical features of young women with hypergonadotropic amenorrhea. *Fertil Steril* 53(5):804, 1990.

- Both groups show diminished bone densities, although 2/3 of women with karyotypically normal POF have a bone mineral density (BMD) one standard deviation below the mean of similar aged women despite having taken standard hormone replacement therapy (Anasti, 1998).
- Progesterone withdrawal bleed is a poor screening test unless patient fails to withdraw after initial response.

ETIOLOGY
Ovarian Follicle Depletion
- Deficient initial follicle number
  - Pure gonadal dysgenesis
  - Thymic aplasia/hypoplasia
  - Idiopathic
- Accelerated follicle atresia
  - X-chromosome related
    ⇨ X mosaics = most common anomaly (45,XO/46,XX; 46,XX/47,XXX)
    ⇨ Turner syndrome
    ⇨ X deletions
  - Galactosemia
  - Iatrogenic (chemotherapy = cyclophosphamide; radiation treatments ≥600 cGy)
  - Viral agents
  - Autoimmunity
  - Oocyte-specific cell-cycle regulation defect
  - Surgical extirpation (need 40% of one ovary to have normal ovulatory function)
  - Idiopathic

PREMATURE OVARIAN FAILURE

Ovarian Follicle Dysfunction
- Enzyme deficiencies
  - 17α-Hydroxylase
  - 17-20 Desmolase
  - Cholesterol desmolase
  - Galactose-1-phosphate uridyltransferase
- Autoimmunity
- Lymphocytic oophoritis
  - Gonadotropin receptor–blocking immunoglobulin (Ig) G antibodies
  - Antibodies to gonadotropins
- Signal defects
  - Abnormal gonadotropin
  - Abnormal gonadotropin receptor
  - Abnormal G protein
- Gene mutations: inhibin α gene, 7% incidence (Shelling et al., 2000)
- Iatrogenic (previous ovarian surgery)
- Idiopathic (resistant ovary syndrome)

DIAGNOSTIC TESTS (Liewan and Santoro, 1997)
- History and physical
- Karyotype if onset <30 yrs old and primary amenorrhea (Y-chromosome necessitates gonadectomy to prevent gonadoblastoma; 50% of **gonadoblastomas** give rise to dysgerminomas).
- Consider karyotype if <60 cm tall, because individual could be a mosaic.

All Patients

2-Hr glucose tolerance test (GTT)
Thyroid-stimulating hormone (TSH), antithyroperoxidase antibodies
Dual-energy x-ray absorptiometry (DXA) scan for bone densitometry
Complete blood cell count (CBC) with peripheral smear (pernicious anemia)
Adrenal antibody test (titer <1:10 is normal) with adrenocorticotropic hormone (ACTH) stimulation test to confirm diagnosis (**Addison's disease;** signs and symptoms: hyperpigmentation of gums and hand skinfolds, loss of pubic/axillary hair): 1 μg cosyntropin IM (cortisol should be >18 μg/dL at 30 or 60 mins) (Bakalov et al., 2002)
Ca^{2+}, PO_4 (hypoparathyroidism)

If Signs and Symptoms Warrant
- Total serum protein; albumin/globulin ratio (**IgA deficiency,** if frequent respiratory tract infections)

PREMATURE OVARIAN FAILURE

- Magnetic resonance imaging (MRI) of sella turcica if signs and symptoms of central nervous system (CNS) mass lesion (rule out **pituitary tumor**)
- 27% of POF associated with hypothyroidism; 2.5% associated with diabetes
- Progression of deficits (in general): **TPA** = *t*hyroid, *p*ancreas, *a*drenal

TREATMENT (Anasti, 1998)

- Estrogen treatment: begin with 0.3 mg Premarin for 1 yr or once patient has bleeding, then add progestin; may become pregnant, therefore offer 20 µg ethinyl estradiol oral contraceptive (OC) (Mircette, Alesse) (Taylor et al., 1996).
- Alternative regimen: transdermal estradiol and medroxyprogesterone (Provera)
- Pregnancy may occur in 10% of patients with POF (secondary amenorrhea), as there is episodic ovarian function in approximately 50% (as judged by elevated estradiol levels) and approximately 20% of these women will ovulate (as noted by serum progesterone >5 ng/mL).
- No prospectively proven treatment restores ovulation (gonadotropins may exacerbate autoimmune ovarian failure via synergizing with interferon (IFN)-γ to increase major histocompatibility complex (MHC) class II expression on granulosa cells).
- Fertility counseling:
  - Time to allow for spontaneous remission
  - Adoption
  - Ovum donation
- FSH rebound using gonadotropin-releasing hormone agonist (GnRH-a) (Lupron, 1 mg/day SC) for 33.2 days (on average) to get FSH <25 mIU/mL; wait 1 day, then recombinant human FSH (rhFSH) at 2 amps/day × 6 days. Need to add luteal phase support. However, **no pregnancies** were reported (Rosen et al., 1992).
  - Conclusions:
    ⇨ Ovulation can occur.
    ⇨ Luteal phase support necessary

32. Genetic Testing

INCIDENCE OF ABNORMAL CHROMOSOMES
- 60–70% of all 1st trimester abortions; 6–11% of all stillborns.
- Sex chromosomal aneuploidy incidence: 1 in 400
- Chance of repeat sex chromosomal aneuploidy: 1% until her age-related risk >1%
  - Note: Previous fetus with 47,XYY or 45,XO has no ↑ risk with subsequent pregnancy.

DIAGNOSIS
- Chorionic villus sampling: 10–12 wks' estimated gestational age (EGA)
- Amniocentesis: >15 wks (ideally, 15–20 wks' EGA)
- The vast majority of aneuploidies are due to errors in chromosome segregation at the first meiotic division in the oocyte (thus, they are maternal in origin).
- Gamete donor screening tests:
  - Rho(D) type
  - Hemoglobinopathies if warranted
  - Rubella
  - Cystic fibrosis
  - Canavan disease (high risk: Ashkenazi Jews, 1 in 40 is a carrier)
  - Karyotype if personal history, family history of recurrent loss; unexplained mental retardation or birth defects
  - Tay-Sachs disease (high risk: Ashkenazi Jews, 1 in 30 is a carrier, French-Canadian, Cajun)

CYSTIC FIBROSIS (Gene Tests Web Site: http://www.genereviews.org)
- Autosomal-recessive disorder; gene (cystic fibrosis transmembrane regulator [CFTR]) located on chromosome 7q

GENETIC TESTING

- >1200 Mutations reported; current recommendation is to screen individuals of European white and Ashkenazi Jewish descent for 25 common mutations; available for other ethnic groups:

Ethnicity	CF Carrier Frequency		Chance for a Child with CF If		
	Before Test	Negative Test	One Parent Negative, Other Untested	One Parent Negative, Other Positive	Both Negative
Ashkenazi Jewish	1 in 29	1 in 930	1 in 107,880	1 in 3720	1 in 3,459,600
European white	1 in 29	1 in 140	1 in 16,240	1 in 560	1 in 78,400

CF, cystic fibrosis.

- CF detection rates by ethnicity:

Ethnicity	Detection Rate (%)
European white	90
African American	69
Hispanic	72
Asian American	Not available

- Clinical symptoms of CF include (but not limited to):
  - **Chronic sinopulmonary disease**
    ⇨ Chronic cough and sputum production, chronic wheeze and air trapping, obstructive lung disease on lung function tests, persistent colonization with CF pathogens, chronic chest radiograph abnormalities, digital clubbing
  - **Gastrointestinal/nutritional abnormalities**
    ⇨ Malabsorption/pancreatic insufficiency, distal intestinal obstructive syndrome, rectal prolapse, recurrent pancreatitis, meconium ileus, chronic hepatobiliary disease, failure to thrive, hypoproteinemia, fat-soluble vitamin deficiencies
  - **Obstructive azoospermia**
  - **Salt-loss syndromes**
    ⇨ Acute salt depletion, chronic metabolic alkalosis
- Key points while screening for CF:
  - Two carriers have 25% chance of an affected child with each pregnancy.
  - Severity, age of onset, and organs affected not predictable

- Preimplantation and prenatal genetic testing available for pregnancies at risk
- The 5T allele reduces amount of CFTR protein produced (quantitative alteration).
- Implications of large size of gene and number of mutations:
  ⇨ Detection is not 100%.
  ⇨ Negative test does not rule out CF/carrier status but reduces likelihood.
  ⇨ Possibility of an unidentified mutation exists even after extensive testing.
  ⇨ Identification of one mutation does not rule out possibility of second unidentified mutation.
- CF and congenital bilateral absence of the vas deferens (CBAVD) (Chillon et al., 1995)
  - 19% of men with CBAVD have two CF mutations.
  - 33% have one identified CF mutation and one 5T allele.
  - 20% have one identified CF mutation.
  - 1% have two 5T alleles.
  - 27% have no identified CF mutation with/without one 5T allele.
  - Most laboratories screen for the 16–32 mutations that account for the greatest proportion of cases; >1200 CF gene mutations reported.

GENETIC TESTING

RISK OF A LIVE-BORN INFANT WITH A GENETIC DIAGNOSIS

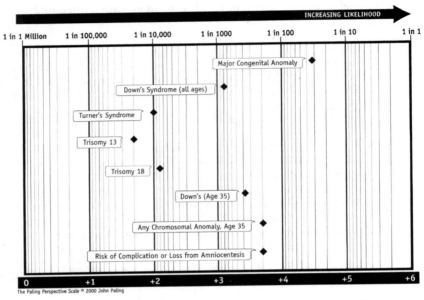

Source: Reproduced with permission from Stallings SP, Paling JE. New tool for presenting risk in obstetrics and gynecology. *Obstet Gynecol* 98:345, 2001.

- Risk of Down syndrome and chromosomal abnormalities at live birth, according to maternal age:

Maternal Age (Yrs)	47,+21	Risk of Any Chromosomal Abnormality
20	1 in 1667	1 in 527
25	1 in 1200	1 in 476
30	1 in 952	1 in 385
35	1 in 378	1 in 192
40	1 in 106	1 in 66
45	1 in 30	1 in 21

Source: Adapted from Hook EB, Cross PK, Schreinemachers DM. Chromosomal abnormality rates at amniocentesis and in live-born infants. *JAMA* 249(15):2034, 1983.

CARRIER TESTING FOR COMMON GENETIC DISEASE BASED ON ETHNICITY

Ethnic Groups	Common Diseases	Carrier Frequency	Testing Methodology
African Americans	Sickle cell anemia	1 in 10	CBC and quantitative hemoglobin electro-phoresis
	Sickle C disease	1 in 50	
	α-Thalassemia	1 in 30	
	β-Thalassemia	1 in 75	
Ashkenazi Jews	Tay-Sachs disease	1 in 30	Biochemical testing
	Canavan disease	1 in 40	Molecular testing
	Cystic fibrosis	1 in 29	Molecular testing
	Gaucher disease	1 in 15	Molecular testing
	Dysautonomia	1 in 32	Molecular testing
Asians	α-Thalassemia	1 in 20	CBC and quantitative hemoglobin electro-phoresis
	β-Thalassemia	1 in 50	
Caribbean	Sickle cell anemia	1 in 12 to 1 in 30	CBC and quantitative hemoglobin electro-phoresis
	α-Thalassemia	1 in 30	
	β-Thalassemia	1 in 50 to 1 in 75	
Whites (non-Jewish)	Cystic fibrosis	1 in 29	Molecular testing
French Canadian	Tay-Sachs disease	1 in 30	Molecular testing
Hispanic	Sickle cell anemia	1 in 30 to 1 in 200	CBC and quantitative hemoglobin electro-phoresis
	α-Thalassemia	Variable	
	β-Thalassemia	1 in 30 to 1 in 75	
Indian/Pakistani	Sickle cell anemia	1 in 50 to 1 in 100	CBC and quantitative hemoglobin electro-phoresis
	α-Thalassemia	Variable	
	β-Thalassemia	1 in 30 to 1 in 50	
Mediterranean (Italian/Greek)	Sickle cell anemia	1 in 30 to 1 in 50	CBC and quantitative hemoglobin electro-phoresis
	α-Thalassemia	1 in 30 to 1 in 50	
	β-Thalassemia	1 in 20 to 1 in 30	
Middle-Eastern (Arabic)	Sickle cell anemia	1 in 50 to 1 in 100	CBC and quantitative hemoglobin electro-phoresis
	α-Thalassemia	Variable	
	β-Thalassemia	1 in 50	
South-East Asians	α-Thalassemia	1 in 20	CBC and quantitative hemoglobin electro-phoresis
	β-Thalassemia	1 in 30	

CBC, complete blood cell count.
Note: Numbers may not be exact and are estimates only.
Source: Adapted from March of Dimes.

GENETIC TESTING

MALE FACTORS

- 10–15% of men with obstructive azoospermia have cystic fibrosis/CBAVD.
- 24% of men with azoospermia or severe oligozoospermia (<1 × 10^6/mL) have some genetic abnormality (Dohle et al., 2002).
- 10–15% of men with azoospermia and 3–10% of men with severe oligozoospermia (<1 × 10^6/mL) have microdeletions of sections of the Y chromosome.
- **Y microdeletions** (Foresta et al., 2001; McElreavey et al., 2000):
  - Y microdeletions are the most common genetic cause of male infertility due to spermatogenic failure; important to delineate before testicular sperm aspiration (TESA)/intracytoplasmic sperm injection (ICSI).
  - Clinical picture: severe oligozoospermia (<1 × 10^6/mL; 4.4%), azoospermia (8.1%), infertile males (0.4%), ICSI candidates (4%); normal physical findings and normal concentration of gonadotropins (Dohle et al., 2002)
  - These microdeletions are too small to be detected on a karyotype but can be identified with molecular techniques (polymerase chain reaction [PCR]).
  - Most deletions occur on the long arm of the Y chromosome (Yq11) in the azoospermic factor (*AZF*) region.
  - Nonoverlapping segments in *AZF* region: *AZFa*, *AZFb*, and *AZFc*; these contain multiple genes important for spermatogenesis.
    - ⇨ **DAZ** (deleted in azoospermia) is in *AZFc*.
  - Distribution of frequencies for *AZF* deletions:

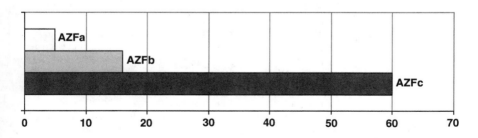

  - ⇨ Deletions involving two or three regions: 14%
  - ⇨ Deletions not involving *AZFa, b,* or *c*: 5%
  - No clear genotype–phenotype correlation: phenotype defined on the basis of semen analysis and testis histology:
    - ⇨ *AZFa–c* deletions → **absent spermatozoa**
    - ⇨ *AZFa* deletions: prognosis for sperm retrieval poor
    - ⇨ *AZFb* deletions: prognosis for sperm retrieval poor

GENETIC TESTING

⇨ *AZFc* deletions: may have sperm in ejaculate with severe oligozoospermia; others may be azoospermic but produce sufficient numbers to allow sperm recovery from testicular biopsy.

- Y microdeletions currently not associated with other known health problems, although limited information is available regarding phenotypes of sons of affected males. There is a concern that males with Y microdeletion may be at higher risk for offspring 45,X/46,XY karyotypes due to instability of the deleted Y chromosome (see Sex Chromosome Abnormalities table below) (Siffroi et al., 2000).

FEATURES OF COMMON SEX CHROMOSOME ABNORMALITIES

Karyotype; Name	Expected Phenotype
47,XXY; Klinefelter syndrome	1 in 500 newborn males.
	Most common cause of hypogonadism and infertility.
	Normal at birth, normal genitalia.
	Normal puberty, testicular size reduced, need for testosterone supplementation beginning in adolescence and through adulthood, infertility, risk for gynecomastia.
	Heterosexual orientation.
	Tall stature, slim, expressive language deficits.
	Risk of learning disabilities, especially in reading; 50% may have dyslexia.
47,XY/47,XXY; Klinefelter mosaic	Usually normal in appearance.
	Fertility possible in many cases.
	Developmental risks reduced consistent with 47,XXY.
47,XXX; Triple X	"Super female."
	1 in 1000 newborn females.
	Normal in appearance, tall stature.
	Normal puberty although poor ovarian function and early menopause.
	Risk for learning disabilities and hyperactivity, risk for depression, variable menses.
	No ↑ incidence of aggression.
45,X; Turner syndrome	At birth, may have congenital lymphedema; risk for cardiac malformations; webbing of neck; kidney malformations.
	Growth delay, short stature, risk for obesity.

continued

GENETIC TESTING

Karyotype; Name	Expected Phenotype
	Ovarian dysgenesis and absence of sexual development; hormone supplementation usually begun in adolescence.
	At risk for otitis media, cerebrovascular disease, hypertension, diabetes mellitus, thyroid disorders, obesity.
	Risk for learning disabilities, especially those involving spatial relations and perception; depression and decreased social skills and self-esteem.
45,X/46,XX; Turner mosaic	Often normal in appearance, may have slightly short stature.
	Fertility possible in many cases; at risk for spontaneous losses and early menopause.
	Developmental risks reduced compared with 45,X.
46,XX/47,XXX; Triple X mosaic	Usually normal in appearance, and fertility is likely.
	Developmental risks reduced compared with 47,XXX.
45,X/46,XY	Mixed gonadal dysgenesis.
	Gonads: one streak gonad (as in 45,X) and one poorly developed testis.
	Varying degrees of male-type genitalia due to varying testicular hormone production.
	Short stature as in 45,X.
	Wide spectrum of phenotype: normal male genitalia to mixed gonadal dysgenesis and ambiguous external genitalia to normal female external genitalia.
47,XYY	1 in 840 newborn males.
	Majority phenotypically normal.
	Accelerated growth in mid childhood; low-normal intelligence quotient, possible learning disability, speech delay common; poor musculature; behavior problems: hyperactivity and tantrums (aggression *not* a problem).
	Heterosexual.
	Puberty delayed by 6 mos.
Fragile X syndrome	X-linked autosomal-dominant inheritance; most common inherited cause of mental retardation.
	Caused by expanded CGG repeat sequence in the FMR1 gene; direct DNA analysis.
	Carrier frequency in women, 1 in 250.
	Almost all males and approximately 1/2 of females with the full mutation have significant mental retardation (1 in 2000 males; 1 in 4000 females).
	Screen those with developmental disability of unknown etiology: Autism.

GENETIC TESTING

Karyotype; Name	Expected Phenotype
	Family history of unexplained mental retardation or fragile X syndrome. Premature ovarian failure (up to $1/4$ are fragile X carriers).
Triploidy 69,XXY or 69,XYY	Rare and usually observed in aborted embryos/fetuses. If liveborn, demise is rapid (newborns with ambiguous genitalia).

Source: Adapted from Linden MG, Bender BG, Robinson A. Intrauterine diagnosis of sex chromosome aneuploidy. *Obstet Gynecol* 87(3):468, 1996.

33. Androgen Replacement Therapy

ANDROGENS
- Majority of androgens are synthesized by the adrenal glands and ovaries:

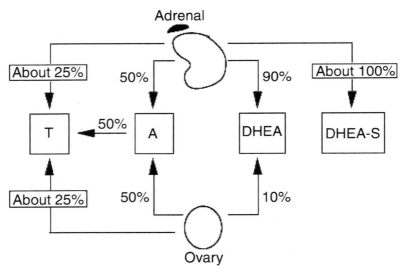

A, androstenedione; DHA, dehydroepiandrosterone; DHEA-S, dehydroepiandrosterone sulfate; T, testosterone. (Source: Adapted from Speroff L, Fritz MA, eds. *Clinical Gynecologic Endocrinology and Infertility* [7th ed]. Philadelphia: Lippincott Williams & Wilkins, 2005:503.)

- Dihydrotestosterone (DHT) is a nonaromatizable androgen.

- Binding affinity for steroids bound by sex hormone–binding globulin (SHBG) is DHT > testosterone (T) > androstenediol > estradiol > estrone (E_1) (Dunn et al., 1981).

Structure	Compound	Relative activity level
	Dihydrotestosterone	300
	Testosterone	100
	Androstenedione	10
	Dehydroepiandrosterone sulfate	5

- Question yet to be definitively answered: Does androgen-replacement treatment affect libido, energy, muscle mass and strength, and bone mineral density (BMD)?
- Androgen levels decline into menopausal transition (↓ from ovaries and adrenal glands)

317

ANDROGEN REPLACEMENT THERAPY

• Postmenopausal androgen production:

	↓ Testosterone (%)	Testosterone (μg/day)
Pre-MP	—	250
Natural MP	28	180
Surgical MP	50	125

MP, menopausal.
Source: Adapted from Snyder PJ. The role of androgens in women. *J Clin Endocrinol Metab* 86(3):1006, 2001.

	Testosterone (μg/day) % ↓	Androstenedione % ↓
Pre-MP ovariectomy	50	50
Natural MP	28	50
Post-MP ovariectomy	50	50

MP, menopausal.
Source: Adapted from Snyder PJ. The role of androgens in women. *J Clin Endocrinol Metab* 86(3):1006, 2001.

- In premenopausal women, ovariectomy results in equal fall in T and androstenedione (50%), suggesting that these two androgens come equally from the ovaries and adrenal glands in premenopausal women.
- In postmenopausal women, the T concentration drops more after an ovariectomy (50%) compared with natural menopause (MP). Therefore, the secretion of T, but not androstenedione, by the ovaries is maintained in MP.
• Total T does not change appreciably until women are very much older (71–95 yrs old).
• In a study examining the relation of remote hysterectomy ± oophorectomy to endogenous sex hormone levels in older women, bilateral salpingo-oophorectomy had little or no effect on circulating estradiol (E_2) levels in older women but was associated with a substantial and sustained reduction in bioavailable T levels. Although T levels were low around the time of MP, an apparent ↑ in

ANDROGEN REPLACEMENT THERAPY

ovarian T production and a return to premenopausal levels occurred in intact women (Laughlin et al., 2000).

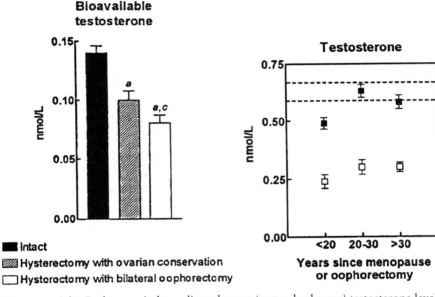

Bioavailable testosterone

Testosterone

■ Intact
▨ Hysterectomy with ovarian conservation
☐ Hysterectomy with bilateral oophorectomy

Years since menopause or oophorectomy

Figure on right: Body mass index–adjusted mean (± standard error) testosterone levels in 438 intact women (*closed squares*) and 123 bilateral salpingooophorectomy women (*open squares*) stratified by years since menopause for intact women and years since surgery. Dotted lines indicate the mean (± standard error) testosterone level for premenopausal women. (Source: Adapted from Laughlin GA, Barrett-Connor E, et al. Hysterectomy, oophorectomy, and endogenous sex hormone levels in older women: the Rancho Bernardo Study. *J Clin Endocrinol Metab* 85[2]:645, 2000.)

- The climacteric ovary is not a major androgen-producing gland (Couzinet et al., 2001):
  - In the absence of adrenal steroids, postmenopausal women have no circulating androgens.
    - ⇨ Absent from postmenopausal ovaries → T, androstenedione (A^4), P450aromatase, follicle-stimulating hormone (FSH) receptor, luteinizing hormone (LH) receptor

ANDROGEN REPLACEMENT THERAPY

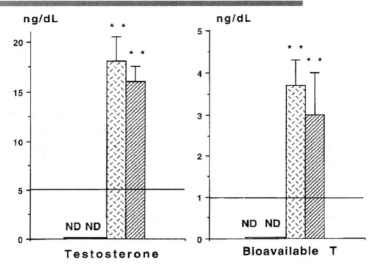

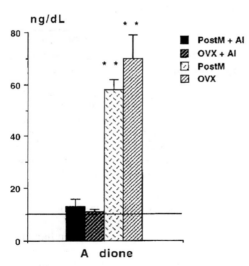

A dione, androstenedione; AI, adrenal insufficiency; PostM, postmenopausal; ND, no difference; OVX, ovariectomized women; T, testosterone. (Source: Reproduced with permission from Couzinet B, Meduri G, Lecce MG, et al. The postmenopausal ovary is not a major androgen-producing gland. *J Clin Endocrinol Metab* 86[10]:5060, 2001.)

ANDROGEN REPLACEMENT THERAPY

DECREASED LIBIDO: ESTRADIOL FIRST
- E_2 first: 90% reported a return of desire after 3–6 mos of E_2 treatment. Clitoral sensitivity returned, and there was return of orgasmic capacity (Sarrel, 1999). Adding androgens did not differ from E_2 alone (statistically).

INDICATIONS FOR ANDROGEN REPLACEMENT THERAPY
- A relationship between a specific free T level and diminished sexual symptoms has not been established (Dennerstein et al., 2002).
- Assays are insensitive at the lower end of normal T.
- Consider in patients with premature ovarian failure (e.g., Turner syndrome).
- Clinical profile most likely to respond to androgen replacement therapy (in a woman who is E_2 replete):
  - Persistent inexplicable fatigue
  - Blunted motivation
  - ↓ Libido
  - ↓ Well-being
  - ↓ Free T (in the lower 1/3 range)

CONTRAINDICATIONS
- Moderate to severe acne
- Clinical hirsutism
- Androgenic alopecia
- Known or suspected androgen-dependent neoplasia

SIDE EFFECTS
- Virilization/hirsutism
- Hoarseness
- Alopecia
- Fluid retention
- Acne
- Unknown if there is a relationship between androgen treatment and breast cancer incidence
- Adverse lipoprotein-lipid effects
- Clitoromegaly

ANDROGEN REPLACEMENT THERAPY
- Oral form only: methyltestosterone (MT) (0.625 mg E_2 + 1.25 mg or 1.25 mg E_2 + 2.5 mg)
  - MT is at least as potent as T.
  - 1936: Mocquot and Moricard (improved hot flashes)

ANDROGEN REPLACEMENT THERAPY

- Androgen replacement therapy decreases high-density lipoprotein (HDL) ($\downarrow$ 20%), triglycerides ($\downarrow$ 30%) (Basaria et al., 2002), and total cholesterol; no change in low-density lipoprotein (LDL)
- Further studies needed to assess the overall cardiovascular (CV) effect.
- For libido: need to restore T levels to at least the upper end of the normal physiologic range for ovulating women (although serum MT levels cannot be measured).
- Studies have demonstrated that androgen replacement therapy increases the bioavailability of androgens and E_2 by $\downarrow$ SHBG.
- Advantages of androgen replacement therapy:

$\uparrow$ Energy
$\uparrow$ Libido
$\uparrow$ Sexuality
$\uparrow$ Well-being
$\downarrow$ Breast tenderness
No change in lipids

- Disadvantages of androgen replacement therapy:

Masculinizing (hirsutism, acne, alopecia, voice, clitoromegaly)
Somatic (fluid retention, bloating)
Serious (hepatocellular, CV, and cancer risks)

ESTROGEN REPLACEMENT THERAPY EFFECTS ON CIRCULATING ANDROGENS (Casson et al., 1997)

- Natural MP does not lead to $\downarrow$ T until approximately 5 yrs post-MP, whereas dehydroepiandrosterone (DHEA) (–75%) and A (–50%) $\downarrow$ at the time of peri-MP.
- With surgical ablation, there is a 50% $\downarrow$ in T.
- T and E_2 are influenced by SHBG, but A^4 and E_1 have *no binding* to SHBG.
- Study: blinded, randomized >2 mg/day of *oral* micronized E_2 vs. placebo (Casson et al., 1997)
  - $\uparrow$ E_2 (8.7 pg/mL $\rightarrow$ 117 pg/mL)
  - $\downarrow$ T by 42%
  - $\uparrow$ SHBG by 160%
- Oral MT may $\uparrow$ lipoproteins and lead to long-term hepatic toxicity.
- Unknown if the above effects are seen with the current low-dose hormone-replacement therapy (HRT).
- This study not done with the addition of progesterone replacement.

ANDROGEN REPLACEMENT THERAPY

TESTOSTERONE PATCH TO IMPROVE SEXUAL FUNCTION
(Shifren et al., 2000)
- Long-term daily use of 300 µg T-patch (in conjunction with estrogen-replacement therapy [ERT]) was effective (as measured by improved sexual frequency, pleasure, and mood) for women >48 yrs old and status post–total abdominal hysterectomy (TAH)/bilateral salpingooophorectomy (BSO) with significantly impaired sexual function at baseline (patch not available as of spring 2005; in phase III clinical trials).

FUTURE
Selective Androgen Receptor Modulators
- Affecting selected proteins named *coactivators* or *corepressors*
- Desired profile of selective androgen receptor modulator (SARM) activity:
  - Enhance libido
  - Bone growth
  - Enhance muscle mass
  - Free of key side effects
  - No effect on liver enzymes

Tibolone
- Synthetic steroid with estrogenic, androgenic, and progestogenic properties (not available in the United States)
- Convincing efficacy for:
  - Hot flashes and sweating: significant reduction (equal to HRT)
  - Osteoporosis: ↓ bone turnover, significantly improves BMD (especially trabecular BMD); no fracture data as yet
- Unproven benefits:
  - Climacteric symptoms
  - Sexual function
  - Endometrium and vaginal bleeding: may not need concomitant progesterone; causes significantly more vaginal bleeding than placebo, but approximately 1/2 as much as combined HRT.
  - Lipids
  - Breast cancer: slows proliferation and increases apoptosis; efficacy unknown

34. Postmenopausal Hormone Therapy

HORMONE REPLACEMENT THERAPY (1950s–1990s) → HORMONE THERAPY (2002 TO PRESENT)

- Although the Women's Health Initiative (WHI) estradiol (E_2)/progestin and estrogen-only studies (see Hormone Therapy Risks and Benefits section) are not perfect, the indications and duration of hormone therapy (HT) have been revised. Many areas are still controversial; the following are general recommendations:

  - **Risks** and **benefits** of these interventions for perimenopausal and naturally and surgically postmenopausal women are now more clearly defined.
  - Unopposed estrogen therapy **does not ↑ breast cancer incidence** (see WHI data below); the role of progestins in combined E_2/progestin HT is still controversial.
  - Data on **prevention and treatment of osteoporosis** with fracture outcomes (not just bone mineral density [BMD]) are more complete for estrogen therapy than for any other treatment option.
  - Role of HT in primary prevention of coronary heart disease (CHD) is controversial; current data suggest that **neither primary nor secondary prevention of CHD is a valid indication** for starting or continuing therapy.
  - Major indications for HT with estrogen ± progestin are relief of **menopausal symptoms** and **prevention/treatment of osteoporosis.**
  - For **symptom relief,** use the lowest effective dose for the shortest time.
  - **Surgical menopause (MP) (bilateral salpingo-oophorectomy [BSO] ± hysterectomy)** and **prevention/treatment of osteoporosis** may be indications for **longer-term treatment** (>2–3 yrs). Use the lowest effective dose; review treatment every few years; and discuss risks, benefits, and alternative treatment options with the patient.
  - **Women currently on long-term HT** who are doing well should not automatically stop treatment but should be reevaluated and individually counseled. Stopping HT causes rapid loss of hip fracture protection (within 5 yrs) (Yates et al., 2004), so women who choose to stop HT need alternative therapy (selective estrogen receptor modulators [SERMs], bisphosphonates) and/or BMD follow-up.

POSTMENOPAUSAL HORMONE THERAPY

COMMON COMPLAINTS AND SYMPTOMS ENCOUNTERED IN THE PERIMENOPAUSE

- Vasomotor symptoms:
  - ↑ Hot flashes from pre-MP (10%) to MP (approximately 50%), but ↓ by 4 yrs after MP (20%).
  - Frequency of hot flashes is associated with ↓ E_2 and ↑ follicle-stimulating hormone (FSH), although this is not supported by definitive data.
- Irregular bleeding:
  - Must rule out endometrial hyperplasia.
    - ⇨ Transvaginal sonography; endometrium >4 mm requires sampling.
    - ⇨ Hysteroscopy or hysterogram (saline or water infusion sonogram) may reveal filling defects (polyps/submucous myomas).
- ↓ BMD:
  - ↑ Bone loss at all sites, but especially trabecular bone
  - ↑ Loss with positive risk factors (smoking, lack of exercise, poor diet, weight)
- Vaginal dryness and urethritis
- Hysterectomy:
  - 55% of all hysterectomies occur between ages 35 and 49 yrs.
  - Highest rate is between 40 and 44 yrs
  - Most common indications:
    - ⇨ Symptomatic fibroids
    - ⇨ Endometriosis
    - ⇨ Atypical hyperplasia or cancer
    - ⇨ Abnormal uterine bleeding

HORMONE THERAPY IN THE PERIMENOPAUSE

- Standard HT is not an adequate contraceptive.
  - Can use low-dose oral contraceptives (OCs) (20 µg ethinyl E_2) as HT for nonsmokers
  - Change to standard HT (oral, transdermal, and so forth) with lower estrogen doses 1–2 yrs after expected time of MP (mean, 51 yrs old).

POSTMENOPAUSAL HORMONE THERAPY

CLASSIC APPROACH TO HORMONE THERAPY (BASED ON OBSERVATIONAL STUDIES ONLY)

1. Estrogen is good for you.
2. Start taking it now.
3. Take it for the rest of your life.

Post–Women's Health Initiative Approach

- Individualize estimates of the benefit to risk ratio for HT.
  - Alleviating menopausal symptoms (no other treatment is as effective, but symptoms were not included in WHI main outcome measures)
  - Bone preserving (annual loss in bone mass after MP: 3–5%).
  - **Risk of breast cancer:** No ↑ risk found with E_2 alone in WHI study; questionable progestin (Provera) effect.
  - Cardioprotective: Observational data (e.g., Nurses' Health Study [NHS]) may well have overstated CHD reduction, *but* younger, healthier patients starting HT closer to MP may still reap benefit vs. older population, smokers, obese patients, and those farther from MP in WHI studies.
  - Memory preservation: weak data; ↓ **cognitive function in WHI studies**

HORMONE THERAPY RISKS AND BENEFITS

Large Observational Studies

Nurses' Health Study

- NHS: 48,470 postmenopausal women, 10-yr prospective cohort study:

Nurses' Health Study: E_2 Users vs. Nonusers	Relative Risk
↑ Breast cancer in current hormone therapy users	1.33 (1.12–1.57)
No significant effect on stroke	0.97 (0.65–1.45)
↓ Rate of CHD events in current E_2 users	0.56 (0.40–0.80)[a]
↓ CHD events in low-CHD-risk women[b]	0.53 (0.31–0.91)[a]
↓ CHD mortality in current/past E_2 users	0.72 (0.55–0.95)[a]

CHD, coronary heart disease; E_2, estradiol.

[a]Not supported by large randomized controlled trials (Women's Health Initiative).

[b]Low CHD risk: excludes smoking, diabetes mellitus, hypertension, ↑ cholesterol, or body mass index >90th percentile.

Source: Adapted from Stampfer MJ, Colditz GA, Willett WC, et al. Postmenopausal estrogen therapy and cardiovascular disease. Ten-year follow-up from the nurses' health study. *N Engl J Med* 325(11):756, 1991; and Colditz GA, Stampfer MJ, Willett WC, et al. Type of postmenopausal hormone use and risk of breast cancer: 12-year follow-up from the Nurses' Health Study. *Cancer Causes Control* 3(5):433, 1992.

POSTMENOPAUSAL HORMONE THERAPY

- NHS CHD data were based on 10 yrs' follow-up (337,854 woman-yrs) and provided a rationale for the widespread use of HT for **primary prevention of CHD** in postmenopausal women.
- The finding of ↑ breast cancer risk in HT users was based on 12 yrs' follow-up (480,665 woman-yrs) and was assessed for subgroups as follows:

Nurses' Health Study: Breast Cancer Risks	Relative Risk
↑ Breast cancer in unopposed E_2 users	1.42 (1.19–1.70)[a]
Breast cancer in E_2 + progestin users	1.54 (0.99–2.39)
Breast cancer in progestin-only users	2.52 (0.66–9.63)

E_2, estradiol.
[a]Not supported by large randomized controlled trials (Women's Health Initiative).
Source: Adapted from Stampfer MJ, Colditz GA, Willett WC, et al. Postmenopausal estrogen therapy and cardiovascular disease. Ten-year follow-up from the nurses' health study. *N Engl J Med* 325(11):756, 1991; and Colditz GA, Stampfer MJ, Willett WC, et al. Type of postmenopausal hormone use and risk of breast cancer: 12-year follow-up from the Nurses' Health Study. *Cancer Causes Control* 3(5):433, 1992.

- **Neither the strong benefit for primary prevention of CHD nor the ↑ breast cancer risk with unopposed E_2 has been supported by later randomized controlled trials** (Heart and Estrogen/Progestin Replacement Study [HERS] and the two WHI studies, see below).

Randomized Controlled Trials
Heart and Estrogen/Progestin Replacement Study
- HERS: 2321 women with CHD and a uterus:

HERS: Estradiol + Progestins vs. Placebo	Hazard Ratio (Confidence Interval)
↑ Venous thromboembolism	2.08 (1.28–3.40)
↑ Biliary tract surgery	1.48 (1.12–1.95)
No significant effect on cancers	1.19 (0.95–1.50)
No significant effect on hip, wrist, other fractures	? Need ≥10-yr estrogen therapy
Similar rate of coronary heart disease events	0.96 (0.77–1.19)

Source: Adapted from Grady D, Herrington D, Bittner V, et al. Cardiovascular Disease Outcomes During 6.8 Years of Hormone Therapy: Heart and Estrogen/Progestin Replacement Study Follow-up (HERS II). *JAMA* 288(1):49, 2002; and Hulley S, Furberg C, Barrett-Connor E, et al. Noncardiovascular Disease Outcomes During 6.8 Years of Hormone Therapy: Heart and Estrogen/Progestin Replacement Study Follow-up (HERS II). *JAMA* 288(1):58, 2002.

Raloxifene Use for the Heart (RUTH) (Pending)
- **RUTH:** 10,000 postmenopausal women with CHD, results expected in 2005

POSTMENOPAUSAL HORMONE THERAPY

Women's Health Initiative

- **WHI E_2 + progestin:** 16,608 postmenopausal women without CHD: effect of E_2 + progestin in women *without* CHD; results at 5.2 yrs:

Parameter	Hazard Ratio (Confidence Interval)	Absolute Risk[a]
↑ Invasive breast cancer	1.26 (1.00–1.59)	+8
↑ Coronary heart disease events	1.29 (1.02–1.63)	+7
↑ Stroke	1.41 (1.07–1.85)	+8
↑ Pulmonary embolism	2.13 (1.39–3.25)	+8
Endometrial cancer	0.83 (0.47–1.47)	No difference
↓ Colorectal cancer	0.63 (0.43–0.92)	−6
↓ Hip fracture	0.66 (0.45–0.98)	−5
↓ Vertebral fracture[b]	0.66 (0.44–0.98)	−6
↓ Other osteoporotic fracture[b]	0.77 (0.69–0.86)	−39

[a]Absolute risk: number of excess events per 10,000 woman-yrs of treatment.
[b]Not included in global index of main outcomes.
Source: Adapted from Rossouw JE, Anderson GL, Prentice RL, et al. Risks and benefits of estrogen plus progestin in healthy postmenopausal women: principal results from the Women's Health Initiative randomized controlled trial. *JAMA* 288(3):321, 2002.

- **WHI E_2 alone:** 10,739 postmenopausal women without CHD; halted in February, 2004. Results from 6.8 yrs' mean follow-up:

Parameter	Hazard Ratio (Confidence Interval)	Absolute Risk[a]
↑ Stroke	1.39 (1.10–1.77)	+12
Invasive breast cancer	0.77 (0.59–1.01)	No difference
Coronary heart disease	0.91 (0.75–1.12)	No difference
Pulmonary embolism	1.34 (0.87–2.06)	No difference
Colorectal cancer	1.08 (0.75–1.55)	No difference
↓ Hip fracture	0.61 (0.41–0.91)	−6

[a]Absolute risk: number of excess events per 10,000 woman-yrs of treatment.
Source: Adapted from Anderson GL, Limacher M, Assaf AR, et al.; Women's Health Initiative Steering Committee. Effects of conjugated equine estrogen in postmenopausal women with hysterectomy: the Women's Health Initiative randomized controlled trial. *JAMA* 291(14):1701, 2004.

- **Women's Health Initiative Memory Study (WHIMS)** found adverse effects of conjugated equine estrogen (CEE) on cognitive function and ↑ dementia and ↑ mild cognitive impairment in both E_2/medroxyprogesterone acetate (MPA) and E_2-alone studies (Shumaker et al., 2004; Espeland et al., 2004), but these findings are based on a subset of WHI patients, as cognitive performance was not one of the primary outcome measures of the WHI study.

328

POSTMENOPAUSAL HORMONE THERAPY

Why the Discrepancy between Observational and Randomized Controlled Trials?

- Why did large observational studies (NHS) show ↓ CHD and ↑ breast cancer incidence in HT users, but these findings were not substantiated in recent large randomized controlled trials (HERS, two WHI studies)?

In Favor of Hormone Therapy

- Primary vs. secondary prevention
- Differences exist between the NHS population and the WHI subjects (e.g., mean age in NHS, 57 yrs old vs. WHI E_2/progestin study, 63 yrs old). WHI subjects thus started HT at an average of 12 yrs post-MP, in contrast with women in the NHS, who commenced hormones in the peri-menopausal or early postmenopausal periods consistent with both primary prevention goals and with typical clinical practice.
- WHI studies combine a smaller (<20% of the study) primary prevention group of patients in their early 50s at the start of the study with a much larger secondary prevention group of patients in their late 50s to late 70s. In the E_2/MPA WHI study, only 33% of subjects and control subjects were 50–59 yrs old, and only 16–17% were within 5 yrs of the MP at enrollment (Naftolin et al., 2004).
- Despite their large overall size, the WHI trials are **severely underpowered** to detect a CHD reduction resulting from HT started in 50- to 54-yr-olds soon after the MP (Naftolin et al., 2004).

In Favor of the Women's Health Initiative Conclusions

- Observational studies like NHS suffer from the *healthy user effect*, in which nurses using HT were more likely to have confounding positive lifestyle factors, such as being less likely to smoke, leading to apparently ↓ CHD in HT users without a direct causative effect. Also, ↑ breast examinations/↑ mammography use may have ↑ breast cancer diagnosis in HT users for the NHS participants.
- NHS excluded silent myocardial infarction, whereas these were included in WHI data (Col and Pauker, 2003). Biases in the classification of deaths by unblinded investigators may have occurred in the NHS study.
- RCT data are less subject to confounding and bias such as the effects listed above.

HORMONE THERAPY ADMINISTRATION AND DOSING

- Traditional estrogens used in HT
  - Bioequivalent formulations:
    - ⇨ **0.625 mg conjugated estrogens: CEE (Premarin), plant-derived conjugated estrogens** (Cenestin), **esterified estrogen** (Estratab)
    - ⇨ **1 mg micronized E_2** (Estrace)
    - ⇨ **0.005 mg (5 μg) oral ethinyl E_2** (OCs)
    - ⇨ **0.05 mg/day 17β-E_2** (patches)

329

POSTMENOPAUSAL HORMONE THERAPY

- Lower estrogen doses for HT
  - Women's Health, Osteoporosis, Progestin, Estrogen (HOPE) study, a randomized controlled trial (Utian et al., 2001), found that lower daily doses of CEE of 0.3 mg or 0.45 mg produced comparable symptom relief to standard doses (0.625 mg/day).
  - Both CEE doses were effective in increasing spine and hip BMD (Lindsay et al., 2002).
  - 14 µg/day transdermal 17β-E_2 weekly patch (Menostar) preserves BMD without endometrial hyperplasia (Ettinger et al., 2004).

Progestins and Natural Progesterone

- **Progestins greatly reduce the risk of endometrial hyperplasia/endometrial carcinoma associated with estrogen therapy** (but not down to zero).
- **Most data exist for MPA (WHI E_2/MPA arm).** The progestin component may be responsible for some of the adverse effects in the combined HT study that were not found by the E_2-alone arm. However, large studies of other progestins are lacking.
- **Possible disadvantages of adding progestins:**
  - $\uparrow$ Breast cancer risk? (suggested by WHI data but not proven)
  - Adverse effect on lipid profiles ($\uparrow$ low-density lipoprotein, $\downarrow$ high-density lipoprotein; may reduce E_2 benefits)
  - Impaired glucose tolerance (rarely clinically significant)
- **Cyclic vs. continuous combined therapy** (for women without hysterectomy):
  - Cyclic therapy usually consists of 10–12 days/month of progestin/progesterone (P_4) followed by a withdrawal bleed.
    - ⇨ May be better tolerated in the peri-MP than continuous combined therapy ($\downarrow$ breakthrough bleeding)
  - Continuous combined therapy adds a daily dose of progestin/P_4 to estrogen therapy
    - ⇨ May be via the same administration route as E_2 (i.e., oral CEE and MPA [Prempro], oral E_2/norethindrone acetate [NETA; Activella], or transdermal E_2/progestin [see below])
    - ⇨ Some combinations require two routes, e.g., transdermal E_2 patches/levonorgestrel intrauterine system (LNG-IUS).
  - **MPA (Provera)**
    - ⇨ Standard doses are 5 or 10 mg/day × 10–14 days/month for cyclic HT; 2.5 or 5.0 mg/day for standard-dose continuous combined HT. Low-dose MPA (1.5 mg/day) is used with CEE 0.3 or 0.45 mg/day for continuous combined HT.
  - **NETA:** Aygestin alone, FemHRT with ethinyl E_2
    - ⇨ Standard doses are 5 or 10 mg/day × 10–14 days/month for cyclic HT; 1.0–2.5 mg/day for standard-dose continuous combined HT.

330

POSTMENOPAUSAL HORMONE THERAPY

- Micronized P_4 (Prometrium)
  - ⇨ Identical to natural P_4 (bioequivalent HT). May cause drowsiness; give q.h.s.
  - ⇨ Standard doses are 200 or 300 mg/day × 10–14 days/month for cyclic HT; 100–200 mg/day for standard-dose continuous combined HT.
- LNG-IUS (Mirena)
  - ⇨ Induces endometrial atrophy and amenorrhea; lasts for 5 yrs (off-label use)
  - ⇨ Randomized trial of 200 women receiving E_2 with the LNG-IUS vs. oral E_2/NETA found equal efficacy for endometrial protection and higher continuation rates with the LNG-IUS over 2 yrs' follow-up (Boon et al., 2003).

Transdermal Hormone Therapy Patches

- Doses range from 0.015–0.1 mg/day of E_2. 0.05 and 0.1 mg/day doses are most commonly used; typically, start with 0.05 mg/day.
  - Avoiding first-pass liver metabolism is beneficial for patients with ↑ triglyceridemia but loses the favorable effects of E_2 on cholesterol profile (E_2 ↓ LDL, ↑ HDL).
- Once-weekly application:
  - E_2 alone: Climara, Menostar, generic
  - Combination E_2/progestin: E_2/LNG patch, 0.045 mg E_2/day (Climara Pro)
- Twice-weekly application:
  - E_2 alone: Alora, Esclim, Estraderm, Vivelle, Vivelle-Dot, generic
  - Combination E_2/progestin: E_2/NETA patch, E_2 0.05 mg/day, progestin doses 0.14 or 0.25 mg/day (CombiPatch)

NEWER HORMONE THERAPY FORMULATIONS AND ROUTES

Estring

- Estring: low-dose (2 mg) E_2 vaginal ring (Femring, below, or NuvaRing, a vaginal contraceptive ring containing both ethinyl E_2 and the progestin etonogestrel). Worn continuously for 3 mos = 0.0075 mg (7.5 µg) E_2/day → serum E_2 level: approximately 8–11 pg/mL.
  - Indicated only for urogenital symptoms from vulvovaginal atrophy
  - Low serum E_2 levels: does not relieve hot flashes. Low systemic side effects.
  - Systemic E_2 dose should be too low to produce **endometrial hyperplasia**.
  - Unlikely to have withdrawal bleeds with progestins due to low E_2 dose

Femring

- Femring: higher-dose (12 or 24 mg) E_2 vaginal ring. Two strengths: 0.05 and 0.1 mg/day. Worn continuously for 3 mos → serum E_2 level: ~41 pg/mL with 0.05 mg/day, ~76 pg/mL with 0.1 mg/day.

POSTMENOPAUSAL HORMONE THERAPY

- Indicated for both vasomotor symptoms and urogenital symptoms
- Significant serum E_2 levels: systemic effects comparable to oral/transdermal HT
- Need to add cyclic or continuous progestins in women without hysterectomy

EstroGel

- EstroGel: E_2 0.06% transdermal gel (used in Europe, available in the United States from 2004). Dose: 1.25 g gel/day = 0.75 mg E_2/day $\rightarrow$ $\uparrow$ serum E_2 level: ~28–30 pg/mL
  - Indicated for moderate-severe vasomotor symptoms ± vaginal atrophy
  - Avoids first-pass metabolism by the liver (like E_2 patches)
  - Combine with continuous or cyclic progestin/P_4 for women with a uterus.

Tibolone

- Tibolone: synthetic steroid with estrogenic, androgenic, and progestogenic properties (used in Europe; not available in the United States)
  - Convincing efficacy for
    - ⇨ Hot flashes and sweating: significant reduction (equal to HT)
    - ⇨ Osteoporosis: ↓ bone turnover, significantly improves BMD (especially trabecular BMD); no fracture data as yet pending completion of the Long-Term Intervention on Fractures with Tibolone (LIFT) study
  - Unproven benefits:
    - ⇨ Climacteric symptoms
    - ⇨ Sexual function
    - ⇨ Endometrium and vaginal bleeding: may not need concomitant progestin; causes significantly more vaginal bleeding than placebo, but approximately 1/2 as much as combined HT.
    - ⇨ Lipids
    - ⇨ Breast cancer: slows proliferation and increases apoptosis; efficacy unknown

A. Hormone Therapy

Active Ingredients	Drug Name	Company	Typical Daily Dosage Choices
Estrogens			
CEEs	Premarin	Wyeth-Ayerst	0.3, 0.625, 0.9, 1.25, 2.5 mg/ continuous daily dosing or cyclic dosing
17β Estradiol (oral)	Estrace	Warner Chilcott	0.5, 1.0, 2.0 mg/continuous daily dosing
17β Estradiol (transdermal)	Climera	Berlex	0.025, 0.05, 0.075, 0.1 mg weekly patch
	Alora	Watson	0.05, 0.075, 0.1 mg/change patch 2×/wk
	Esclim	Women First	0.025, 0.0375, 0.05, 0.075, 0.1 mg/change patch 2×/wk
	Estraderm	Novartis	0.05, 0.1 mg/change patch 2×/wk
	Vivelle dot	Novartis	0.0375, 0.05, 0.075, 0.1 mg/ change patch 2×/wk
Estropipate	Ogen	Pharmacia	0.625, 1.25, 2.5 mg/continuous daily dosing or cyclic dosing
	Ortho-EST	Women First	0.625, 1.25 mg/continuous daily dosing or cyclic dosing
Esterified estrogens	Estratab	Solvay	0.3, 0.625, 2.5 mg/continuous daily dosing
	Menest	Monarch	0.3, 0.625, 1.25, 2.5 mg/cyclic dosing (3 wks on therapy, 1 wk off)
Synthetic conjugated estrogens	Cenestin	Duramed/ Solvay	0.625, 0.9, 1.25 mg/continuous daily dosing
Oral estrogen-progestin combination therapy			
CEEs and MPA	PremPro	Wyeth-Ayerst	0.625 mg CEE plus 2.5 mg MPA, 0.625 mg CEE plus 5 mg MPA
	PremPhase	Wyeth-Ayerst	0.625 mg CEE days 1–14, 0.625 mg CEE plus 5 mg MPA days 15–28
EE and NE	Fem HRT	Parke-Davis	5 μg EE plus 1 mg NE; continuous daily dosing

continued

POSTMENOPAUSAL HORMONE THERAPY

Active Ingredients	Drug Name	Company	Typical Daily Dosage Choices
Micronized estradiol and norgestimate	Ortho-Prefest	Ortho-McNeil	1 mg 17β estradiol (continuous) and 0.09 mg norgestimate (pulsed in 3-day cycles)
Micronized estradiol and NE	Activella	Pharmacia	1 mg 17β estradiol and 0.5 mg NE; continuous daily dosing
Combination oral estrogen and testosterone			
CEEs and MT	Estratest	Solvay	1.25 mg CEE plus 2.5 mg MT; cyclic dosing (3 wks on therapy, 1 wk off)
	Estratest-HS		0.625 mg CEE plus 1.25 mg MT; cyclic dosing (3 wks on therapy, 1 wk off)
Transdermal combination therapy			
17β Estradiol and NE	CombiPatch	Aventis	0.05 mg 17β estradiol and 0.14 mg NE or 0.05 mg 17β estradiol and 0.25 mg NE; change patch 2×/wk
Vaginal estrogen therapy			
CEE	Premarin	Wyeth-Ayerst	0.625 mg/g; daily
17β Estradiol	Estrace	Warner-Chilcott	0.1 mg/g; daily then 1–3×/wk
Estropipate	Ogen	Pharmacia	1.5 mg/g; daily
Dienestrol	Ortho Dienestrol	Ortho-McNeil	0.1 mg/g; daily then 1–3×/wk
Estradiol	Vagifem	Pharmacia	25 μg tablets daily for 2 wks then 2×/wk
Vaginal estrogen ring			
Estradiol	Estring	Pharmacia	2 mg reservoir; replace every 90 days

CEE, conjugated equine estrogen; EE, ethinyl estradiol; MPA, medroxyprogesterone acetate; MT, methyltestosterone; NE, norethindrone acetate. (Source: Reproduced with permission from Gordon JD, Rydfors JT, et al., eds. *Obstetrics Gynecology and Infertility* [5th ed]. Arlington, VA: Scrub Hill Press, Inc. 2001.)

35. Postmenopausal Osteoporosis

DEFINITION
- Low bone mass and microarchitectural deterioration with consequent ↑ bone fragility and susceptibility to fracture
- Osteoporosis (OP) most frequently found in postmenopausal white women, although it can occur in any age group.
- Approximately 10–15% of women who take estrogen lose bone.
- Diagnosis: bone densitometry

PREVALENCE AND INCIDENCE
- 13–18% in women >50 yrs of age (Looker et al., 1997)
- >1.3 million osteoporotic fractures/year in the United States

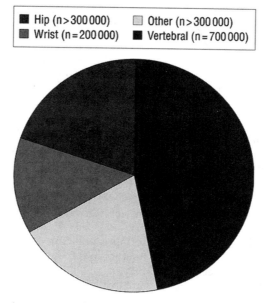

■ Hip (n > 300 000)   ☐ Other (n > 300 000)
■ Wrist (n = 200 000)   ■ Vertebral (n = 700 000)

Annual incidence of osteoporotic fractures in the United States. (Source: Reproduced with permission from Ettinger MP. Aging bone and osteoporosis: strategies for preventing fractures in the elderly. *Arch Intern Med* 163[18]:2237, 2003.)

335

POSTMENOPAUSAL OSTEOPOROSIS

- 8 million women: OP (United States)
- 20 million women: osteopenia (United States)
- 250,000 hip fractures
- Postmenopausal women lose approximately 3% cortical and 8% trabecular bone/year.

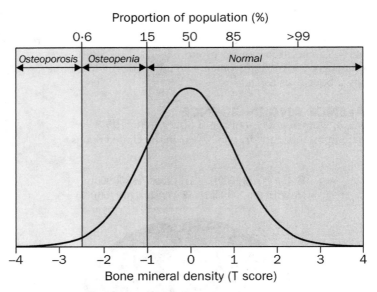

Proportion of population (%)

Distribution of bone mineral density in healthy women aged 30–40 years. (Source: Reproduced with permission from Kanis JA. Diagnosis of osteoporosis and assessment of fracture risk. *Lancet* 359[9321]:1929, 2002.)

SCREENING

- Controversial but justified for the following reasons:
  - Common disease
  - Associated with high morbidity, mortality, and cost
    - ⇨ Estimated cost of osteoporotic fracture in the United States for 1995 was $13.8 billion (Ray et al., 1997).
  - Accurate and safe diagnostic tests are available.
  - Effective treatments are available.
  - Risk factors for OP in postmenopausal women:

336

⇨ History of fracture as an adult, history of fragility fracture in a 1st-degree relative, low body weight (less than approximately 57.7 kg [127 lb]), current smoking, use of oral glucocorticoids for >3 mos, impaired vision due to risk of falling, estrogen deficiency at an early age (<45 yrs), poor health/frailty, recent falls, low calcium intake (lifelong), low physical activity, and alcohol >2 drinks per day

PATHOGENESIS

- Mismatch between bone resorption and bone formation
- Mechanisms of the microarchitectural disruption are not clear.
- ↑ Remodeling itself may cause structural weakening, which may account for the independent association of high bone turnover with fracture risk.
- Age-related bone loss begins in the 4th or 5th decades → slow loss of cortical and trabecular bone → continues in the 9th and 10th decades.
- Menopause-related bone loss begins soon after the onset of menopause and the estrogen deficiency that accompanies it → rapid acceleration of bone loss, particularly trabecular bone.
- Mechanism by which lack of estrogen leads to ↑ bone loss in women is not well understood:
  - Direct effect on osteoclast function and changes in the release of certain cytokines (i.e., interleukin [IL]-1, IL-6, tumor necrosis factor [TNF]-α, prostaglandin [PG] E_2)

DIAGNOSIS

- Silent disease until complicated by stress fracture
- Clinically, vertebral fracture can be suspected in patients with back pain, vertebral deformities by physical examination (kyphosis), or loss of height.
- After a hip fracture, nearly 1 in 6 patients aged 50 to 55 yrs and more than 1/2 of those older than 90 yrs are discharged from the hospital to a nursing home (Walker-Bone et al., 2001).
- Standard x-rays do not detect OP until approximately 40% of bone mass is lost.
- Gold standard of bone mineral density (BMD): **dual energy x-ray absorptiometry (DXA)** of the spine and hip:
  - Assesses cortical and cancellous bone; BMD ↑ 3–6% in the 1st year of bisphosphonate therapy.
  - DXA can be used to monitor response to treatment.
  - **DXA T score: number of standard deviations (SDs) above or below the average BMD for a healthy 30-yr-old woman.**

POSTMENOPAUSAL OSTEOPOROSIS

- **DXA Z score:** number of SDs above or below the average BMD for age- and sex-method controls; a Z score below –1 indicates a value in the lowest 25% of the reference range (risk of fractures doubled).
- Note: Z scores rather than T scores should be used for healthy **premenopausal** women.
- Biochemical markers:
  - Assess cancellous bone only.
  - Provide monitoring information; subject to diurnal variation.
  - Change in markers seen as early as 1–3 mos into therapy.
  - Some clinicians recommend checking markers at 3 mos.

Serum markers of bone **formation**	Alkaline phosphatase, osteocalcin
Serum markers of bone **resorption**	C-telopeptide (CTx)
Urine markers of bone **resorption**	N-telopeptide (NTx), deoxypyridinoline

- **T score:** compares the patient with mean peak bone mass levels as a difference in SD score from a 30-yr-old reference point:

T Score	World Health Organization Classification
Greater than or equal to –1	Normal
–1 to –2.5	Osteopenia
Less than –2.5	Osteoporosis

  - –1 SD: twofold ↑ hip fractures
  - –2 SD: fourfold ↑ hip fractures
  - –3 SD: eightfold ↑ hip fractures

POSTMENOPAUSAL OSTEOPOROSIS

- The lowest T score of posteroanterior (PA) spine, femoral neck, total hip, tro-chanter, or the 33% radius, if measured, should be selected.

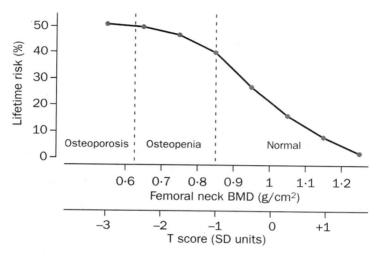

Lifetime risk of hip fractures in women aged 50 yrs according to bone mineral density (BMD) or T score at the hip. SD, standard deviation. (Source: Reproduced with permission from Kanis JA. Diagnosis of osteoporosis and assessment of fracture risk. *Lancet* 359[9321]:1929, 2002.)

- A 50-yr-old woman has a 40% lifetime risk of an osteoporotic fracture.
- $1/3$ of women >80 yrs old sustain a hip fracture, and 15–20% die from complications.
- Obtain DXA if
  - Postmenopausal (approximately 10% of women taking estradiol [E_2] lose bone)
  - Endocrine diseases (hyperthyroidism, hyperprolactinemia with amenorrhea) (Colao et al., 2000)
  - Secondary amenorrhea (>1 yr)
  - Anorexia nervosa ($\downarrow$ follicle-stimulating hormone [FSH], luteinizing hormone [LH], triiodothyronine [T_3]; $\uparrow$ reverse T_3 [rT_3], cortisol)
  - Malabsorption disorders
  - Medications (anticonvulsants, glucocorticoids, excessive levothyroxine sodium [Synthroid], prolonged gonadotropin-releasing hormone [GnRH]-agonist)

POSTMENOPAUSAL OSTEOPOROSIS

- Tests to evaluate other (nonmenopausal) etiologies:
  - Complete blood count (CBC), creatinine
  - Thyroid-stimulating hormone (TSH)
  - Electrolytes
  - Liver function tests
  - Ca^{2+}, PO_4, alkaline phosphatase
  - Premenopausal with amenorrhea not due to polycystic ovary syndrome (PCOS):
    - ⇨ E_2, FSH
  - Base on clinical situation:
    - ⇨ Intact parathyroid hormone (PTH) with calcium
    - ⇨ 24-Hr urine free cortisol
    - ⇨ 25-Hydroxy-vitamin D (osteomalacia)
    - ⇨ Evaluation for occult malignancy (including multiple myeloma, bony metastasis)
- In response to treatment of OP, markers respond faster and more dramatically than bone density.
  - A 30% or greater reduction in bone turnover is desirable to confirm a response to therapy.

TREATMENT
- T score less than or equal to −2.0: all women
- T scores of −1.5 to −2.0: prevention strategies and treatment for women with risk factors (family history, prior fracture, smokers, <128 lb, high bone turnover)
- Combined therapy (e.g., estrogen + alendronate) is synergistic (Greenspan et al., 2003).
- Preventive measures for OP:

Drug	Dose
Calcium carbonate, calcium citrate	1000–1500 mg/day (calcium citrate has fewer side effects)
Vitamin D	400–800 IU/day
Exercise[a]	Weight bearing (e.g., walking ≥40 mins/session, ≥4 sessions/wk

[a]Data from Kemmler W, Lauber D, et al. Benefits of 2 years of intense exercise on bone density, physical fitness, and blood lipids in early postmenopausal osteopenic women: results of the Erlangen Fitness Osteoporosis Prevention Study (EFOPS). *Arch Intern Med* 164(10):1084, 2004.

POSTMENOPAUSAL OSTEOPOROSIS

- Nonpharmacologic treatments include diet (adequate intake of calories to avoid malnutrition, calcium, and vitamin D), weight-bearing exercise, and smoking cessation.
- Estrogen/progestin therapy is no longer a first-line approach for the treatment of OP in postmenopausal women because of increased risk of breast cancer, stroke, venous thromboembolism (VTE), and perhaps coronary disease (Women's Health Initiative [WHI]).
- Bisphosphonates reduce bone turnover and increase BMD:

Drug	Half-Life
Alendronate (Fosamax)	10 yrs
Risedronate (Actonel)	3 wks

- Antifracture efficacy of various treatments based on placebo-controlled randomized trials:

Drug	Vertebral Fractures	Hip Fractures
Raloxifene	+++	++
Bisphosphonates	+++	++
Calcitonin (nasal)	+	0
Parathyroid hormone	+++	NA
Vitamin D derivatives	±	0
Estrogen[a]	+	0
Strontium ranelate	++	NA
Fluoride	±	−
Statins[a]	0	0

+++, strong evidence; ++, good evidence; +, some evidence; ±, equivocal; 0, no effects; −, negative effects; NA, none available.
[a]Evidence derived mainly from observational studies.

POSTMENOPAUSAL OSTEOPOROSIS

- Medicines:

Drug	Dose	Comments	Side Effects
Raloxifene (Evista)	60 mg/day	Lowers low-density lipoprotein; no effect on high-density lipoprotein Long-term effects on cardiovascular disease (RUTH study, 2005) and breast cancer not yet known	Hot flashes Muscle cramps Venous thromboembolism
Bisphosphonates			
Alendronate (Fosamax)	T: 10 mg/day or 70 mg/wk	Nonspecific gastrointestinal symptoms often related to Ca^{2+}, not the drug ↑ Ca^{2+}/vitamin D intake to avoid hypocalcemia Encouraging clinical trials (Reid et al., 2002)	Esophageal irritation/erosion Muscle pain Uveitis
Risedronate (Actonel)	P: 5 mg/day T and P: 5 mg/day or 35 mg/wk		
Zoledronic acid (Zometa)	4 mg IV once/yr		
Calcitonin (Miacalcin)	200 IU, 1 intranasal spray/day	Anecdotal evidence of reducing bone pain in acute fracture	Nasal stuffiness or rhinitis
Teriparatide (rPTH) (Forteo)	20 µg SC 1/day	Approved by the U.S. Food and Drug Administration for "high risk"[a] fracture groups	Nausea, headache, hypercalcemia ? Risk of osteosarcoma with high dose
Vitamin D (Calcitriol)	0.25 µg PO 2/day	Least favorite choice due to lack of proven consistent benefit	Hypercalcemia Hypercalciuria Renal insufficiency

P, prevention; T, treatment.
[a]"High risk": those with previous osteoporotic fractures, multiple risk factors for fractures, or failed previous therapy.

- Contraindications:

Drug	Contraindications
Raloxifene (Evista)	History of venous thromboembolism
Bisphosphonates	Hypocalcemia Esophageal stricture Unable to remain upright after dosing
Calcitonin (Miacalcin)	Hypocalcemia Renal failure Allergy to calcitonin

- Evidence for the effect of pharmacologic therapy on OP-related outcomes by patient group:

Therapy	Patient Group	
	Postmenopause, Any	Postmenopause + Osteoporosis
Calcium + vitamin D	↑ BMD [A]	↓ Hip fracture [A] (if patient vitamin D deficient)
Alendronate	↑ BMD [A]	↓ Spine and hip fracture [A]
Risedronate	↑ BMD [A]	↓ Spine and hip fracture [A]
Raloxifene	↑ BMD [A]	↓ Spine fracture [A] (trend: ↓ non-spine fracture [A])
Estrogen	↑ BMD [A]	↓ Spine and hip fracture [C]
Calcitonin	↑ BMD [A]	↓ Spine fracture [A]

BMD, bone mineral density.
Note: Levels of evidence reflect the best available literature in support of an intervention or test: A, randomized controlled trials; B, controlled trials, no randomization; C, observational trials; D, opinion of expert panel.

MONITORING RESPONSE TO THERAPY: SEVERAL APPROACHES

1. DXA scan after 1 yr of therapy:
   - Single site measurement can be misleading; hence, both spine and hip mineral density should be measured.
   - If significant ↓ at both sites → modify therapy.
   - If loss at one site and no change or ↓ at the other site → repeat in 1 yr.
2. DXA after 2 yrs of therapy:
   - For most, this provides the most meaningful information.
   - May delay detection of poor response
3. DXA + biochemical markers of bone turnover
   - Recommended approach

POSTMENOPAUSAL OSTEOPOROSIS

- Measure at baseline and repeat measurement of markers in 6 mos.
- If marker ↓ significantly (i.e., >50% of urine N-telopeptide [NTx] and >30% for serum C-telopeptide [CTx]) → therapy is having desired effect → repeat DXA after 2 yrs
4. No monitoring
    - No evidence that outcome can be improved in those who do not respond to therapy
- Effective antiresorptive treatments induce a ↓ in bone turnover that reaches plateau within 1–3 mos for oral bisphosphonates and usually up to 6 mos for various types of estrogen, raloxifene, and nasal calcitonin, depending on the potency and route of administration of the drug and on the marker (Delmas, 2000). Changes in bone turnover markers produced by raloxifene and calcitonin are generally smaller than those produced by the bisphosphonates and hormone therapy (HT) (Delmas, 2000).

IN DEVELOPMENT
- Growth hormone and insulin-like growth factor-I (IGF-I) stimulate bone growth and osteoblast activity.
    - Beneficial for women with growth hormone deficiency; results have been conflicting for women who do not have growth hormone deficiency.
- Hydroxymethylglutaryl coenzyme A reductase inhibitors (statins): prospective studies needed
    - Metaanalysis did not support a protective effect with statin use for hip fracture or nonspine fracture; controlled trials are needed (Bauer et al., 2004).
- 3rd-generation bisphosphonates:
    - Ibandronate
- Fluoride:
    - Slow-release fluoride: under U.S. Food and Drug Administration review; ↑ bone formation
- Strontium ranelate, an orally active drug, dissociates bone resorption (which is increased in OP) from bone formation (which is reduced but continues in OP).
    - Strontium ranelate (2 g PO/day) therapy seems to be safe and efficacious and results in an early and sustained reduction in the risk of vertebral fractures among postmenopausal women with OP (randomized controlled trial [RCT]) (Meunier et al., 2004).
- Selective estrogen receptor modulators:
    - Idoxifene
- Bone morphogenetic protein
- Potassium bicarbonate
- Cytokines

344

A. Osteoporosis Therapy

Agents	Dosage	Comments
Estrogen	0.625 mg conjugated equine estrogen or estradiol 1 mg	Greatest benefit relative to cost Reduces new fractures by 50% Bone density drops rapidly after hormone replacement therapy discontinued
Alendronate (Fosamax)	Prevention: 5 mg daily or 35 mg weekly Treatment: 10 mg daily or 70 mg weekly	Take with 6–8 oz water Do not eat or drink for the following 30 mins Do not lie down for at least 30 mins Reduces new fractures by 50% 3-wk half-life, so no rapid drop in bone density after stopping drug
Risedronate (Actonel)	Prevention and treatment: 5 mg daily	Take with 6–8 oz water Do not eat or drink for the following 30 mins Do not lie down for at least 30 mins Reduces new fractures by 50% 3-wk half-life, so no rapid drop in bone density after stopping drug
Calcitonin Nasal Spray (Miacalcin)	200 IU/day (1 spray)	Alternate nostrils daily Can be taken any time Has bone analgesic qualities Reduces new fractures by 30%
Raloxifene (Evista)	Prevention: 60 mg daily	Can be taken at any time Reduces new fractures by 30%

POSTMENOPAUSAL OSTEOPOROSIS

Agent	Mechanism of Action	Effect on Bone	Effect on Fractures	Recommended for	Risks	Comments
Calcium	Increased availability	Deficiency causes loss; supplements reduce loss.	Reduction in fracture risk by use of calcium with vitamin D	Adolescents, lactating women, hypoestrogenic women, osteoporosis risk factors including age	Should not exceed 2000 mg daily; hypercalcuria, hypercalcemia.	Revised daily requirement.
Vitamin D	Increased intestinal absorption of calcium	Direct effect unknown; increases bone mass when combined with calcium.	Reduction in fracture risk by use of calcium with vitamin D	Institutionalized elderly and women over 70	Hypercalcuria and hypercalcemia with increased doses.	Overdose in elderly can lead to renal failure.
Estrogen	Reduces bone resorption by inhibiting osteoclasts	Slows bone loss, increases bone mass slightly; affects all types of bone.	Documented reduction of all fractures; as high as 50% reduction of hip fractures	First-line choice for prevention in absence of contraindications; indicated for proven osteoporosis or abnormal bone density	Uterine bleeding, endometrial hyperplasia, endometrial cancer.	Additional cardiovascular and other benefits have been described.
Alendronate	Reduces bone resorption by inhibiting osteoclasts	Slows bone loss, increases bone mass.	Significant reduction (48%) in new vertebral fractures	Treatment of osteoporosis (10 mg dose); prevention of repeat vertebral fractures	Not recommended for patients with renal insufficiency or upper gastrointestinal problems.	Use as a preventative in normal population (5 mg dose).

Calcitonin	Reduces bone resorption by inhibiting osteoclasts	Increases vertebral bone mass.	Significant reduction in new vertebral fractures	Alternative to estrogen therapy	Development of neutralizing antibodies; effect unknown.	Objection to injections now avoided by intranasal spray; absorption is variable.
Raloxifene	Reduces bone resorption by inhibiting osteoclasts	Slight increase in bone mass over 2–3 yrs.	—	Prevention of osteoporosis	—	Low rate of uterine bleeding.
Progestins	Reduces bone resorption by inhibiting osteoclasts	Slows bone loss.	Long-term study of progestins alone unavailable	Women on estrogen replacement therapy unless uterus surgically absent; not recommended as sole agent	Dosage required to positively affect bone causes reduction in high-density lipoprotein and increases in low-density lipoprotein.	—
Fluoride	Deposited and concentrated in bone; slowly reabsorbed	Increases bone mass in continuous manner; new bone is structurally abnormal.	No demonstrated reduction in vertebral fractures; may increase nonvertebral fractures	Not recommended in the United States	New bone may be weaker and increase fracture risk.	Slow-release formulations may improve effectiveness of fluoride.

continued

POSTMENOPAUSAL OSTEOPOROSIS

Agent	Mechanism of Action	Effect on Bone	Effect on Fractures	Recommended for	Risks	Comments
Etidronate	Inhibits bone resorption by reducing ability of osteoclasts to resorb bone	Increases bone mass; reduces bone remodeling.	Reduction not clearly demonstrated	Not FDA approved for this purpose	Inhibits mineralization at slightly higher doses; long-term effects unknown.	Approved for osteoporosis treatment in Canada.
Tamoxifen	Assumed to be an antiabsorptive agent with an effect of a weak estrogen	Laboratory evidence of reduced bone loss in rats.	No long-term data	Not recommended as an agent specific for osteoporosis prevention	Endometrial carcinoma incidence is reportedly increased.	Level of protection against osteoporosis unknown; other agents should be added.

Source: Reproduced with permission from American College of Obstetricians and Gynecologists. Educational Bulletin no. 246. Washington, DC: American College of Obstetricians and Gynecologists, 1998.

36. Hot Flashes

INCIDENCE
- Overall incidence:
  - Premenopausal: 25%
  - Late perimenopausal: 69%
  - Late postmenopause: 39%

BACKGROUND
- Usually a sensation of heat, sweating, flushing, dizziness, palpitations, irritability, anxiety, and/or panic
- Classic hot flash (HF): head-to-toe sensation of heat, culminating in perspiration
- Large cross-cultural variability in prevalence:

%	Culture
0	Mayan women in Mexico
18	Chinese factory workers in Hong Kong
70	North American women (black women > white women)
80	Dutch women

- Despite these vast differences, some trends are seen:
  - HFs usually last 0.5–5.0 yrs (but may last up to 15 yrs); one study reported that among women who had experienced moderate to severe HFs, 58% persisted at 5 yrs, 12% at 8 yrs, and 10% at 15 yrs out.
  - Generally more severe in women who undergo surgical menopause; one study reported that 100% of patients undergoing surgical menopause had vasomotor symptoms, and 90% of them had continuing symptoms for 8.5 yrs. It is postulated that slower, continuous reductions on gonadal steroid levels result in downward regulation of hormone receptors in the hypothalamus in women undergoing natural (vs. surgical) menopause.
  - Recent finding challenges dogma that HFs cause sleep disturbances: no correlation between the HFs and sleep disturbance (Freedman and Roehrs, 2004)
  - HFs have been associated with a diminished sense of well-being (likely as a result of fatigue, irritability, poor concentration, anxiety-type symptoms).
  - Premenopausal/early perimenopausal women with symptoms may be more likely to report a ↓ sense of well-being than late perimenopausal and late postmenopausal women.
  - Some studies estimate that approximately 50% of breast cancer survivors list HF as their most prominent complaint.

HOT FLASHES

ETIOLOGY
- Speculative but believed to be related to estrogen withdrawal (not seen in 45,XO patients)
- Estrogen modulates the firing rate of thermosensitive neurons in the preoptic area of the hypothalamus in response to thermal stimulation in the rat.
- Responsiveness of arterioles to catecholamines is greater in women with HFs than in those without HFs. Estrogen enhances α_2-adrenergic activity, and estrogen withdrawal may therefore lead to vasomotor flushes as a result of $\downarrow \alpha_2$-adrenergic activity.
- Women who experience HFs have a significantly smaller thermoneutral zone than women without HF (0.0° C vs. 0.4° C, respectively); small elevations in core body temperature have been shown to precede most HFs.
- Other causes: thyroid disease, epilepsy, infection, insulinoma, pheochromocytoma, carcinoid syndromes, leukemia, pancreatic tumors, autoimmune disorders, and mast-cell disorders

TREATMENT OPTIONS

Intervention	Notes
Lifestyle modification	
Core body temperature	$\downarrow$ Air temperature $\rightarrow \downarrow$ HFs.
	Advice: fan, dress in layers, cold food/drinks.
Exercise	Observational studies: physically active women $\rightarrow \downarrow$ HFs.
	No RCTs.
BMI	$\uparrow$ BMI $\rightarrow \uparrow$ HFs.
	Unknown if losing weight $\downarrow$ HFs.
Smoking	Associated with $\uparrow$ HFs.
Relaxation techniques	Paced respiration (slow, controlled, diaphragmatic breathing) $\rightarrow \downarrow$ HFs.
Nonprescription substances	
Soy	Only slight $\downarrow$ HFs, likely no effect (RCT).
Red clover–derived isoflavones	Slight to no effect.
	Long-term safety unknown.
Black cohosh	No effect.
	Long-term safety unknown.
Dong quai	No effect.
	Contraindicated in women using warfarin.
Evening primrose oil	No effect.
Ginseng	No effect.

Intervention	Notes
Licorice	Avoid with MAOIs, anticoagulants, or stimulants.
	No effect.
	Large doses → pseudoprimary aldosteronism.
Chinese herb mixtures	No effect.
Vitamin E	Little to no effect.
Flaxseed	40 g/day led to 38% ↓ HF frequency in randomized trial (yet to be published).
Topical P	Topical P mixed with vitamin E + aloe vera (Pro-Gest) at 20 mg/day ↓ HFs 83% vs. 19% for placebo group (RCT).
	Other RCTs show no effect.
Acupuncture	No effect.
Magnet therapy	No effect.

Prescription substances
Hormonal

Estrogen	Estrogen or estrogen + P ↓ HF frequency 77% compared with placebo.
	Conjugated equine estrogen, 0.400–0.625 mg/day.
	17β-Estradiol, 0.5–1.0 mg/day (PO).
	17β-Estradiol, 0.025–0.075 mg/day (patch).
	Estradiol acetate, 0.05–0.10 mg/day (vaginal ring).
	If uterus is present, add P:
	MPA, 2.5 mg/day.
	Norethindrone, 0.35 mg/day.
	Norethindrone acetate, 5 mg/day.
	Norgestrel, 0.075 mg/day.
	Micronized P, 100–200 mg/day.
	Contraindications: hormone-sensitive cancer, liver disease, history of venous thromboembolism, confirmed cardiovascular disease.
Progestogen	Depot medroxyprogesterone acetate, 150 mg/mo IM.
	↓ HF frequency 90% compared with 25% for placebo.
	MPA, 20 mg/day PO.
	↓ HF significantly and without adverse effect on bone mineral density and less uterine bleeding.
	Megestrol acetate, 20 mg b.i.d.
	↓ HF frequency 85% compared with 21% for placebo.

continued

HOT FLASHES

Intervention	Notes
Estrogen + progestin patch	Contraindications: concern regarding effect on breast cancer. **Climara Pro** once-a-week patch. 45 µg/day estradiol + 15 µg/day levonorgestrel. Two randomized trials showing ↓ HF frequency/ severity. Effect seen as early as 1 wk.
OCs	Low-dose OC (20 µg ethinyl estradiol). Smokers >35 yrs should not use OCs.
Androgen-estrogen	0.625 or 1.250 mg esterified estrogens + 1.25 or 2.50 mg methyltestosterone. May be no better than estrogen alone. Long-term effects unknown.
Nonhormonal options	
Antidepressants	Effect seen as early as 1–2 weeks.
Venlafaxine (Effexor XR)	75 mg/day; ↓ HFs in breast cancer patients by 60%.
Fluoxetine (Prozac)	20 mg/day; avoid MAOI, thioridazine, warfarin.
Paroxetine (Paxil CR)	12.5 mg/day; same cautions as for Prozac.
Anticonvulsants	
Gabapentin (Neurontin)	100 mg/day up to 300 mg t.i.d.; ↓ HFs by 45% vs. 29% (Guttuso et al., 2003). Adverse effects: dizziness, lightheadedness, and peripheral edema. Contraindications: hypersensitivity to gabapentin.
Antihistamines	
Cetirizine (Zyrtec)	10 mg/day; ↓ HF frequency by 40% vs. 9% for placebo.

BMI, body mass index; HF, hot flash; MAOI, monoamine oxidase inhibitor; MPA, medroxyproges-terone; OC, oral contraceptive; P, progesterone; RCT, randomized controlled trial.
Source: Adapted from North American Menopause Society. Treatment of menopause-associated vasomotor symptoms: position statement of The North American Menopause Society. *Menopause* 11(1):11, 2004.

Estrogens

- Numerous studies have shown the effectiveness of estrogen therapy for HFs. This occurs regardless of route (patch vs. PO) and appears to be dose dependent.
- Overall, estradiol (E_2) treatment is estimated to reduce HFs by 50% in naturally menopausal women and by 70% in surgically menopausal women.

- Important points (Bachmann, 1999):
  - Reduction in HFs did not occur immediately (therefore, a treatment should be used for 4–6 wks before trying something new).
  - Placebo gives only an initial, nonlasting effect.

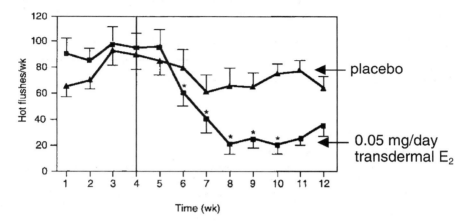

E_2, estradiol. (Source: Reproduced with permission from Bachmann GA. Vasomotor flushes in menopausal women. *Am J Obstet Gynecol* 180[3 Pt 2]:S312, 1999.)

Antihypertensives

- Reported to ↓ frequency in postmenopausal women by 4%.
- Tamoxifen-induced HFs in breast cancer patients: after 8 wks of treatment with oral clonidine (0.1 mg/day), HF frequency ↓ 38% compared to 24% with placebo.

Antidepressants (Gottlieb, 2000; Loprinzi et al., 2000)

- **Venlafaxine (Effexor) (75 mg/day):** A small percentage of patients experience side effects such as ↓ appetite, nausea, mouth dryness. ↓ Libido, however, was not seen with this dose of Effexor as has been seen with other studies using anti-depressants against HFs.
- **Fluoxetine (Prozac) (20 mg/day):** In a pilot trial of 30 women, ↓ HF frequency by 67%, severity by 75%; the most common side effect was somnolence (although percentage not noted); 25 of 30 chose to continue therapy after the trial.
- **Paroxetine (Paxil CR) (12.5 mg/day):** ↓ HF frequency by 62% vs. 38% for placebo (Stearns et al., 2003); Paxil is investigational at present.

HOT FLASHES

Clonidine

- Similar degree of efficacy as vitamin E or maybe a bit more; this benefit from clonidine, which is a bit better than that ascribed to a placebo, comes with some significant toxic effects (mouth dryness, dizziness, drowsiness, and sleeping difficulties); this can limit its utility and patient acceptance, which may the reason why only 13 of the intervention patients (39%) continued to use it in one study.

RECOMMENDATIONS (North American Menopause Society, 2004)

Lifestyle changes:
   Keep core body temperature as cool as possible.
   Regular exercise
   Paced respiration
Nonprescription treatment:
   Vitamin E (800 IU/day)
   Dietary isoflavones (40–80 mg/day)
   Avoid: progesterone creams, dong quai, black cohosh, evening primrose oil, ginseng, licorice, Chinese herb mixtures, acupuncture, magnet therapy
Prescription therapies, hormonal options for short durations (allow 2–3 mos):
   0.5–1.0 mg/day 17β-estradiol
   0.30–0.45 mg/day conjugated estrogen
   0.025–0.075 mg/day 17β-estradiol patch
   1.25–2.50 g 17β-estradiol gel
   0.05–0.10 mg/day estradiol acetate ring
   Note: If uterus present, need progestogen added (progestogen-intrauterine device)
   Combination oral contraceptives
Prescription therapies, nonhormonal options (quick benefit):
   Antidepressants (taper off slowly):
      75 mg/day venlafaxine (Effexor XR)
      20 mg/day fluoxetine (Prozac)
      12.5 mg/day paroxetine (Paxil CR)
   Gabapentin, 100 mg/day–300 mg t.i.d.
   10 mg/day cetirizine (Zyrtec)

37. Transvaginal Ultrasound in Reproductive Endocrinology and Infertility

BASIC PRINCIPLES OF SCANNING

- Develop a routine to systematically scan all pelvic structures.
- Each structure must be scanned in two planes perpendicular to one another.
- Transducer's position should be monitored during insertion. Once the probe has been properly inserted, the operator should observe the screen at all times, and the position of the probe is determined by optimal visualization of the pelvic viscera. The orientation of the probe is controlled by angulation (accomplished by up and down movement of the transducer handle) and rotation:
  - The probe can be rotated 90 degrees around its axis to obtain sagittal and coronal plane images.
  - The probe can be angled in any plane to direct the plane of image.
  - Deeper insertion or withdrawal can be used to bring the area of interest within the focal zone of the transducer.
- The scan area needs to be thought of as a pie-shaped area emanating from the transducer:

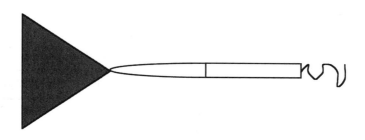

TRANSVAGINAL ULTRASOUND

- Rotation of the transducer changes the spatial orientation of that pie between longitudinal and coronal planes:

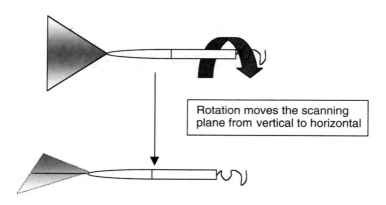

Rotation moves the scanning plane from vertical to horizontal

- Angling the probe (moving the probe up or down) allows for proper orientation of the probe with respect to the pelvic structures, depending on their position (e.g., anteversion, retroversion) within the pelvis:

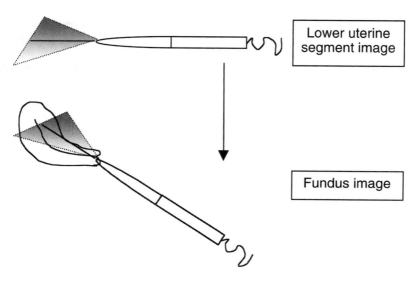

Lower uterine segment image

Fundus image

- The right to left orientation of the image in the coronal plane is controlled in two ways:
  1. Image direction button on the machine itself
  2. Direction of rotation from the sagittal plane
     - For example, if the image direction is set on the machine in such a way that the bladder is in the upper left corner while scanning in the sagittal plane, rotation of the probe 90 degrees clockwise will maintain the right to left orientation (patient's left will be displayed on the left of the screen). Rotation of the probe 90 degrees counterclockwise will change that orientation, and now patient's left will be displayed on the right of the screen (Callen, 2000).

OVARIAN RESERVE ASSESSMENT

- Ovarian aging is associated with a decline in number of ovarian follicles as well as a possible deterioration of oocyte quality (Toner, 2003). Direct measurement of oocyte quantity is not possible at this time; however, ovarian reserve tests reflect the size of the remaining follicular pool:
  - **Antral follicles** 2–8 mm in diameter can be measured on day 2 or 3 of menstrual cycle.
  - **Antral follicle counts** are a reproducible measure of remaining follicle pool and are directly correlated with likelihood of pregnancy after assisted reproductive technology (ART) treatments and inversely correlated with cancellation rates. No antral follicle count, however, can be used as an absolute predictor of pregnancy or cancellation during ART treatments. An antral follicle count of <4 is associated with a high (41–69%) cancellation rate. There is a negative linear correlation between antral follicle counts and gonadotropin dose required to achieve response (Chang et al., 1998; Frattarelli et al., 2000; Frattarelli et al., 2003).
  - **Antral follicle numbers** decrease with advancing chronologic age. The rate of this decline is biphasic, with mean yearly decline of 4.8% in women <37 yrs of age and increasing to a mean of 11.7% thereafter (Scheffer et al., 1999).

TRANSVAGINAL ULTRASOUND

IN-CYCLE MONITORING OF OVARIAN RESPONSE

(Schwimer and Lebovic, 1984)

- Both size and number of follicles are measured during monitoring for ART treatments.
- A follicle of ≥18 mm is believed to contain a mature oocyte and is used as a marker of when human chorionic gonadotropin (hCG) is to be administered.

	Optimal Response
Ovulation induction	1 Follicle >18 mm
Controlled ovarian hyperstimulation	3 Follicles >18 mm

Antral Follicle Count and Multiple Pregnancy Rate

- Factors linked to ↑ risk of multiple pregnancies in controlled ovarian hyperstimulation (COH) cycles:
  - Age of the female patient
  - Estradiol levels
  - Total number of follicles developed: The use of ultrasound (US) has been proposed not only to assess follicular size, but to determine follicle number to reduce multiple pregnancy rates.
- Several recent publications failed, however, to show a relationship between follicle counts and multiple pregnancies. A large metaanalysis that reviewed 3608 COH cycles showed that triplet implantations were increased threefold when more than six follicles >12 mm were noted on US in patients <35 yrs old. Follicle counts can therefore be used as a crude estimate of an ↑ risk of multifetal gestation in young patients. A total count of large and intermediate-size follicles needs to be used in that assessment. Follicle counts have not been helpful in minimizing the risk of twin gestation regardless of age (Dickey et al., 1991; Dickey et al., 2001; Valbuena et al., 1996).

ULTRASOUND ASSESSMENT OF THE ENDOMETRIUM IN OVULATION INDUCTION

- Endometrial thickness is best assessed in the longitudinal/sagittal axis of the uterus, encompassing the thickness of both anterior and posterior endometrial layers. (Note: The figure below is a transverse image to illustrate the layers, although the proper measurement of endometrial thickness should be in the longitudinal/sagittal axis.)

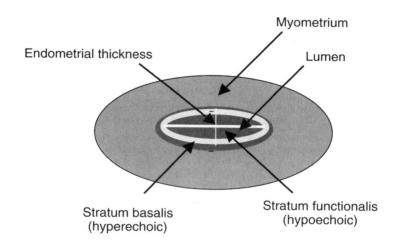

TRANSVAGINAL ULTRASOUND

- Endometrial thickness increases slowly in early follicular phase but can thicken by 1–2 mm daily in the late follicular phase. (Note: The figures below are transverse images illustrating the change in endometrial lining, although the proper measurement of endometrial thickness should be in the longitudinal/sagittal axis.)

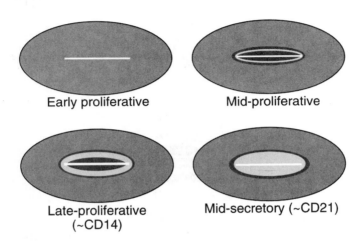

Early proliferative	Mid-proliferative
Late-proliferative (~CD14)	Mid-secretory (~CD21)

- Thickness of 6 mm appears to represent a critical threshold for achieving pregnancy. No significant improvements in pregnancy rates are seen when endometrial thickness exceeds 6 mm (Dickey et al., 1993).
- A distinct multilayer pattern typically develops within the endometrium in the late follicular phase, commonly referred to as *triple-line* or *trilaminar pattern*. The endometrial patterns are generally divided into three categories:

Pattern A: three hyperechoic lines separated by hypoechoic region
Pattern B: intermediate pattern where three lines are visible, but the intervening endometrium is somewhat hyperechoic.
Pattern C: homogeneous hyperechoic endometrium throughout

⇨ The uniformly hyperechoic endometrium pattern has been associated with lower implantation rates and poor likelihood of pregnancy (Coulam et al., 1994; Fanchin et al., 2000; Potlog-Nahari et al., 2003).

❖ 447 patients, retrospective analysis, blastocyst transfer (pattern B on day of hCG is associated with ↓ pregnancy rate):

Pattern (No.)	Clinical Pregnancy Rate (%)
A (376)[a]	68
B (66)[a]	47
C (5)	60
B + C (71)	48

[a]P <.001

Source: Adapted from Potlog-Nahari C, Catherino WH, McKeeby JL, et al. A suboptimal endometrial pattern is associated with a reduced likelihood of pregnancy after a day 5 embryo transfer. *Fertil Steril* 83(1):235, 2005.

IMPACT OF ULTRASOUND GUIDANCE AT EMBRYO TRANSFER ON OUTCOME

- Recently, transabdominal US has been used during embryo transfers for guidance of the catheter through the cervical canal and to determine the depth of embryo placement within the uterine cavity.
- Many studies have evaluated the impact of this approach with mixed results. The recent metaanalysis of published studies concluded that US-guided embryo transfer significantly increased implantation rates (Buckett, 2003).
  - Proposed theories to explain this improvement include:
    ⇨ Confirmation of appropriate placement
    ⇨ Ease of transfer due to guidance through the cervical canal
    ⇨ Placement of embryos in the uterine cavity but away from uterine fundus
  - One recent study supported the last theory by demonstrating that clinical pregnancy rates improved with increasing distance between the catheter tip and fundus and by demonstrating US to be superior to clinical touch alone in estimating this distance accurately (Pope et al., 2004).

SONOHYSTEROGRAPHY

- US technique whereby 10–15 cc of sterile saline is introduced into the uterine cavity via a balloon-tipped catheter. The saline acts as a contrast medium within the uterine cavity and allows for enhanced visualization of endometrial contour.
- A recent metaanalysis examining 2278 procedures compared sonohysterography (SHG) to hysteroscopy as the gold standard for assessment of endometrial lesions (de Kroon et al., 2003):
  - SHG sensitivity: 95% (confidence interval [CI], 0.83–0.97)
  - SHG specificity: 88% (CI, 0.85–0.92)

TRANSVAGINAL ULTRASOUND

⇨ The procedure was more likely to be successfully accomplished in pre-menopausal vs. postmenopausal women; 93.0% (CI, 92–94) vs. 86.5% (CI, 83.2–89.8).

- When compared to hysterosalpingography (HSG), SHG had greater sensitivity for detecting polypoid lesions (100% vs. 50%) and uterine malformations (77.8% vs. 44.0%). Its sensitivity in detection of intrauterine adhesions was equal to that of an HSG (75%) (Soares et al., 2000).
- The use of SHG significantly enhances the diagnostic capability of transvaginal US alone for both submucosal myomas and endometrial polyps. One study demonstrated that, in 114 patients evaluated for abnormal bleeding, the use of SHG permitted identification of 16 (**14%**) additional lesions in those patients in whom the screening US was **normal** (Laifer-Narin et al., 2002). SHG should therefore be included in a standard protocol for evaluation of abnormal uterine bleeding.

POSTMENOPAUSAL VAGINAL BLEEDING

- Postmenopausal vaginal bleeding (PMB) is a high-risk clinical condition in which diagnostic evaluation is indicated. Pelvic US with measurement of mid-sagittal endometrial thickness (two layers) has been proposed as a screening tool to determine who may benefit from more invasive evaluation. Hormone-replacement therapy (HRT) (sequential and continuous-combined regimens) does influence endometrial thickness (Affinito et al., 1998); however, it is generally recommended that the endometrial thickness cutoff at which invasive testing is used is not adjusted even if HRT is used.
- The endometrial thickness that should be used as an indication for invasive testing is controversial. When a cutoff level of ≥5 mm is used, the US sensitivity to detect endometrial cancer equals that of nontargeted endometrial biopsy (Gull et al., 2003; Gupta et al., 2002).
- The use of an endometrial thickness cutoff of >4 mm improves the sensitivity of US to detect endometrial cancer to 100%, at a cost of a low positive predictive value of only 25% (Goldstein et al., 2001).
- See diagnostic algorithms for pre- and postmenopausal bleeding in Chapter 8, Abnormal Uterine Bleeding.

38. Hysteroscopy

RESECTOSCOPE HYSTEROSCOPY SETTINGS

Electrode	Current	Watts
VaporTrode (all three types)	Pure cut	200
	Coag	75
Loop	Pure cut	90–120
	Coag	75
Roller ball coag	Pure cut	100–200
	Coag	75

Coag, coagulation.

- Hysteroscopic myomectomy resection: Use VaporTrode cutting and, to clean instrument head, use coagulation setting.

HYSTEROSCOPY FLUIDS
- Pressure:
  - 40–50 mm Hg to open the uterine cavity (Baker and Adamson, 1998)
  - 70–75 mm Hg usually adequate for surgery
  - Set pump pressure at the patient's mean arterial pressure (MAP); ask anesthesiologists for the patient's MAP; for every foot above the uterus → 10 mm Hg.

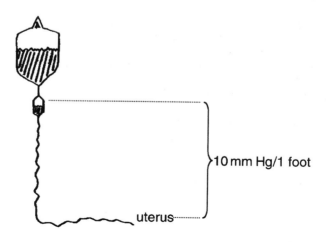

HYSTEROSCOPY

- Avoid Trendelenburg's position: By tipping the head down, the heart is below the operative field, and a negative pressure gradient is created, thus predisposing to emboli.
- Mechanism to ↓ fluid absorption and to extrude the myoma into the cavity:
  - 5 U vasopressin in 100 mL normal saline (**0.05 U/mL**): inject 10 mL (20 mL total) into the cervical stroma at 4- and 8-o'clock positions (Phillips et al., 1996)
- Fluids:

Solution	Complication
Hypotonic, electrolyte-free solutions (osm)	Hypotonic fluid overload
Glycine 1.5% (200)	
Sorbitol/mannitol (178)	
Mannitol 5% (280)	
Isotonic, electrolyte-containing solutions (osm)	Isotonic fluid overload
Normal saline (308)	
Lactated Ringer solution (273)	

- Lactated Ringer (LR) solution for diagnostic hysteroscopy
- 32% Dextran (Hyskon): nonconductive/immiscible with blood; side effect: anaphylaxis (uncommon)
- Glycine, sorbitol, or mannitol: 1000-cc deficit → stop and evaluate before progressing; possible use of Lasix (consider sending laboratory tests: electrolytes, renal panel; Na^+ ↓ 10 mEq/L for every 1 L absorbed)
- Distinguishing between fluid overload and gas embolus:
  - ↓ CO_2 for both, but the diastolic blood pressure rises with ↑ fluid volume.
- Treatment for gas embolus:
  - Leave the hysteroscope in place (preventing further air access).
  - 100% supplemental oxygen
  - Left lateral decubitus position
  - Catheterization of the subclavian vein or right internal jugular vein to suck out the air from the right atrium
- Treatment for **hyponatremia** (Na^+ <120):
  - O_2
  - Hypocalcemia may accompany; therefore, check Ca^{2+}, K^+, Na^+
  - **3% NaCl** to ↑ Na^+ by 1 mmol/L/hr
- Maximum doses of lidocaine for 60-kg woman: 270 mg (without epinephrine), 420 mg (with epinephrine)

ASHERMAN SYNDROME AND INTRAUTERINE ADHESIONS

- Those with normal-appearing endometrium above the level of obstruction on transvaginal ultrasound are likely to have successful hysteroscopic treatment and resumption of menses (Schlaff and Hurst, 1995).
- LR solution pressure may require up to 200 mm Hg to break adhesive disease.
- Postoperative prevention of adhesions (courtesy of Dr. Michael DiMattina, Dominion Fertility, Arlington, Virginia):
  - Intrauterine splint:
    - ⇨ Place a **No. 14–16 Foley catheter** into the mid- to upper cavity.
    - ⇨ Inflate with 4–8 cc of sterile water, depending on the size of the cavity.
    - ⇨ Attach to a leg drainage bag without tension.
    - ⇨ Maintain for 5–7 days.
  - Medical therapy:
    - ⇨ **Estradiol valerate, 5 mg IM,** before discharge (lasts for 5–10 days and circumvents nausea with oral estrogen)
    - ⇨ **Doxycycline, 100 mg PO b.i.d.,** until the catheter is removed
    - ⇨ **Nonsteroidal antiinflammatory drug** for the first 48–72 hours postoperative to alleviate pain from catheter and possibly diminish inflammation that can led to adhesion formation
    - ⇨ Conjugated estrogens (Premarin), 2.5 mg/day, starting 7 days after surgery for 30 days
    - ⇨ Medroxyprogesterone (Provera), 10 mg/day, starting on day 20 of the Premarin therapy for 10 days

39. Laparoscopy

RECOMMENDED LAPAROSCOPIC EQUIPMENT
Equipment
- Mono- and bipolar cords
- Uterine manipulator with access for chromopertubation
- Laparoscope
  - 5 mm and 10 mm sizes
  - 0 degrees, 12 degrees, 30 degrees available
- Camera head
- Light cable
- CO_2 tubing
- Veress needle
  - Standard length: 11.5 cm
  - Long: 17 cm
- Trocars: Sizes vary from 5 to 15 mm.

Instruments (Length Usually 35 cm)
- Suction/irrigator assembly
- Metal probe
- Fine- and blunt-tip forceps
- Atraumatic forceps
- Monopolar shears
- Scissors: curved, serrated, hook
- Kleppinger bipolar instrument or equivalent
- Microlaparoscopy set of instruments (3-mm instruments): best for performing reparative tubal surgery

PATIENT PREPARATION AND POSITIONING
Bowel Preparation
- Consider in all patients or those with a history of endometriosis (especially with bowel-related symptoms) or adhesions, previous exploratory laparotomy, history of pelvic inflammatory disease/tuboovarian abscess (TOA), and history of multiple laparoscopies.
- Types: Fleets Phosphosoda, magnesium citrate, GoLYTELY

Positioning
- Modified lithotomy:
  - Hips extended and thighs parallel to the abdomen; this facilitates access to upper pelvic/abdominal structures and tissue removal.

- Make sure legs are well positioned and protected (see Positioning Injuries below).
  - Shoulder brace
  - Sequential compression devices for the lower extremities
- Sacrum: Avoid undue pressure leading to coccydynia.
- Foley catheter for bladder decompression and proper placement of suprapubic port
- Arms adducted and pronated to side and tucked to the patient's side
  - Protect fingers, hands, and elbows with foam cushions.
- Patient supine (0 degrees) for initial Veress needle insertion and primary trocar
- Steep Trendelenburg (20–30 degrees) during the case

Positioning Injuries

Brachial plexus

  Caused by outstretched arm or direct compression by shoulder braces during steep Trendelenburg

  Result: sensory loss over radial 2/3 of hand, wrist drop if severe

Ulnar nerve

  Caused by supination of arm if tucked to the side or pronation if outstretched on arm board

  Result: sensory loss of ulnar 1/2 of 4th/5th fingers, claw hand if severe

Peroneal nerve

  Compression of the lateral head of the fibula

  Result: sensory loss over the lateral aspect of the lower leg, foot drop

Femoral nerve

  Exaggerated dorsal lithotomy or stretch injury

  Result: sensory loss to anterior thigh, inability to raise leg

Ergonomics

- Table height at waist level and position yourself so that elbows are comfortably flexed at 90 degrees and shoulders are at resting position
- Monitor located centrally between the legs or, ideally, two monitors placed at the outside of the patient's knees to minimize neck strain

Anesthetic Considerations

- General anesthesia used for all procedures except perhaps tubal ligation
- Orogastric tube to $\downarrow$ possibility of trocar injury to the stomach and $\downarrow$ small bowel distention
- CO_2 and Trendelenburg position may lead to splinting of the diaphragm $\rightarrow$ difficulty maintaining ventilation $\rightarrow$ hypercapnia

LAPAROSCOPY

ABDOMINAL ENTRY TECHNIQUE (VERESS NEEDLE)

- Injection of 5 mL 0.25% bupivacaine at the trocar site before incision results in ↓ postoperative pain (Ke et al., 1998).
- Intraabdominal pressure should be <8–10 mm Hg except in obese patients.
- Veress needle preparation:
  - Check to ensure the spring-loaded obturator is working before use.
  - Stopcock should be open and gas tubing unconnected so that once the negative pressure in the abdomen is encountered, room air enters the abdomen, and bowel and omentum fall away from the tip of the Veress needle.
- Veress needle **double-click**: puncture of (a) rectus sheath and (b) peritoneum
- Confirmation:
  - First withdraw with a syringe:
    - ⇨ **Blood?** Consider vessel injury; need to open immediately if large vessel injury and consult vascular surgery.
    - ⇨ **Bile?** Consider small intestine or gallbladder injury.
    - ⇨ **Bowel** (feculent)? **Do not remove Veress needle**; otherwise, difficult to identify bowel perforation; consult general surgery or consider laparoscopic repair after obtaining alternate entry site and accessory trocar placement
  - Inject approximately 1 mL normal saline (NS) to remove any possible skin/subcutaneous tissue from Veress tip.
  - Drop test with NS as a sign of intraabdominal negative pressure
  - *Schriock sign:* Initially, intraabdominal pressure reading is a few mm Hg higher to account for a surfactant-like effect requiring some pressure to separate the bowel from the abdominal wall.
  - If entry pressure is >8–10 mm Hg:
    - ⇨ Usually incorrect placement in the preperitoneal/subfascial compartment (or a viscus), potentially leading to subcutaneous emphysema
- Once intraperitoneal access is obtained:
  - Insufflate with low-flow CO_2 (1 L/min) and percuss over the liver (lose liver dullness—tympanic—after 0.5 L has been insufflated).
  - ↑ CO_2 to high flow (2.0–2.5 L/min) once reassured of placement.
  - Inspect viscera and retroperitoneal structures before requesting Trendelenburg.
  - Operate with CO_2 pressure at 12–15 mm Hg (may need ↑ in obese patients).

ALTERNATE ENTRY TECHNIQUES
Alternate Access Sites
Left Upper Quadrant (Palmer's Point)
- Midclavicular
- 2 cm below costal margin
- Orogastric tube in place
- **Not recommended** if history of hepatosplenomegaly or gastric surgery

Posterior Vaginal Fornix
- Trendelenburg, long Veress needle, tenaculum on posterior cervix
- Maintain midline entry.
- Remove under direct visualization.
- **Not recommended** if cul-de-sac mass, fixed uterine retroversion, rectovaginal endometriosis, or prior vaginal vault surgery

Transfundal
- Approach vaginally, Trendelenburg, long Veress needle, tenaculum on anterior cervix
- Maintain midline entry of uterus.
- Antevert uterus on entry; remove under direct visualization.
- **Not recommended** if multiple myomas, fixed retroversion, or high risk for uterine adhesions

Direct Entry (No Veress Needle)
- Advantages: shortened operating time and ↓ risks associated with the Veress
- Incision large enough to accommodate trocar and avoid skin dystocia
- Elevate abdominal wall; insert trocar directly, aiming toward the sacral hollow.
  - Maintain abdominal elevation until peritoneal confirmation.
- Remove obturator and insert laparoscope to confirm placement.
- If the omentum has been perforated, carefully withdraw laparoscope/trocar in a perpendicular fashion, and omentum should fall off trocar sleeve.

Direct Entry Using Laparoscope
- Laparoscope is placed within primary trocar during entry (Visiport, Optiview).

Open Entry (Hasson)
- Skin held up by Allis clamps, incision of skin, reposition of Allis clamps at skin edges, S-retractors placed, dissect to the fascial layer, small Kocher clamps on the fascia, incise fascia carefully, place sutures on lateral edges, enter peritoneum, bluntly enlarge, blunt trocar placed and CO_2 insufflation started, tie sutures to cannula, close fascia with stay sutures, check for fascial defects (may need to place additional suture).

LAPAROSCOPY
ACCESSORY TROCAR INSERTION
Transillumination
- Helps visualize the superficial epigastric vessels
- If unable to see (obese patients), stay 6–8 cm from the midline (avoids the rectus sheath).
- Make appropriate skin incision along transverse lines of the lower abdominal skin tension (Langer's lines).
- Slow, steady rotational motion with insertion technique
- Perpendicular to skin and subcutaneous tissue

COMPLICATIONS
Trocar Bleeding
- Abdominal wall: superficial or deep epigastric or deep circumflex vessels
  - Repair under direct visualization.
  - **Endoclose device:** Place needle and suture on one side of bleeding vessel; release suture and reenter the needle on the other side of bleeding vessel and pull up suture out of the abdomen.
  - **Keith needle:** Same idea but must bring needle back up through trocar (grasp suture instead of needle to facilitate removal)
  - **30-cc Foley balloon:** Temporary tamponade
  - **Cautery:** Only if superficial peritoneal vessels
- Pelvic/aortic vasculature
  - Perform immediate laparotomy, apply pressure, and consult vascular surgery
  - Most common vessel injury: right common iliac

Organ Damage
- Bladder: Repair in layers, may consult urology.
- Bowel: Do not remove trocar/Veress needle! Consult general surgery.

Venous Bleeding
- ↓ Intraabdominal pressure to 8 mm Hg to help visualize.
- Remember mean venous pressure.
- Visualize under irrigation and low CO_2 pressure.

ELECTROSURGERY
Cut (30–50 W)
- High current, low-voltage (continuous) waveform
- Rapidly elevates tissue temperature, producing vaporization or dissection of tissue with the least effect on coagulation (hemostasis)

- Noncontact means of dissection
  - Activate electrode before touching tissue!
- If energy source left in place, the maximum temperature and width of thermal spread increase with time.

Blend Waveforms

- Interrupts current and increases voltage (noncontinuous)
- Mix between cut and coagulation
- Requires more time to dissect than cut, producing ↑ thermal spread at the same power setting

Coagulation/Fulguration (30–50 W)

- High-voltage, low-current (noncontinuous) waveform
- Delivers long electrical sparks to tissue
- Superficial eschar produced with minimal depth of necrosis
- Noncontact modality

Monopolar Principles

- Grounding pad
  - Required to help direct the current back to the generator
  - Must be applied correctly to avoid burn at the pad site
- Direct coupling
  - Energy transfer achieved by means of physical contact.
    ⇨ Activated electrode makes unintentional contact with another metal device (e.g., laparoscope, trocar)
- Capacitive coupling
  - Transfer of energy from one circuit to another by means of the mutual capacitance between circuits
    ⇨ Induction of stray current to a surrounding conductor through the intact insulation of an active electrode
    ⇨ Avoid metal/plastic trocars; use only all metal or all plastic with monopolar electrosurgery.
- Insulation failure
  - Break in insulation provides an alternate pathway for conduction of energy.

Bipolar Principles

- Combines an active electrode with a return electrode in same hand piece
- Eliminates capacitive coupling and alternate current pathways
- Medium-current, low-voltage (continuous) waveform
- Strategies to ↓ thermal injury:
  - Apply current in a pulsatile fashion.
  - Irrigate surrounding tissue.
  - Minimize tissue volume.

LAPAROSCOPY

Complications
- Thermal injuries to the bowel: incidence of 1.3 in 1000
  - Usually manifest 2–3 days postoperatively if not identified at the time of laparoscopy
  - Persistent and relatively extreme trocar site pain closest to the bowel injury (local irritation from bowel contents?) (Bishoff et al., 1999)
  - Other possible symptoms: ileus, abdominal pain, abdominal rigidity, leukocytosis with a left shift, fever, and large-volume fluid requirements followed by tachycardia and hypotension

Ultrasonic Energy
Harmonic Scalpel/Autosonic Scalpel
- Ultrasound energy converted to mechanical energy by linear oscillation
- 2-mm lateral spread
- Settings:
  - Level 3
    - ⇨ Vascular adhesions (shears)
    - ⇨ Ovarian cyst (hook)
    - ⇨ Oophorectomy (shears)
  - Level 5
    - ⇨ Avascular adhesions (hook or shears)
    - ⇨ Ablation endometriosis (ball)
    - ⇨ Myometrial incisions

LAPAROSCOPIC MYOMECTOMY
- Laparoscopic needle to infiltrate subserosa until blanched with vasopressin
  - Dose: vasopressin (Pitressin): 20 U in 50 cc NS
- Myoma incision
  - Make incision horizontal to ↓ bleeding and facilitate closure.
  - Instruments:
    - ⇨ Harmonic scalpel
    - ⇨ Monopolar needle: creates ↑ smoke, use suction to clear
- Laparoscopic myoma screw or 5- to 10-mm tenaculum for manipulation of myoma
- Onion-skinning technique
  - Cut on the myoma and not into the myometrial tissue
  - ↓ Blood loss and facilitates closure of the defect
- Specimen removal
  - Electromorcelator (Gynecare: 12 mm; Storz: 12, 15 mm) or
  - Mini-lap incision for removal

- Closure
  - Slow absorbable suture (PDS, Maxon, Vicryl, Polysorb)
  - Intracorporeal needle holders or extracorporeal knot pusher or mini-lap incision

ECTOPIC PREGNANCY

- May find $\uparrow$ intraabdominal pressure on entry if large hemoperitoneum
- If large hemoperitoneum, consider using 10-mm suction irrigation (Yankauer) to facilitate faster removal of blood clots.
- Linear salpingotomy
  - May inject the mesentery with dilute vasopressin
  - Linear (1–2 cm) incision with monopolar needle or shears on the antimesenteric border
    ⇨ Make incision approximately 0.5 cm from the proximal site of distended tube.
  - Hydrodissection as needed
  - Healing by secondary intention
  - If large incision, consider 5-0 or 6-0 delayed absorbable suture.
  - Specimen removal
    ⇨ Babcock forceps, EndoCatch bag, remove from 10–12 port
  - Need to follow serial weekly β-human chorionic gonadotropin (β-hCG) to <2 mIU/mL (rule out persistent ectopic pregnancy)
  - If unable to remove all of ectopic tissue, consider methotrexate.
- Salpingectomy
  - Reserved for severely damaged tube, ruptured tube, or undesired future fertility
  - Electrocoagulate mesosalpinx as close to fallopian tube as possible.
    ⇨ Avoid compromising ovarian blood supply.
  - Follow serial weekly β-hCG to <2 mIU/mL, especially if ovulation induction agents used.
  - Partial salpingectomy if **isthmic** ectopic

LAPAROSCOPIC CYSTECTOMY

- Sharp shears, curved or straight; lasers used as well
  - Make small incision to separate ovarian cortex from the cyst wall.
  - May use monopolar needle, but $\uparrow$ chance of cyst rupture.
- Traction–countertraction
  - Pull tissues apart in a slow motion, holding near the plane of dissection.
  - Hydrodissection with suction irrigator may help.
  - Electrocoagulation of small bleeders, but keep to minimum to preserve maximal ovarian function

LAPAROSCOPY

- Repair
  - Usually not needed secondary to involution of ovary
  - If large defect, suture with 4-0 absorbable suture
- Specimen removal
  - EndoCatch bag: Decompress cyst under direct visualization.
  - Enlarge trocar incision as needed.
  - Posterior colpotomy (Ghezzi et al., 2002)

A. Pelvic Anatomy (Ureters) during Laparoscopy

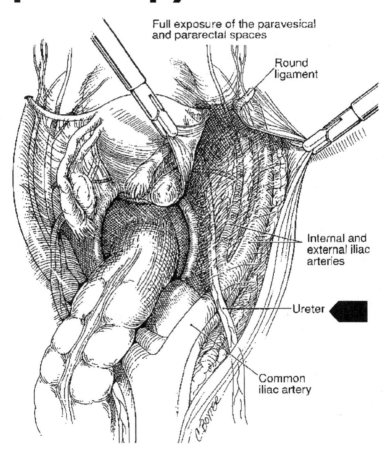

Full exposure of the paravesical and pararectal spaces

Round ligament

Internal and external iliac arteries

Ureter

Common iliac artery

(Source: Reproduced with permission from Nezhat CR, Nezhat FR, et al. *Operative Gynecologic Laparoscopy: Principles and Techniques.* New York: McGraw-Hill, 1995.)

375

40. Journal Club Guide

REFERENCE
• Title of article, authors, journal, site(s) of research

BACKGROUND INFORMATION ON THE TOPIC
• Review of the literature suggesting the purpose of the article and how it contributes to the field of knowledge in the specific area

HYPOTHESIS
• Research question (explicitly stated or implied)
• To what population will the findings apply? (relevance of the study)

METHODS/STUDY DESIGN
• Type of study (i.e., descriptive, cross-sectional, cohort, case-control, randomized controlled trial [RCT], metaanalysis, and so forth)
• Selection of study subjects (i.e., How were the subjects chosen? Are there any potential sources of bias? Were the groups similar at the start of the trial? Confounding variables can be controlled for in an RCT [e.g., stratification].)
• Were patients, health workers, and study personnel "blind" to treatment?
• Inclusion/exclusion criteria
• Bias that may have been introduced (ascertainment bias? what was exposure?)
• Control subjects
• Adequate randomization: concealed? *SNOSE* (sequentially numbered, opaque, sealed envelopes)?
• Adequate compliance?
• Outcomes to be measured (are they clearly defined?)
• Types of measurements used
• Were all subjects analyzed in the groups to which they were allocated?
• Was follow-up sufficiently long and complete?

RESULTS
• Statistical analysis used
• Levels of significance used/achieved
• Power analysis
• Findings (review the results in detail)
  ▪ How large was the treatment effect?

CONCLUSIONS
- Stated conclusions
- Do the authors answer the question posed in the hypothesis?
- Are the conclusions justified by the analysis presented?

INTERPRETATION
- Internal validity/external validity (i.e., How does this study apply to the population sampled and to your clinical practice?)
- Clinical vs. statistical significance
- Were all clinically important outcomes considered?
- Are the likely treatment benefits worth the potential harms and costs?
- What alternative treatments are available?
- Is this a significant contribution to the literature?
- Is this study reproducible?

CONSTRUCTION SUGGESTIONS
- How could this study be improved?
- Alternative study design to address this question (make a suggestion about another approach to answering this question)
- Does this study suggest the need for future research in this area?

QUALITY OF EVIDENCE

I. Evidence obtained from at least one properly designed, randomized controlled trial.

II-1. Evidence obtained from well-designed controlled trials without randomization.

II-2. Evidence obtained from well-designed cohort or case-control studies, preferably from more than one center or research group.

II-3. Evidence obtained from multiple time series with or without the intervention. Dramatic results in uncontrolled experiments could also be regarded as this type of evidence.

III. Opinions of respected authorities, based on clinical experience, descriptive studies, or reports of expert committees.

SENSITIVITY AND SPECIFICITY
- A rule of thumb is that the sensitivity and specificity of a good test should add up to ≥1.50, and those of a very good test should add up to ≥1.80 (Griffith and Grimes, 1990).

JOURNAL CLUB GUIDE

STATISTICS

	2 Groups		>2 Groups		Measure of Association
	Related	Independent	Related	Independent	
Nominal	McNemar test	Chi^2, Fisher exact test[a]	Cochran Q test	Chi^2	—
Ordinal	Wilcoxon signed rank test	Mann-Whitney U	Friedman 2-way, ANOVA	Kruskal-Wallis test	Spearman rank correlation
Interval	Paired t-test	Unpaired t-test	ANOVA	ANOVA[b]	Pearson correlation, linear regression

ANOVA, analysis of variance.

Note: **Nominal:** e.g., surgical complications; **Ordinal:** nonparametric, e.g., endometriosis stages; **Interval:** normal distribution, continuous variables, e.g., blood pressure. **Parametric distribution:** normally distributed, randomly selected.

[a]Use if there are small numbers (<5 in a cell).

[b]Post-hoc: Scheffé's or Tukey test.

- Number needed to treat (NNT): the number needed to *obtain* or *avoid* a single additional outcome

$$NNT = 1/EER - CER$$

  - Where EER = experimental group event rate and CER = control group event rate

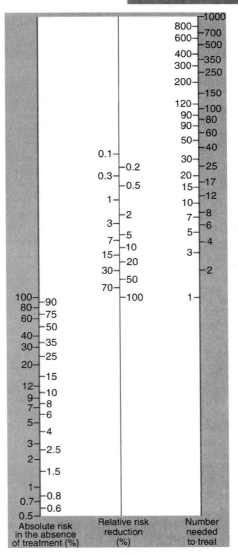

Number needed to treat nomogram. (Source: Reproduced with permission from Chatellier G, Zapletal E, Lemaitre D, et al. The number needed to treat: a clinically useful nomogram in its proper context. *BMJ* 312[7028]:426, 1996.)

References

Abdalla H, Thum MY. An elevated basal FSH reflects a quantitative rather than qualitative decline of the ovarian reserve. *Hum Reprod* 19(4):893, 2004.

Abdel Gadir A, Alnaser HMI, et al. The response of patients with polycystic ovarian disease to human menopausal gonadotropin therapy after ovarian electrocautery or a luteinizing hormone-releasing hormone agonist. *Fertil Steril* 57:309, 1992.

Abdel Gadir A, Mowafi RS, et al. Ovarian electrocautery versus human menopausal gonadotrophins and pure follicle stimulating hormone therapy in the treatment of patients with polycystic ovarian disease. *Clin Endocrinol (Oxf)* 33(5):585, 1990.

Aboulghar M, Evers JH, et al. Intra-venous albumin for preventing severe ovarian hyperstimulation syndrome. *Cochrane Database Syst Rev* (2):CD001302, 2002.

Adam Z, Poulin F, et al. Increased risk of neural tube defects after recurrent pregnancy losses. *Am J Med Genet* 55(4):512, 1995.

Advincula AP, Song A. Chronic pelvic pain. In Sanfilippo J, Smith R, eds. *Primary Care in Obstetrics & Gynecology A Handbook for Clinicians.* New York: Springer, 2004.

Affinito P, Palomba S, et al. Ultrasonographic measurement of endometrial thickness during hormonal replacement therapy in postmenopausal women. *Ultrasound Obstet Gynecol* 11(5):343, 1998.

Ailawadi RK, Jobanputra S, et al. Treatment of endometriosis and chronic pelvic pain with letrozole and norethindrone acetate: a pilot study. *Fertil Steril* 81(2):290, 2004.

Ailawadi M, Lorch SA, et al. Cost-effectiveness of presumptively medically treating women at risk for ectopic pregnancy compared with first performing a dilatation and curettage. *Fertil Steril* 83(2):376, 2005.

Aitken RJ, Clarkson JS, et al. Analysis of the relationship between defective sperm function and the generation of reactive oxygen species in cases of oligozoospermia. *J Androl* 10(3):214, 1989.

Akande VA, Hunt LP, et al. Differences in time to natural conception between women with unexplained infertility and infertile women with minor endometriosis. *Hum Reprod* 19(1):96, 2004.

Alberman E. The epidemiology of repeated abortion. In Beard RW, Sharp F. *Early Pregnancy Loss: Mechanisms and Treatment.* New York: Springer-Verlag, 1988:9.

Amar AP, Couldwell WT, et al. Predictive value of serum prolactin levels measured immediately after transsphenoidal surgery. *J Neurosurg* 97(2):307, 2002.

Amer SA, Li TC, et al. Ovulation induction using laparoscopic ovarian drilling in women with polycystic ovarian syndrome: predictors of success. *Hum Reprod* 19(8):1719, 2004.

REFERENCES

American College of Obstetricians and Gynecologists. Educational Bulletin no. 246. Washington, DC: American College of Obstetricians and Gynecologists, 1998.

The American Fertility Society. The American Fertility Society classifications of adnexal adhesions, distal tubal occlusion, tubal occlusion secondary to tubal ligation, tubal pregnancies, mullerian anomalies and intrauterine adhesions. *Fertil Steril* 49(6):944, 1988.

American Psychiatric Association. *Diagnostic and Statistical Manual of Mental Disorders* (4th ed, text revision). Washington, DC: American Psychiatric Association, 2004:367.

American Society for Reproductive Medicine. Revised American Society for Reproductive Medicine classification of endometriosis: 1996. *Fertil Steril* 67(5):817, 1997.

Anasti JN. Premature ovarian failure: an update. *Fertil Steril* 70(1):1, 1998.

Andersen AG, Als-Nielsen B, et al. Time interval from human chorionic gonadotrophin (HCG) injection to follicular rupture. *Hum Reprod* 10(12):3202, 1995.

Anderson GL, Limacher M, et al.; Women's Health Initiative Steering Committee. Effects of conjugated equine estrogen in postmenopausal women with hysterectomy: the Women's Health Initiative randomized controlled trial. *JAMA* 291(14):1701, 2004.

Apter D, Viinikka L, et al. Hormonal pattern of adolescent menstrual cycles. *J Clin Endocrinol Metab* 47(5):944, 1978.

Arici A, Byrd W, et al. Evaluation of clomiphene citrate and human chorionic gonadotropin treatment: a prospective, randomized, crossover study during intrauterine insemination cycles. *Fertil Steril* 61(2):314, 1994.

Association of Professors of Gynecology and Obstetrics Clinical management of abnormal uterine bleeding. Association of Professors of Gynecology and Obstetrics educational series on women's health issues, 2002.

Awonuga A, Govindbhai J. Is waiting for an endogenous luteinizing hormone surge and/or administration of human chorionic gonadotrophin of benefit in intrauterine insemination? *Hum Reprod* 14(7):1765, 1999.

Ayvaliotis B, Bronson R, et al. Conception rates in couples where autoimmunity to sperm is detected. *Fertil Steril* 43(5):739, 1985.

Bachmann GA. Vasomotor flushes in menopausal women. *Am J Obstet Gynecol* 180(3 Pt 2):S312, 1999.

Bachmann GA, Kemmann E. Prevalence of oligomenorrhea and amenorrhea in a college population. *Am J Obstet Gynecol* 144(1):98, 1982.

Bagratee JS, Khullar V, et al. A randomized controlled trial comparing medical and expectant management of first trimester miscarriage. *Hum Reprod* 19(2):266, 2004.

Baillargeon JP, Jakubowicz DJ, et al. Effects of metformin and rosiglitazone, alone

REFERENCES

and in combination, in nonobese women with polycystic ovary syndrome and normal indices of insulin sensitivity. *Fertil Steril* 82(4):893, 2004.

Baird DT. A model for follicular selection and ovulation: lessons from superovulation. *J Steroid Biochem* 27(1–3):15, 1987.

Bajekal N, Li TC. Fibroids, infertility and pregnancy wastage. *Hum Reprod Update* 6(6):614, 2000.

Bakalov VK, Vanderhoof VH, et al. Adrenal antibodies detect asymptomatic auto-immune adrenal insufficiency in young women with spontaneous premature ovarian failure. *Hum Reprod* 17(8):2096, 2002.

Baker VL, Adamson GD. Minimum intrauterine pressure required for uterine distention. *J Am Assoc Gynecol Laparosc* 5(1):51, 1998.

Balasch J, Creus M, et al. Lack of endometriosis in patients with repeated abortion. *Hum Reprod* 3(2):263, 1988.

Balasch J, Creus M, et al. Visible and non-visible endometriosis at laparoscopy in fertile and infertile women and in patients with chronic pelvic pain: a prospective study. *Hum Reprod* 11(2):1163, 1996.

Balasch J, Creus M, et al. Pentoxifylline versus placebo in the treatment of infertility associated with minimal or mild endometriosis: a pilot randomized clinical trial. *Hum Reprod* 12(9):2046, 1997.

Bancsi LF, Broekmans FJ, et al. Predictors of poor ovarian response in in vitro fertilization: a prospective study comparing basal markers of ovarian reserve. *Fertil Steril* 77(2):328, 2002.

Barbieri RL. Hormone treatment of endometriosis: the estrogen threshold hypothesis. *Am J Obstet Gynecol* 166:740, 1992.

Barnhart K, Dunsmoor-Su R, et al. Effect of endometriosis on in vitro fertilization. *Fertil Steril* 77(6):1148, 2002.

Barnhart K, Osheroff J. Follicle stimulating hormone as a predictor of fertility. *Curr Opin Obstet Gynecol* 10(3):227, 1998.

Barnhart K, Sammel MD, et al. Decline of serum human chorionic gonadotropin and spontaneous complete abortion: defining the normal curve. *Obstet Gynecol* 104(5):975, 2004a.

Barnhart KT, Sammel MD, et al. Symptomatic patients with an early viable intrauterine pregnancy: HCG curves redefined. *Obstet Gynecol* 104(1):50, 2004b.

Basaria S, Nguyen T, et al. Effect of methyl testosterone administration on plasma viscosity in postmenopausal women. *Clin Endocrinol (Oxf)* 57(2):209, 2002.

Bateman BG, Taylor PT, Jr. Reproductive considerations during abdominal surgical procedures in young women. *Surg Clin North Am* 71(5):1053, 1991.

Bates G.W, Jr., Hill JA. Autoimmune ovarian failure. *Infertil Reprod Med Clinics NA* 13(1):65, 2002.

Bauer DC, Mundy GR, et al. Use of statins and fracture: results of 4 prospective studies and cumulative meta-analysis of observational studies and controlled trials. *Arch Intern Med* 164(2):146, 2004.

Bayram N, van Wely M, et al. Using an electrocautery strategy or recombinant follicle stimulating hormone to induce ovulation in polycystic ovary syndrome: randomised controlled trial. *BMJ* 328(7433):192, 2004.

Beck LE, Gevirtz R, Mortola JF. The predictive role of psychosocial stress on symptom severity in premenstrual syndrome. *Psychosom Med* 52(5):536, 1990.

Beerendonk CC, van Dop PA, et al. Ovarian hyperstimulation syndrome: facts and fallacies. *Obstet Gynecol Surv* 53(7):439, 1998.

Belker AM, Thomas AJ, Jr., et al. Results of 1,469 microsurgical vasectomy reversals by the Vasovasostomy Study Group. *J Urol* 145(3):505, 1991.

Belli SH, Graffigna MN, et al. Effect of rosiglitazone on insulin resistance, growth factors, and reproductive disturbances in women with polycystic ovary syndrome. *Fertil Steril* 81(3):624, 2004.

Beretta P, Franchi M, et al. Randomized clinical trial of two laparoscopic treatments of endometriomas: cystectomy versus drainage and coagulation. *Fertil Steril* 70(6):1176, 1998.

Berube S, Marcoux S, et al. Fecundity of infertile women with minimal or mild endometriosis and women with unexplained infertility. The Canadian Collaborative Group on Endometriosis. *Fertil Steril* 69(6):1034, 1998.

Bishoff JT, Allaf ME, et al. Laparoscopic bowel injury: incidence and clinical presentation. *J Urol* 161(3):887, 1999.

Bissonnette F, Lapensee L, et al. Outpatient laparoscopic tubal anastomosis and subsequent fertility. *Fertil Steril* 72(3):549, 1999.

Blake D, Proctor M, et al. Cleavage stage versus blastocyst stage embryo transfer in assisted conception. *The Cochrane Database of Systematic Reviews* Issue 2, 2002.

Blumenfeld Z, Avivi I, et al. Prevention of irreversible chemotherapy-induced ovarian damage in young women with lymphoma by a gonadotrophin-releasing hormone agonist in parallel to chemotherapy. *Hum Reprod* 11(8):1620, 1996.

Boer-Meisel ME, te Velde ER, et al. Predicting the pregnancy outcome in patients treated for hydrosalpinx: a prospective study. *Fertil Steril* 45(1):23, 1986.

Bonduelle M, Aytoz A, et al. Incidence of chromosomal aberrations in children born after assisted reproduction through intracytoplasmic sperm injection. *Hum Reprod* 13(4):781, 1998a.

Bonduelle M, Wilikens A, et al. A follow-up study of children born after intracytoplasmic sperm injection (ICSI) with epididymal and testicular spermatozoa and after replacement of cryopreserved embryos obtained after ICSI. *Hum Reprod* 13[Suppl 1]:196, 1998b.

Boon J, Scholten PC, et al. Continuous intrauterine compared with cyclic oral progestin administration in perimenopausal HRT. *Maturitas* 46(1):69, 2003.

REFERENCES

Boue A, Boue J, et al. Cytogenetics of pregnancy wastage. *Adv Hum Genet* 14:1, 1985.

Boue JG, Boue A. Increased frequency of chromosomal anomalies in abortions after induced ovulation. *Lancet* 1(7804):679, 1973.

Breitkopf DM, Frederickson RA, et al. Detection of benign endometrial masses by endometrial stripe measurement in premenopausal women. *Obstet Gynecol* 104(1):120, 2004.

Brenner B, Sarig G, et al. Thrombophilic polymorphisms are common in women with fetal loss without apparent cause. *Thromb Haemost* 82(1):6, 1999.

Brinton LA, Gridley G, et al. Cancer risk after a hospital discharge diagnosis of endometriosis. *Am J Obstet Gynecol* 176(3):572, 1997.

Braunstein GD, Grodin JM, et al. Secretory rates of human chorionic gonadotropin by normal trophoblast. *Am J Obstet Gynecol* 15;115(4):447, 1973.

Brown DL, Felker RE, et al. Serial endovaginal sonography of ectopic pregnancies treated with methotrexate. *Obstet Gynecol* 77:406, 1991.

Brzezinski AA, Wurtman JJ, et al. d-Fenfluramine suppresses the increased calorie and carbohydrate intakes and improves the mood of women with premenstrual depression. *Obstet Gynecol* 76(2):296, 1990.

Buckett WM. A meta-analysis of ultrasound-guided versus clinical touch embryo transfer. *Fertil Steril* 80(4):1037, 2003.

Burrow GN, Wortzman G, et al. Microadenomas of the pituitary and abnormal sellar tomograms in an unselected autopsy series. *N Engl J Med* 304(3):156, 1981.

Buster JE, Pisarska MD. Medical management of ectopic pregnancy. *Clinical Obstet Gynecol* 42(1):23, 1999.

Buttram VC, Jr. Mullerian anomalies and their management. *Fertil Steril* 40(2):159, 1983.

Buttram VC, Jr., Reiter RC. Abdominal myomectomy and subsequent fertility. *Fertil Steril* 36:433, 1981.

Buyalos RP, Daneshmand S, et al. Basal estradiol and follicle-stimulating hormone predict fecundity in women of advanced reproductive age undergoing ovulation induction therapy. *Fertil Steril* 68(2):272, 1997.

Buyalos RP, Ghosh K, et al. Infertile women of advanced reproductive age. Variability of day 3 FSH and E2 levels. *J Reprod Med* 43(12):1023, 1998.

Callen PW. *Ultrasonography in Obstetrics and Gynecology*. San Francisco: WB Saunders, 2000.

Camus E, Poncelet C, et al. Pregnancy rates after in-vitro fertilization in cases of tubal infertility with and without hydrosalpinx: a meta-analysis of published comparative studies. *Hum Reprod* 14(5):1243, 1999.

Carr B, Breslau N, et al. Oral contraceptive pill, GnRH agonists, or use in combination for treatment of hirsutism. *J Clin Endocrinol Metab* 60(4): 1169, 1995.

384

REFERENCES

Carrington BM, Hricak H, et al. Mullerian duct anomalies: MR imaging evaluation. *Radiology* 176(3):715, 1990.

Casper RF. Treatment of premenstrual dysphoric disorder. UpToDate Patient Information Web site: http://www.utdol.com. Accessed February, 2005

Casson PR, Elkind-Hirsch KE, et al. Effect of postmenopausal estrogen replacement on circulating androgens. *Obstet Gynecol* 90(6):995, 1997.

Castelbaum AJ, Wheeler J, et al. Timing of the endometrial biopsy may be critical for the accurate diagnosis of luteal phase deficiency. *Fertil Steril* 61(3):443, 1994.

Catarci T, Fiacco F, et al. Empty sella and headache. *Headache* 34(10):583, 1994.

Centers for Disease Control and Prevention. *2001 Assisted Reproductive Technology Success Rates*, December 2003.

Chan AF, Mortola JF, et al. Persistence of premenstrual syndrome during low-dose administration of the progesterone antagonist RU 486. *Obstet Gynecol* 84(6):1001, 1994.

Chang MY, Chiang CH, et al. Use of the antral follicle count to predict the outcome of assisted reproductive technologies. *Fertil Steril* 69(3):505, 1998.

Chatellier G, Zapletal E, et al. The number needed to treat: a clinically useful nomogram in its proper context. *BMJ* 312(7028):426, 1996.

Cheung AP. Ultrasound and menstrual history in predicting endometrial hyperplasia in polycystic ovary syndrome. *Obstet Gynecol* 98(2):325, 2001.

Chillon M, Casals T, et al. Mutations in the cystic fibrosis gene in patients with congenital absence of the vas deferens. *N Engl J Med* 332(22):1475, 1995.

Chipchase J, James D. Randomised trial of expectant versus surgical management of spontaneous miscarriage. *Br J Obstet Gynaecol* 104(7):840, 1997.

Choudhury SR, Knapp LA. Human reproductive failure II: immunogenetic and interacting factors. *Hum Reprod Update* 7(2):135, 2001.

Christiansen OB, Pedersen B, et al. A randomized, double-blind, placebo-controlled trial of intravenous immunoglobulin in the prevention of recurrent miscarriage: evidence for a therapeutic effect in women with secondary recurrent miscarriage. *Hum Reprod* 17(3):809, 2002.

Chuong CJ, Dawson EB, et al. Vitamin A levels in premenstrual syndrome. *Fertil Steril* 54(4):643, 1990a.

Chuong CJ, Dawson EB, et al. Vitamin E levels in premenstrual syndrome. *Am J Obstet Gynecol* 163(5 Pt 1):1591, 1990b.

Ciccarelli E, Camanni F. Diagnosis and drug therapy of prolactinoma. *Drugs* 51(6):954, 1996.

Ciotta L, Cianci A, et al. Clinical and endocrine effects of finasteride, a 5 α-reductase inhibitor, in women with idiopathic hirsutism. *Fertil Steril* 64(2): 299, 1995.

Clarke GN, Elliott PJ, et al. Detection of sperm antibodies in semen using the

REFERENCES

immunobead test: a survey of 813 consecutive patients. *Am J Reprod Immunol Microbiol* 7(3):118, 1985.

Clifford K, Rai R, et al. An informative protocol for the investigation of recurrent miscarriage: preliminary experience of 500 consecutive cases. *Hum Reprod* 9(7):1328, 1994.

Cnattingius S, Signorello LB, et al. Caffeine intake and the risk of first-trimester spontaneous abortion. *N Engl J Med* 343(25):1839, 2000.

Col NF, Pauker SG. The discrepancy between observational studies and randomized trials of menopausal hormone therapy: did expectations shape experience? *Ann Intern Med* 139(11):923, 2003.

Colao A, Di Sarno A, et al. Withdrawal of long-term cabergoline therapy for tumoral and nontumoral hyperprolactinemia. *N Engl J Med* 349(21):2023, 2003.

Colao A, Di Somma C, et al. Prolactinomas in adolescents: persistent bone loss after 2 years of prolactin normalization. *Clin Endocrinol (Oxf)* 52(3):319, 2000.

Colditz GA, Stampfer MJ, et al. Type of postmenopausal hormone use and risk of breast cancer: 12-year follow-up from the Nurses' Health Study. *Cancer Causes Control* 3(5):433, 1992.

Cole LA. Phantom hCG and phantom choriocarcinoma. *Gynecol Oncol* 71(2):325, 1998.

Cole LA, Khanlian SA, et al. Accuracy of home pregnancy tests at the time of missed menses. *Am J Obstet Gynecol* 190(1):100, 2004.

Condon JT. The premenstrual syndrome: a twin study. *Br J Psychiatry* 162:481, 1993.

Cooper DS. Subclinical hypothyroidism. *New Engl J Med* 345(4):260, 2001.

Corenblum B, Donovan L. The safety of physiological estrogen plus progestin replacement therapy and with oral contraceptive therapy in women with pathological hyperprolactinemia. *Fertil Steril* 59(3):671, 1993.

Coulam CB, Adamson SC, et al. Incidence of premature ovarian failure. *Obstet Gynecol* 67:604, 1986.

Coulam CB, Bustillo M, et al. Ultrasonographic predictors of implantation after assisted reproduction. *Fertil Steril* 62(5):1004, 1994.

Coutifaris C, Myers ER, et al. Histological dating of timed endometrial biopsy tissue is not related to fertility status. *Fertil Steril* 82(5):1264, 2004.

Coutinho EM, Mascarenhas I, et al. Comparative study on the efficacy, acceptability, and side effects of a contraceptive pill administered by the oral and the vaginal route: an international multicenter clinical trial. *Clin Pharmacol Ther* 54(5):540, 1993.

Couzinet B, Meduri G, et al. The postmenopausal ovary is not a major androgen-producing gland. *J Clin Endocrinol Metab* 86(10):5060, 2001.

Craig LB, Ke RW, et al. Increased prevalence of insulin resistance in women with a history of recurrent pregnancy loss. *Fertil Steril* 78(3):487, 2002.

Creinin MD. Laboratory criteria for menopause in women using oral contraceptives. *Fertil Steril* 66(1):101, 1996.

Creinin MD, Schwartz JL, et al. Early pregnancy failure—current management concepts. *Obstet Gynecol Surv* 56(2):105, 2001.

Creus M, Penarrubia J, et al. Day 3 serum inhibin B and FSH and age as predictors of assisted reproduction treatment outcome. *Hum Reprod* 15(11):2341, 2000.

Csapo AI, Pulkkinen M. Indispensability of the human corpus luteum in the maintenance of early pregnancy. Luteectomy evidence. *Obstet Gynecol Surv* 33(2):69, 1978.

Curtis KM, Chrisman CE, et al. Contraception for women in selected circumstances. *Obstet Gynecol* 99(6):1100, 2002.

Dabirashrafi H, Bahadori M, et al. Septate uterus: new idea on the histologic features of the septum in this abnormal uterus. *Am J Obstet Gynecol* 172(1 Pt 1):105, 1995.

Daly DC, Walters CA, et al. A randomized study of dexamethasone in ovulation induction with clomiphene citrate. *Fertil Steril* 41(6):844, 1984.

Danforth DR, Roberts A, et al. Follicular preservation during cyclophosphamide treatment: GnRH agonist vs. antagonist. *J Soc Gynecol Investig* 10(2 [Suppl]):135A, 2003.

Daniell JF, Miller W. Polycystic ovaries treated by laparoscopic laser vaporization. *Fertil Steril* 51(2):232, 1989.

Daniely M, Aviram-Goldring A, et al. Detection of chromosomal aberration in fetuses arising from recurrent spontaneous abortion by comparative genomic hybridization. *Hum Reprod* 13(4):805, 1998.

Davis OK, Berkeley AS, et al. The incidence of luteal phase defect in normal, fertile women, determined by serial endometrial biopsies. *Fertil Steril* 51(4):582, 1989.

Davis RO, Katz DF. Computer-aided sperm analysis: technology at a crossroads. *Fertil Steril* 59(5):953, 1993.

Daya S, Ward S, et al. Progesterone profiles in luteal phase defect cycles and outcome of progesterone treatment in patients with recurrent spontaneous abortion. *Am J Obstet Gynecol* 158(2):225, 1988.

de Kroon CD, de Bock GH, et al. Saline contrast hysterosonography in abnormal uterine bleeding: a systematic review and meta-analysis. *BJOG* 110(10):938, 2003.

De Placido G, Alviggi C, et al. Serum concentrations of soluble human leukocyte class I antigens and of the soluble intercellular adhesion molecule-1 in endometriosis: relationship with stage and non-pigmented peritoneal lesions. *Hum Reprod* 13(11):3206, 1998.

REFERENCES

De Souza MJ, Miller BE, et al. High frequency of luteal phase deficiency and anovulation in recreational women runners: blunted elevation in follicle-stimulating hormone observed during luteal-follicular transition. *J Clin Endocrinol Metab* 83(12):4220, 1998.

Deaton JL, Gibson M, et al. A randomized, controlled trial of clomiphene citrate and intrauterine insemination in couples with unexplained infertility or surgically corrected endometriosis. *Fertil Steril* 54(6):1083, 1990.

Deaton JL, Honore GM, et al. Early transvaginal ultrasound following an accurately dated pregnancy: the importance of finding a yolk sac or fetal heart motion. *Hum Reprod* 12(12):2820, 1997.

Delemarre-van de Waal HA. Regulation of puberty. *Best Pract Res Clin Endocrinol Metab* 16(1):1, 2002.

Delmas PD. Markers of bone turnover for monitoring treatment of osteoporosis with antiresorptive drugs. *Osteoporos Int* 11[Suppl 6]:S66, 2000.

Dennerstein L, Randolph J, et al. Hormones, mood, sexuality, and the menopausal transition. *Fertil Steril* 77[Suppl 4]:S42, 2002.

D'Hooghe TM, Debrock S, et al. Endometriosis and subfertility: is the relationship resolved? *Semin Reprod Med* 21(2):243, 2003.

D'Hooghe, TM, Hill JA. Killer cell activity, statistics, and endometriosis. *Fertil Steril* 64(1):226, 1995.

Dias Pereira G, Hajenius PJ, et al. Fertility outcome after systemic methotrexate and laparoscopic salpingostomy for tubal pregnancy. *Lancet* 353(9154):724, 1999.

Dickey RP, Olar TT, et al. Relationship of follicle number, serum estradiol, and other factors to birth rate and multiparity in human menopausal gonadotropin-induced intrauterine insemination cycles. *Fertil Steril* 56(1):89, 1991.

Dickey RP, Olar TT, et al. Relationship of endometrial thickness and pattern to fecundity in ovulation induction cycles: effect of clomiphene citrate alone and with human menopausal gonadotropin. *Fertil Steril* 59(4):756, 1993.

Dickey RP, Taylor SN, et al. Relationship of follicle numbers and estradiol levels to multiple implantation in 3,608 intrauterine insemination cycles. *Fertil Steril* 75(1):69, 2001.

DiSaia PJ, Creasman WT. Epithelial ovarian cancer. In *Clinical Gynecologic Oncology*. St. Louis: Mosby Year Book, 1997:529.

Dizerega GS, Barber DL, et al. Endometriosis: role of ovarian steroids in initiation, maintenance, and suppression. *Fertil Steril* 33(6):649, 1980.

Djahanbakhch O, McNeily AS, et al. Changes in plasma levels of prolactin, in relation to those of FSH, oestradiol, androstenedione and progesterone around the preovulatory surge of LH in women. *Clin Endocrinol (Oxf)* 20:463, 1984.

Dohle GR, Halley DJ, et al. Genetic risk factors in infertile men with severe oligozoospermia and azoospermia. *Hum Reprod* 17(1):13, 2002.

Donnelly ET, McClure N, et al. Cryopreservation of human semen and prepared sperm: effects on motility parameters and DNA integrity. *Fertil Steril* 76(5):892, 2001.

Donnez J, Dolmans MM, et al. Livebirth after orthotopic transplantation of cryopreserved ovarian tissue. *Lancet* 364(9443):1405, 2004.

Donnez J, Nisolle M, et al. Peritoneal endometriosis and "endometriotic" nodules of the rectovaginal septum are two different entities. *Fertil Steril* 66:362, 1996.

Dorflinger LJ. Relative potency of progestins used in oral contraceptives. *Contraception* 31(6):557, 1985.

Dorman JS, Burke JP, et al. Temporal trends in spontaneous abortion associated with Type 1 diabetes. *Diabetes Res Clin Pract* 43(1):41, 1999.

Dorn C, Mouillet JF, et al. Insulin enhances the transcription of luteinizing hormone-beta gene. *Am J Obstet Gynecol* 191(1):132, 2004.

Dubowy RL, Feinberg RF, et al. Improved endometrial assessment using cyclin E and p27. *Fertil Steril* 80(1):146, 2003.

Duggan MA, Brashert P, et al. The accuracy and interobserver reproducibility of endometrial dating. *Pathology* 33(3):292, 2001.

Dunaif A. Insulin resistance and the polycystic ovary syndrome: mechanism and implications for pathogenesis. *Endocr Rev* 18(6):774, 1997.

Dunaif A, Zia J, et al. Excessive insulin receptor serine phosphorylation in cultured fibroblasts and in skeletal muscle. A potential mechanism for insulin resistance in the polycystic ovary syndrome. *J Clin Invest* 96(2):801, 1995.

Dunn JF, Nisula BC, et al. Transport of steroid hormones: binding of 21 endogenous steroids to both testosterone-binding globulin and corticosteroid-binding globulin in human plasma. *J Clin Endocrinol Metab* 53(1):58, 1981.

Dunson DB, Colombo B, et al. Changes with age in the level and duration of fertility in the menstrual cycle. *Hum Reprod* 17(5):1399, 2002.

Eagleson CA, Gingrich MB, et al. Polycystic ovarian syndrome: evidence that flutamide restores sensitivity of the gonadotropin-releasing hormone pulse generator to inhibition by estradiol and progesterone. *J Clin Endocrinol Metab* 85(11):4047, 2000.

Ecochard R, Gougeon A. Side of ovulation and cycle characteristics in normally fertile women. *Hum Reprod* 15(4):752, 2000.

Edmonds DK, Lindsay KS, et al. Early embryonic mortality in women. *Fertil Steril* 38(4):447, 1982.

Elias KA, Weiner RI. Direct arterial vascularization of estrogen-induced prolactin-secreting anterior pituitary tumors. *Proc Natl Acad Sci U S A* 81(14):4549, 1984.

Elting MW, Korsen TJ, et al. Women with polycystic ovary syndrome gain regular menstrual cycles when ageing. *Hum Reprod* 15(1):24, 2000.

Empson M, Lassere M, et al. Recurrent pregnancy loss with antiphospholipid antibody: a systematic review of therapeutic trials. *Obstet Gynecol* 99(1):135, 2002.

REFERENCES

Endo T, Kitajima Y, et al. Low-molecular-weight dextran infusion is more effective for the treatment of hemoconcentration due to severe ovarian hyperstimulation syndrome than human albumin infusion. *Fertil Steril* 82(5):1449, 2004.

Erick M. Hyperemesis gravidarum: a practical management strategy. *OBG Management*, November 2000: 25–35.

Erickson GF, Magoffin DA, et al. The ovarian androgen producing cells: a review of structure/function relationships. *Endocr Rev* 6(3):371, 1985.

Eskenazi B, Wyrobek AJ, et al. The association of age and semen quality in healthy men. *Hum Reprod* 18(2):447, 2003.

Espeland MA, Rapp SR, et al. Conjugated equine estrogens and global cognitive function in postmenopausal women: Women's Health Initiative Memory Study. *JAMA* 291(24):2959, 2004.

Ettinger B, Ensrud KE, et al. Effects of ultralow-dose transdermal estradiol on bone mineral density: a randomized clinical trial. *Obstet Gynecol* 104(3):443, 2004.

Ettinger MP. Aging bone and osteoporosis: strategies for preventing fractures in the elderly. *Arch Intern Med* 163(18):2237, 2003.

Evers JL, Collins JA. Assessment of efficacy of varicocele repair for male subfertility: a systematic review. *Lancet* 361(9372):1849, 2003.

Facchinetti F, Borella P, et al. Oral magnesium successfully relieves premenstrual mood changes. *Obstet Gynecol* 78(2):177, 1991.

Falcone T, Attaran M, et al. Ovarian function preservation in the cancer patient. *Fertil Steril* 81(2):243, 2004.

Fanchin R, Righini C, et al. New look at endometrial echogenicity: objective computer-assisted measurements predict endometrial receptivity in in vitro fertilization-embryo transfer. *Fertil Steril* 74(2):274, 2000.

Farhi J, Ashkenazi J, et al. Effect of uterine leiomyomata on the results of in-vitro fertilization treatment. *Hum Reprod* 10(10):2576, 1995.

Farley TM, Meirik O, et al. Cardiovascular disease and combined oral contraceptives: reviewing the evidence and balancing the risks. *Hum Reprod Update* 5(6):721, 1999.

Farquhar CM, Lethaby A, et al. An evaluation of risk factors for endometrial hyperplasia in premenopausal women with abnormal menstrual bleeding. *Am J Obstet Gynecol* 181(3):525, 1999.

Fassnacht M, Schlenz N, et al. Beyond adrenal and ovarian androgen generation: increased peripheral 5 alpha-reductase activity in women with polycystic ovary syndrome. *J Clin Endocrinol Metab* 88(6):2760, 2003.

Fedele L, Bianchi S, et al. Superovulation with human menopausal gonadotropins in the treatment of infertility associated with minimal or mild endometriosis: a controlled randomized study. *Fertil Steril* 58(1):28, 1992.

Fedele L, Bianchi S, et al. Residual uterine septum of less than 1 cm after hysteroscopic metroplasty does not impair reproductive outcome. *Hum Reprod* 11(4):727, 1996a.

Fedele L, Bianchi S, et al. Ultrastructural aspects of endometrium in infertile women with septate uterus. *Fertil Steril* 65(4):750, 1996b.

Fedele L, Bianchi S, et al. Transrectal ultrasonography in the assessment of rectovaginal endometriosis. *Obstet Gynecol* 91:444, 1998.

Feicht CB, Johnson TS, et al. Secondary amenorrhoea in athletes. *Lancet* 2(8100): 1145, 1978.

Feigenbaum SL, Downey DE, et al. Transsphenoidal pituitary resection for preoperative diagnosis of prolactin-secreting pituitary adenoma in women: long term follow-up. *J Clin Endocrinol Metab* 81(5):1711, 1996.

Felemban A, Tan SL, et al. Laparoscopic treatment of polycystic ovaries with insulated needle cautery: a reappraisal. *Fertil Steril* 73(2):266, 2000.

Fernandez E, La Vecchia C, et al. Oral contraceptives and colorectal cancer risk: a meta-analysis. *Br J Cancer* 84(5):722, 2001.

Ferriman D, Gallway JD. Clinical assessment of body hair growth in women. *J Clin Endocrinol Metab* 21:1440, 1961.

Fertility Plus Web Site: http://www.fertilityplus.org. Accessed February, 2005.

Filicori M, Cognigni GE. Roles and novel regimens of luteinizing hormone and follicle-stimulating hormone in ovulation induction. *J Clin Endocrinol Metab* 86(4):1437, 2001.

Filicori M, Santoro N, et al. Characterization of the physiological pattern of episodic gonadotropin secretion throughout the human menstrual cycle. *J Clin Endocrinol Metab* 62(6):1136, 1986.

Fishel SB, Edwards RG, et al. Human chorionic gonadotropin secreted by preimplantation embryos cultured in vitro. *Science* 223(4638):816, 1984.

Foka ZJ, Lambropoulos AF, et al. Factor V Leiden and prothrombin G20210A mutations, but not methylenetetrahydrofolate reductase C677T, are associated with recurrent miscarriages. *Hum Reprod* 15(2):458, 2000.

Foma F, Gulmezoglu AM. Surgical procedures to evacuate incomplete abortion (Cochrane Review). In *The Cochrane Library*. Chichester, UK: John Wiley and Sons, 2003.

Foresta C, Moro E, et al. Prognostic value of Y deletion analysis. The role of current methods. *Hum Reprod* 16(8):1543, 2001.

Foulk RA, Martin MC, et al. Hyperreactio luteinalis differentiated from severe ovarian hyperstimulation syndrome in a spontaneously conceived pregnancy. *Am J Obstet Gynecol* 176(6):1300; discussion, 1302, 1997.

Frank RT. The hormonal causes of premenstrual tension. *Arch Neurol Psychiatr* 26:1052, 1931.

Frank RT. Formation of artificial vagina without operation. *Am J Obstet Gynecol* 35:1053, 1938.

REFERENCES

Frattarelli JL, Lauria-Costab DF, et al. Basal antral follicle number and mean ovarian diameter predict cycle cancellation and ovarian responsiveness in assisted reproductive technology cycles. *Fertil Steril* 74(3):512, 2000.

Frattarelli JL, Levi AJ, et al. A prospective assessment of the predictive value of basal antral follicles in in vitro fertilization cycles. *Fertil Steril* 80(2):350, 2003.

Freedman RR, Roehrs TA. Lack of sleep disturbance from menopausal hot flashes. *Fertil Steril* 82(1):138, 2004.

Freeman EW, Kroll R, et al.; PMS/PMDD Research Group. Evaluation of a unique oral contraceptive in the treatment of premenstrual dysphoric disorder. *J Womens Health Gend Based Med* 10(6):561, 2001.

Friedler S, Margalioth EJ, et al. Incidence of post-abortion intra-uterine adhesions evaluated by hysteroscopy—a prospective study. *Hum Reprod* 8(3):442, 1993.

Friedman AJ, Daly M, et al. Recurrence of myomas after myomectomy in women pretreated with leuprolide acetate depot or placebo. *Fertil Steril* 58(1):205, 1992.

Friedman SA, de Groot CJM, et al. Plasma cellular fibronectin as a measure of endothelial cell injury in preeclampsia and intrauterine growth retardation. Proceedings of the 8th World Congress on Hypertension in Pregnancy. Presented in Buenos Aires, November 1992: 54.

Frisch RE, McArthur JW. Menstrual cycles: fatness as a determinant of minimum weight for height necessary for their maintenance or onset. *Science* 185(4155): 949, 1974.

Fritz B, Hallermann C, et al. Cytogenetic analyses of culture failures by comparative genomic hybridisation (CGH)-Re-evaluation of chromosome aberration rates in early spontaneous abortions. *Eur J Hum Genet* 9(7):539, 2001.

Fruzzetti F, Bersi C, et al. Treatment of hirsutism: comparisons between different antiandrogens with central and peripheral effects. *Fertil Steril* 71:445, 1999.

Fujimoto VY, Clifton DK, et al. Variability of serum prolactin and progesterone levels in normal women: the relevance of single hormone measurements in the clinical setting. *Obstet Gynecol* 76(1):71, 1990.

Garcia-Velasco JA, Arici A, et al. Macrophage derived growth factors modulate Fas ligand expression in cultured endometrial stromal cells: a role in endometriosis. *Mol Hum Reprod* 5(7):642, 1999.

Garcia-Velasco JA, Mahutte NG, et al. Removal of endometriomas before in vitro fertilization does not improve fertility outcomes: a matched, case-control study. *Fertil Steril* 81(5):1194, 2004.

Gene Tests Web Site: http://www.genereviews.org. Accessed February, 2005.

George L, Mills JL, et al. Plasma folate levels and risk of spontaneous abortion. *JAMA* 288(15):1867, 2002.

Ghazeeri G, Kutteh WH, et al. Effect of rosiglitazone on spontaneous and clomiphene citrate-induced ovulation in women with polycystic ovary syndrome. *Fertil Steril* 79(3):562, 2003.

Ghezzi F, Beretta P, et al. Recurrence of ovarian endometriosis and anatomical location of the primary lesion. *Fertil Steril* 75(1):136, 2001.

Ghezzi F, Raio L, et al. Vaginal extraction of pelvic masses following operative laparoscopy. *Surg Endosc* 16(12):1691, 2002.

Givens JR. Polycystic ovaries—a sign, not a diagnosis. *Semin Reprod Endocrinol* 34:67, 1984.

Gjønnæss H. Polycystic ovarian syndrome treated by ovarian electrocautery through the laparoscope. *Fertil Steril* 41(1):20, 1984.

Gjønnæss H. Late endocrine effects of ovarian electrocautery in women with polycystic ovary syndrome. *Fertil Steril* 69(4):697, 1998.

Glasow A, Breidert M, et al. Functional aspects of the effect of prolactin (PRL) on adrenal steroidogenesis and distribution of the PRL receptor in the human adrenal gland. *J Clin Endocrinol Metab* 81(8):3103, 1996.

Glick H, Endicott J, et al. Premenstrual changes: are they familial? *Acta Psychiatr Scand* 88(3):149, 1993.

Glueck CJ, Phillips H, et al. Continuing metformin throughout pregnancy in women with polycystic ovary syndrome appears to safely reduce first-trimester spontaneous abortion: a pilot study. *Fertil Steril* 75(1):46, 2001.

Glueck CJ, Wang P, et al. Metformin therapy throughout pregnancy reduces the development of gestational diabetes in women with polycystic ovary syndrome. *Fertil Steril* 77(3):520, 2002a.

Glueck CJ, Wang P, et al. Pregnancy outcomes among women with polycystic ovary syndrome treated with metformin. *Hum Reprod* 17(11):2858, 2002b.

Gnoth C, Godehardt D, et al. Time to pregnancy: results of the German prospective study and impact on the management of infertility. *Hum Reprod* 18(9):1959, 2003.

Golan A, Ron-El R, et al. Ovarian hyperstimulation syndrome: an update review. *Obstet Gynecol Surv* 44:430, 1989.

Golbus MJ. Chromosome aberrations and mammalian reproduction. In Mastroianni L, Biggers JD, eds. *Fertilization and Embryonic Development In Vitro*. New York: Plenum Press, 1981.

Goldstein RB, Bree RL, et al. Evaluation of the woman with postmenopausal bleeding: Society of Radiologists in Ultrasound–Sponsored Consensus Conference statement. *J Ultrasound Med* 20(10):1025, 2001.

Gordon JD, Rydfors JT, et al., eds. *Obstetrics Gynecology and Infertility* (5th ed). Arlington, VA: Scrub Hill Press, Inc., 2001.

Gottlieb N. Nonhormonal agents show promise against hot flashes. *J Natl Cancer Inst* 92(14):1118, 2000.

Gougeon A. Dynamics of follicular growth in the human: a model from preliminary results. *Hum Reprod* 1(2):81, 1986.

Grady D, Herrington D, et al. Cardiovascular disease outcomes during 6.8 years

REFERENCES

of hormone therapy: Heart and Estrogen/Progestin Replacement Study Follow-up (HERS II). *JAMA* 288(1):49, 2002.

Gravholt CH, Fedder J, et al. Occurrence of gonadoblastoma in females with Turner syndrome and Y chromosome material: a population study. *J Clin Endocrinol Metab* 85(9):3199, 2000.

Green J, Berrington de Gonzalez A, et al. Risk factors for adenocarcinoma and squamous cell carcinoma of the cervix in women aged 20–44 years: the UK National Case-Control Study of Cervical Cancer. *Br J Cancer* 89(11):2078, 2003.

Green LK, Harris RE. Uterine anomalies. Frequency of diagnosis and associated obstetric complications. *Obstet Gynecol* 47(4):427, 1976.

Greene R, Dalton K. The premenstrual syndrome. *Br Med J* i:1007, 1953.

Greenspan SL, Resnick NM, et al. Combination therapy with hormone replacement and alendronate for prevention of bone loss in elderly women: a randomized controlled trial. *JAMA* 289(19):2525, 2003.

Greer IA. Exploring the role of low-molecular-weight heparins in pregnancy. *Semin Thromb Hemost* 28[Suppl 3]:25, 2002.

Griffin JE, Edwards C, et al. Congenital absence of the vagina. *Ann Intern Med* 85:224, 1976.

Griffith CS, Grimes DA. The validity of the postcoital test. *Am J Obstet Gynecol* 162(3):615, 1990.

Groome NP, Illingworth PJ, et al. Measurement of dimeric inhibin B throughout the human menstrual cycle. *J Clin Endocrinol Metab* 81(4):1401, 1996.

Guermandi E, Vegetti W, et al. Reliability of ovulation tests in infertile women. *Obstet Gynecol* 97:92, 2001.

Guidelines on the number of embryos transferred. The Practice Committee of the Society for Assisted Reproductive Technology and the American Society for Reproductive Medicine. *Fertil Steril* 82[Suppl 1]:S1, 2004.

Gull B, Karlsson B, et al. Can ultrasound replace dilation and curettage? A longitudinal evaluation of postmenopausal bleeding and transvaginal sonographic measurement of the endometrium as predictors of endometrial cancer. *Am J Obstet Gynecol* 188(2):401, 2003.

Gupta JK, Chien PF, et al. Ultrasonographic endometrial thickness for diagnosing endometrial pathology in women with postmenopausal bleeding: a meta-analysis. *Acta Obstet Gynecol Scand* 81(9):799, 2002.

Gupta S. Weight gain on the combined pill—is it real? *Hum Reprod Update* 6(5):427, 2000.

Guttuso T, Jr., Kurlan R, et al. Gabapentin's effects on hot flashes in postmenopausal women: a randomized controlled trial. *Obstet Gynecol* 101(2):337, 2003.

Guzick D, Wing R, et al. Endocrine consequences of weight loss in obese, hyperandrogenic, anovulatory women. *Fertil Steril* 61(4):598, 1994.

Guzick DS, Carson SA, et al. Efficacy of superovulation and intrauterine insemination in the treatment of infertility. National Cooperative Reproductive Medicine Network. *N Engl J Med* 340(3):177, 1999.

Guzick DS, Overstreet JW, et al. Sperm morphology, motility, and concentration in fertile and infertile men. *N Engl J Med* 345(19):1388, 2001.

Guzick DS, Sullivan MW, et al. Efficacy of treatment for unexplained infertility. *Fertil Steril* 70(2):207, 1998.

Gysler M, March CM, et al. A decade's experience with an individualized clomiphene treatment regimen including its effect on the postcoital test. *Fertil Steril* 37(2):161, 1982.

Hak AE, Pols HA, et al. Subclinical hypothyroidism is an independent risk factor for atherosclerosis and myocardial infarction in elderly women: the Rotterdam Study. *Ann Intern Med* 132(4):270, 2000.

Halbreich U, Smoller JW. Intermittent luteal phase sertraline treatment of dysphoric premenstrual syndrome. *J Clin Psychiatry* 58(9):399, 1997.

Halbreich U, Tworek H. Altered serotonergic activity in women with dysphoric premenstrual syndromes. *Int J Psychiatry Med* 23(1):1, 1993.

Halme J, Becker S, et al. Altered maturation and function of peritoneal macrophages: possible role in pathogenesis of endometriosis. *Am J Obstet Gynecol* 156(4):783, 1987.

Hammond KR, Steinkampf MP, et al. The effect of routine breast examination on serum prolactin levels. *Fertil Steril* 65(4):869, 1996.

Hammond MG, Jordan S, et al. Factors affecting pregnancy rates in a donor insemination program using frozen semen. *Am J Obstet Gynecol* 155(3): 480, 1986.

Hankinson SE, Willett WC, et al. Plasma prolactin levels and subsequent risk of breast cancer in postmenopausal women. *J Natl Cancer Inst* 91(7):629, 1999.

Hansen KR, Morris JL, et al. Reproductive aging and variability in the ovarian antral follicle count: application in the clinical setting. *Fertil Steril* 80(3):577, 2003.

Hansen LM, Batzer FR, et al. Evaluating ovarian reserve: follicle stimulating hormone and oestradiol variability during cycle days 2–5. *Hum Reprod* 11(3):486, 1996.

Hansen M, Bower C, et al. Assisted reproductive technologies and the risk of birth defects—a systematic review. *Hum Reprod* 20(2):328, 2005.

Hansen M, Kurinczuk JJ, et al. The risk of major birth defects after intracytoplasmic sperm injection and in vitro fertilization. *N Engl J Med* 346(10):725, 2002.

Harada M, Osuga Y, et al. Concentration of osteoprotegerin (OPG) in peritoneal fluid is increased in women with endometriosis. *Hum Reprod* 19(10):2188, 2004.

Hardiman P, Pillay OC, et al. Polycystic ovary syndrome and endometrial carcinoma. *Lancet* 361(9371):1810, 2003.

REFERENCES

Harlap S, Shiono PH. Alcohol, smoking, and incidence of spontaneous abortions in the first and second trimester. *Lancet* 2(8187):173, 1980.

Harrison RF, Barry-Kinsella C. Efficacy of medroxyprogesterone treatment in infertile women with endometriosis: a prospective, randomized, placebo-controlled study. *Fertil Steril* 74(1):24, 2000.

Hassold TJ. A cytogenetic study of repeated spontaneous abortions. *Am J Hum Genet* 32(5):723, 1980.

Haynes PJ, Hodgson H, et al. Measurement of menstrual blood loss in patients complaining of menorrhagia. *Br J Obstet Gynaecol* 84(10):763, 1977.

Heard MJ, Pierce A, et al. Pregnancies following use of metformin for ovulation induction in patients with polycystic ovary syndrome. *Fertil Steril* 77(4):669, 2002.

Hecht BR, Bardawil WA, et al. Luteal insufficiency: correlation between endometrial dating and integrated progesterone output in clomiphene citrate-induced cycles. *Am J Obstet Gynecol* 163(6 Pt 1):1986, 1990.

Heck KE, Schoendorf KC, et al. Delayed childbearing by education level in the United States, 1969–1994. *Matern Child Health J* 1(2):81, 1997.

Heinonen PK. Unicornuate uterus and rudimentary horn. *Fertil Steril* 68(2):224, 1997.

Hellmuth E, Damm P, et al. Oral hypoglycaemic agents in 118 diabetic pregnancies. *Diabet Med* 17(7):507, 2000.

Herman-Giddens ME, Slora EJ, et al. Secondary sexual characteristics and menses in young girls seen in office practice: a study from the Pediatric Research in Office Settings network. *Pediatrics* 99(4):505, 1997.

Hickman TN, Namnoum AB, et al. Timing of estrogen replacement therapy following hysterectomy with oophorectomy for endometriosis. *Obstet Gynecol* 91(5 Pt 1):673, 1998.

Hill JA. Recurrent pregnancy loss: male and female factor, etiology and treatment. Frontiers in Reproductive Endocrinology, Washington, DC, Serono Symposia USA, Inc., 2001.

Hill JA, Polgar K, et al. T-helper 1-type immunity to trophoblast in women with recurrent spontaneous abortion. *JAMA* 273(24):1933, 1995.

Hirata J, Kikuchi Y, et al. Endometriotic tissues produce immunosuppressive factors. *Gynecol Obstet Invest* 37(1):43, 1994.

Hobbs L, Ort R, et al. Synopsis of laser assisted hair removal systems. *Skin Therapy Lett* 5(3):1, 2000.

Hock DL, Sharafi K, et al. Contribution of diminished ovarian reserve to hypofertility associated with endometriosis. *J Reprod Med* 46(1):7, 2001.

Hoff JD, Quigley ME, et al. Hormonal dynamics at midcycle: a reevaluation. *J Clin Endocrinol Metab* 57(4):792, 1983.

REFERENCES

Hofmann GE, Khoury J, et al. Recurrent pregnancy loss and diminished ovarian reserve. *Fertil Steril* 74(6):1192, 2000.

Homer HA, Li TC, et al. The septate uterus: a review of management and reproductive outcome. *Fertil Steril* 73(1):1, 2000.

Honda I, Sato T, et al. [Uterine artery embolization for leiomyoma: complications and effects on fertility]. *Nippon Igaku Hoshasen Gakkai Zasshi* 63(6):294, 2003.

Hook EB, Cross PK, et al. Chromosomal abnormality rates at amniocentesis and in live-born infants. *JAMA* 249(15):2034, 1983.

Hornstein MD, Hemmings R, et al. Use of nafarelin versus placebo after reductive laparoscopic surgery for endometriosis. *Fertil Steril* 68(5):860, 1997.

Hornstein MD, Surrey ES, et al. Leuprolide acetate depot and hormonal add-back in endometriosis: a 12-month study. Lupron Add-Back Study Group. *Obstet Gynecol* 91(1):16, 1998.

Hornstein MD, Yuzpe AA, et al. Prospective randomized double-blind trial of 3 versus 6 months of nafarelin therapy for endometriosis associated pelvic pain. *Fertil Steril* 63(5):955, 1995.

Hovatta O. Pregnancies in women with Turner's syndrome. *Ann Med* 31(2):106, 1999.

Howard FM. The role of laparoscopy in chronic pelvic pain: promise and pitfalls. *Obstet Gynecol Surv* 48(6):357, 1993.

Howards SS. Treatment of male infertility. *N Engl J Med* 332(5):312, 1995.

Huang KE. The primary treatment of luteal phase inadequacy: progesterone versus clomiphene citrate. *Am J Obstet Gynecol* 155(4):824, 1986.

Hubacher D, Lara-Ricalde R, et al. Use of copper intrauterine devices and the risk of tubal infertility among nulligravid women. *N Engl J Med* 345(8):561, 2001.

Hughes E, Collins J, et al. Clomiphene citrate for unexplained subfertility in women. *Cochrane Database Syst Rev* (3):CD000057, 2000.

Hull MG, Savage PE, et al. The value of a single serum progesterone measurement in the midluteal phase as a criterion of a potentially fertile cycle ("ovulation") derived form treated and untreated conception cycles. *Fertil Steril* 37(3):355, 1982.

Hulley S, Furberg C, et al. Noncardiovascular disease outcomes during 6.8 years of hormone therapy: Heart and Estrogen/Progestin Replacement Study Follow-up (HERS II). *JAMA* 288(1):58, 2002.

Hurd WW. Criteria that indicate endometriosis is the cause of chronic pelvic pain. *Obstet Gynecol* 92:1029, 1998.

Hurd WW, Whitfield RR, et al. Expectant management versus elective curettage for the treatment of spontaneous abortion. *Fertil Steril* 68(4):601, 1997.

Imani B, Eijkemans MJ, et al. Predictors of patients remaining anovulatory during clomiphene citrate induction of ovulation in normogonadotropic oligoamenorrheic infertility. *J Clin Endocrinol Metab* 83(7):2361, 1998.

REFERENCES

Imani B, Eijkemans MJ, et al. Predictors of chances to conceive in ovulatory patients during clomiphene citrate induction of ovulation in normogonadotropic oligoamenorrheic infertility. *J Clin Endocrinol Metab* 84(5):1617, 1999.

Isik AZ, Gulekli B, et al. Endocrinological and clinical analysis of hyperprolactinemic patients with and without ultrasonically diagnosed polycystic ovarian changes. *Gynecol Obstet Invest* 43(3):183, 1997.

Israel R, Mishell DRJ, et al. Single luteal phase serum progesterone assay as an indicator of ovulation. *Am J Obstet Gynecol* 112(8):1043, 1972.

Jaffe R, Jauniaux E, et al. Maternal circulation in the first-trimester human placenta—myth or reality? *Am J Obstet Gynecol* 176(3):695, 1997.

Jakimiuk AJ, Weitsman SR, et al. Luteinizing hormone receptor, steroidogenesis acute regulatory protein, and steroidogenic enzyme messenger ribonucleic acids are overexpressed in thecal and granulosa cells from polycystic ovaries. *J Clin Endocrinol Metab* 86(3):1318, 2001.

Jakubowicz DJ, Iuorno MJ, et al. Effects of metformin on early pregnancy loss in the polycystic ovary syndrome. *J Clin Endocrinol Metab* 87(2):524, 2002.

Jansen R, Elliott P. Angular and interstitial pregnancies should not be called 'cornual'. *Aust N Z J Obstet Gynaecol* 23(2):123, 1983.

Jansen RP. Surgery-pregnancy time intervals after salpingolysis, unilateral salpingostomy, and bilateral salpingostomy. *Fertil Steril* 34(3):222, 1980.

Jarow JP, Ogle SR, et al. Seminal improvement following repair of ultrasound detected subclinical varicoceles. *J Urol* 155(4):1287, 1996.

Jasonni VM, Raffelli R, et al. Vaginal bromocriptine in hyperprolactinemic patients and puerperal women. *Acta Obstet Gynecol Scand* 70(6):493, 1991.

Jeng GT, Scott JR, et al. A comparison of meta-analytic results using literature vs individual patient data. Paternal cell immunization for recurrent miscarriage. *JAMA* 274(10):830, 1995.

Jenkins S, Olive DL, et al. Endometriosis: pathogenic implications of the anatomic distribution. *Obstet Gynecol* 67:335, 1986.

Jensen I, Rinaldo CH, et al. Human umbilical vein endothelial cells lack expression of the estrogen receptor. *Endothelium* 6(1):9, 1998.

Jirecek S, Lee A, et al. Raloxifene prevents the growth of uterine leiomyomas in premenopausal women. *Fertil Steril* 81(1):132, 2004.

Joffe H, Cohen LS, Harlow BL. Impact of oral contraceptive pill use on premenstrual mood: predictors of improvement and deterioration. *Am J Obstet Gynecol* 189(6):1523, 2003.

Johnson J, Canning J, et al. Germline stem cells and follicular renewal in the postnatal mammalian ovary. *Nature* 428(6979):145, 2004a.

Johnson NP, Farquhar CM, et al. A double-blind randomised controlled trial of laparoscopic uterine nerve ablation for women with chronic pelvic pain. *BJOG* 111(9):950, 2004b.

REFERENCES

Johnson NP, Mak W, et al. Laparoscopic salpingectomy for women with hydrosalpinges enhances the success of IVF: a Cochrane review. *Hum Reprod* 17(3):543, 2002.

Jordan J, Craig K, et al. Luteal phase defect: the sensitivity and specificity of diagnostic methods in common clinical use. *Fertil Steril* 62(1):54, 1994.

Jordan RM, Kendall JW, et al. The primary empty sella syndrome: analysis of the clinical characteristics, radiographic features, pituitary function and cerebrospinal fluid adenohypophysial hormone concentrations. *Am J Med* 62(4):569, 1977.

Jurkovic D, Ross JA, et al. Expectant management of missed miscarriage. *Br J Obstet Gynaecol* 105(6):670, 1998.

Kahsar-Miller MD, Nixon C, et al. Prevalence of polycystic ovary syndrome (PCOS) in first-degree relatives of patients with PCOS. *Fertil Steril* 75(1):53, 2001.

Kamel HS, Darwish AM, et al. Comparison of transvaginal ultrasonography and vaginal sonohysterography in the detection of endometrial polyps. *Acta Obstet Gynecol Scand* 79(1):60, 2000.

Kanis JA. Diagnosis of osteoporosis and assessment of fracture risk. *Lancet* 359(9321):1929, 2002.

Kaplowitz P. Clinical characteristics of 104 children referred for evaluation of precocious puberty. *J Clin Endocrinol Metab* 89(8):3644, 2004.

Kaplowitz PB, Oberfield SE. Reexamination of the age limit for defining when puberty is precocious in girls in the United States: implications for evaluation and treatment. Drug and Therapeutics and Executive Committees of the Lawson Wilkins Pediatric Endocrine Society. *Pediatrics* 104(4 Pt 1):936, 1999.

Katsuragawa H, Kanzaki H, et al. Monoclonal antibody against phosphatidylserine inhibits in vitro human trophoblastic hormone production and invasion. *Biol Reprod* 56(1):50, 1997.

Kaufman RH, Adam E, et al. Continued follow-up of pregnancy outcomes in diethylstilbestrol-exposed offspring. *Obstet Gynecol* 96(4):483, 2000.

Kavtaradze N, Dominguez CE, et al. P-301 Vitamin E and C supplementation reduces endometriosis related pelvic pain. 59th Annual Meeting of the American Society for Reproductive Medicine, San Antonio, TX. *Fertil Steril* 80[Suppl 3]:S221, 2003.

Ke RW, Portera SG, et al. A randomized, double-blinded trial of preemptive analgesia in laparoscopy. *Obstet Gynecol* 92(6):972, 1998.

Khalifa E, Toner JP, et al. Significance of basal follicle-stimulating hormone levels in women with one ovary in a program of in vitro fertilization. *Fertil Steril* 57(4):835, 1992.

Kiddy DS, Hamiton-Fairley D, et al. Improvement in endocrine and ovarian function during dietary treatment of obese women with polycystic ovary syndrome. *Clin Endocrinol (Oxf)* 36:105, 1992.

REFERENCES

Klein JR, Litt IF. Epidemiology of adolescent dysmenorrhea. *Pediatrics* 68(5):661, 1981.

Kodama H, Fukuda J, et al. Characteristics of blood hemostatic markers in a patient with ovarian hyperstimulation syndrome who actually developed thromboembolism. *Fertil Steril* 64:1207, 1995.

Koga K, Osuga Y, et al. Increased concentrations of soluble tumour necrosis factor receptor (sTNFR) I and II in peritoneal fluid from women with endometriosis. *Mol Hum Reprod* 6(10):929, 2000.

Koninckx PR, Mueleman C, et al. Suggestive evidence that pelvic endometriosis is a progressive disease, whereas deeply infiltrating endometriosis is associated with pelvic pain. *Fertil Steril* 55(4):759, 1991.

Kouides PA, Phatak PD, et al. Gynaecological and obstetrical morbidity in women with type I von Willebrand disease: results of a patient survey. *Haemophilia* 6(6):643, 2000.

Kratzer PG, Golbus MS, et al. Corpus luteum function in early pregnancies is primarily determined by the rate of change of human chorionic gonadotropin levels. *Am J Obstet Gynecol* 163(5 Pt 1):1497, 1990.

Kreitmann O, Nixon WE, et al. Induced corpus luteum dysfunction after aspiration of the preovulatory follicle in monkeys. *Fertil Steril* 35(6):671, 1981.

Kriplani A, Agarwal N. Effects of metformin on clinical and biochemical parameters in polycystic ovary syndrome. *J Reprod Med* 49(5):361, 2004.

Kruger TF, Acosta AA, et al. New method of evaluating sperm morphology with predictive value for human in vitro fertilization. *Urology* 30(3):248, 1987.

Kruger TF, Coetzee K. The role of sperm morphology in assisted reproduction. *Hum Reprod Update* 5(2):172, 1999.

Kundsin RB, Driscoll SG, et al. Ureaplasma urealyticum incriminated in perinatal morbidity and mortality. *Science* 213(4506):474, 1981.

Kupfer MC, Schwimer SR, et al. Transvaginal sonographic appearance of endometrioma: spectrum of findings. *J Ultrasound Med* 11:129, 1992.

Kurman RJ, Kaminski PF, et al. The behavior of endometrial hyperplasia. A long-term study of "untreated" hyperplasia in 170 patients. *Cancer* 56(2): 403, 1985.

Kutteh WH. Antiphospholipid antibody-associated recurrent pregnancy loss: treatment with heparin and low-dose aspirin is superior to low-dose aspirin alone. *Am J Obstet Gynecol* 174(5):1584, 1996.

Kutteh WH. Antisperm antibodies. Do antisperm antibodies bound to spermatozoa alter normal reproductive function? *Hum Reprod* 14(10):2426, 1999.

Kutteh WH, Chao CH, et al. Vaginal lubricants for the infertile couple: effect on sperm activity. *Int J Fertil Menopausal Stud* 41(4):400, 1996.

Kutteh WH, Ermel LD. A clinical trial for the treatment of antiphospholipid antibody-associated recurrent pregnancy loss with lower dose heparin and aspirin. *Am J Reprod Immunol* 35(4):402, 1996.

REFERENCES

Laifer-Narin S, Ragavendra N, et al. False-normal appearance of the endometrium on conventional transvaginal sonography: comparison with saline hysterosonography. *AJR Am J Roentgenol* 178(1):129, 2002.

Lanigan SW. Incidence of side effects after laser hair removal. *J Am Acad Dermatol* 49(5):882, 2003.

Lashen H, Fear K, et al. Obesity is associated with increased risk of first trimester and recurrent miscarriage: matched case-control study. *Hum Reprod* 19(7):1644, 2004.

Laufer MR, Ecker JL, et al. Pregnancy outcome following ultrasound-detected fetal cardiac activity in women with a history of multiple spontaneous abortions. *J Soc Gynecol Investig* 1(2):138, 1994.

Laughlin GA, Barrett-Connor E, et al. Hysterectomy, oophorectomy, and endogenous sex hormone levels in older women: the Rancho Bernardo Study. *J Clin Endocrinol Metab* 85(2):645, 2000.

Laughlin GA, Yen SS. Nutritional and endocrine-metabolic aberrations in amenorrheic athletes. *J Clin Endocrinol Metab* 81(12):4301, 1996.

Laughlin GA, Yen SS. Hypoleptinemia in women athletes: absence of a diurnal rhythm with amenorrhea. *J Clin Endocrinol Metab* 82(1):318, 1997.

Lazovic G, Milacic D, et al. Medicaments or surgical therapy of PCOS. *Fertil Steril* 70(3):472 (abst), 1998.

Lebovic DI, Chao VA, et al. IL-1beta induction of RANTES (regulated upon activation, normal T cell expressed and secreted) chemokine gene expression in endometriotic stromal cells depends on a nuclear factor-kappaB site in the proximal promoter. *J Clin Endocrinol Metab* 86(10):4759, 2001a.

Lebovic DI, Mueller MD, et al. Immunobiology of endometriosis. *Fertil Steril* 75(1):1, 2001b.

Legro R, Finegood D, et al. Fasting glucose to insulin ratio is a useful measure of insulin sensitivity in women with polycystic ovary syndrome. *J Clin Endocrinol Metab* 83(8):2694, 1998.

Legro RS, Kunselman AR, et al. Prevalence and predictors of risk for type 2 diabetes mellitus and impaired glucose tolerance in polycystic ovary syndrome: a prospective, controlled study in 254 affected women. *J Clin Endocrinol Metab* 84(1):165, 1999.

Lessey BA, Yeh I, et al. Endometrial progesterone receptors and markers of uterine receptivity in the window of implantation. *Fertil Steril* 65(3):477, 1996.

Lethaby A, Hickey M. Endometrial destruction techniques for heavy menstrual bleeding: a Cochrane review. *Hum Reprod* 17(11):2795, 2002.

Lethaby A, Vollenhoven B, et al. Efficacy of pre-operative gonadotrophin hormone releasing analogues for women with uterine fibroids undergoing hysterectomy or myomectomy: a systematic review. *BJOG* 109(10):1097, 2002.

REFERENCES

Lev-Toaff AS, Coleman BG, et al. Leiomyomas in pregnancy: sonographic study. *Radiology* 164:375, 1987.

Levi AJ, Raynault MF, et al. Reproductive outcome in patients with diminished ovarian reserve. *Fertil Steril* 76(4):666, 2001.

Li DK, Liu L, et al. Exposure to non-steroidal anti-inflammatory drugs during pregnancy and risk of miscarriage: population based cohort study. *BMJ* 327(7411):368, 2003.

Li S, Qayyum A, et al. Association of renal agenesis and mullerian duct anomalies. *J Comput Assist Tomogr* 24(6):829, 2000.

Li TC, Dockery P, et al. How precise is histologic dating of endometrium using the standard dating criteria? *Fertil Steril* 51(5):759, 1989.

Liewan H, Santoro N. Premature ovarian failure: a modern approach to diagnosis and treatment. *Endocrinologist* 7:314, 1997.

Lincoln SR, Ke RW, et al. Screening for hypothyroidism in infertile women. *J Reprod Med* 44(5):455, 1999.

Linden MG, Bender BG, et al. Intrauterine diagnosis of sex chromosome aneuploidy. *Obstet Gynecol* 87(3):468, 1996.

Lindsay R, Gallagher JC, et al. Effect of lower doses of conjugated equine estrogens with and without medroxyprogesterone acetate on bone in early postmenopausal women. *JAMA* 287(20):2668, 2002.

Lippman SA, Warner M, et al. Uterine fibroids and gynecologic pain symptoms in a population-based study. *Fertil Steril* 80(6):1488, 2003.

Lipscomb GH, Bran D, et al. Analysis of three hundred fifteen ectopic pregnancies treated with single-dose methotrexate. *Am J Obstet Gynecol* 178:1354, 1998.

Lipscomb GH, Givens VA, et al. Previous ectopic pregnancy as a predictor of failure of systemic methotrexate therapy. *Fertil Steril* 81(5):1221, 2004.

Lipscomb GH, McCord ML, et al. Predictors of success of methotrexate treatment in women with tubal ectopic pregnancies. *N Engl J Med* 341:1974, 1999a.

Lipscomb GH, Puckett KJ, et al. Management of separation pain after single-dose methotrexate therapy for ectopic pregnancy. *Obstet Gynecol* 93:590, 1999b.

Lipscomb GH, Stovall TG, et al. Nonsurgical treatment of ectopic pregnancy. *N Engl J Med* 343(18):1325, 2000.

Liu HC, Kreiner D, et al. Beta-human chorionic gonadotropin as a monitor of pregnancy outcome in in vitro fertilization-embryo transfer patients. *Fertil Steril* 50(1):89, 1988.

Liu J, Rebar RW, et al. Neuroendocrine control of the postpartum period. *Clin Perinatol* 10(3):723, 1983.

Liu JH, Yen SS. Induction of midcycle gonadotropin surge by ovarian steroids in women: a critical evaluation. *J Clin Endocrinol Metab* 57(4):797, 1983.

Lo JC, Schwitzgebel VM, et al. Normal female infants born of mothers with classic congenital adrenal hyperplasia due to 21-hydroxylase deficiency. *J Clin Endocrinol Metab* 84(3):930, 1999.

Lobo R, Shoupe D, et al. The effects of two doses of spironolactone on serum androgens and anagen hair in hirsute women. *Fertil Steril* 43(2):200, 1985.

Lockhat FB, Emembolu JO, et al. The evaluation of the effectiveness of an intra-uterine-administered progestogen (levonorgestrel) in the symptomatic treatment of endometriosis and in the staging of the disease. *Hum Reprod* 19(1):179, 2004.

Looker AC, Orwoll ES, et al. Prevalence of low femoral bone density in older U.S. adults from NHANES III. *J Bone Miner Res* 12(11):1761, 1997.

Loprinzi CL, Kugler JW, et al. Venlafaxine in management of hot flashes in survivors of breast cancer: a randomised controlled trial. *Lancet* 356(9247): 2059, 2000.

Lord JM, Flight IH, et al. Insulin-sensitising drugs (metformin, troglitazone, rosiglitazone, pioglitazone, D-chiro-inositol) for polycystic ovary syndrome. *Cochrane Database Syst Rev* (3):CD003053, 2003.

Loucks AB, Mortola JF, et al. Alterations in the hypothalamic-pituitary-ovarian and the hypothalamic-pituitary-adrenal axes in athletic women. *J Clin Endocrinol Metab* 68(2):402, 1989.

Luborsky JL, Meyer P, et al. Premature menopause in a multi-ethnic population study of the menopause transition. *Hum Reprod* 18(1):199, 2003.

Lutfallah C, Wang W, et al. Newly proposed hormonal criteria via genotypic proof for type II 3beta-hydroxysteroid dehydrogenase deficiency. *J Clin Endocrinol Metab* 87(6):2611, 2002.

Mahabeer S, Naidoo C, et al. Metabolic profiles and lipoprotein lipid concentrations in non-obese patients with polycystic ovarian disease. *Horm Metab Res* 22(10):537, 1990.

Makris M. Hyperhomocysteinemia and thrombosis. *Clin Lab Haematol* 22(3):133, 2000.

Manners CV. Endometrial assessment in a group of infertile women on stimulated cycles for IVF: immunohistochemical findings. *Hum Reprod* 5(2):128, 1990.

Manning AP, Thompson WG, et al. Towards positive diagnosis of the irritable bowel. *Br Med J* 2(6138):653, 1978.

Many A, Elad R, et al. Third-trimester unexplained intrauterine fetal death is associated with inherited thrombophilia. *Obstet Gynecol* 99(5 Pt 1):684, 2002.

Marchbanks PA, McDonald JA, et al. Oral contraceptives and the risk of breast cancer. *N Engl J Med* 346(26):2025, 2002.

Marcoux S, Maheux R, et al. Laparoscopic surgery in infertile women with minimal or mild endometriosis. *N Engl J Med* 337:217, 1997.

Markee JE. Menstruation in intraocular endometrial transplants in the rhesus monkey. *Contrib Embryol* 177:221, 1940.

REFERENCES

Marshall WA, Tanner JM. Variations in pattern of pubertal changes in girls. *Arch Dis Child* 44(235):291, 1969.

Martin JS, Nisker JA, et al. Future in vitro fertilization pregnancy potential of women with variably elevated day 3 follicle-stimulating hormone levels. *Fertil Steril* 65(6):1238, 1996.

Martinelli I, Mannucci PM, et al. Different risks of thrombosis in four coagulation defects associated with inherited thrombophilia: a study of 150 families. *Blood* 92(7):2353, 1998.

Maruo T, Laoag-Fernandez JB, et al. Effects of the levonorgestrel-releasing intra-uterine system on proliferation and apoptosis in the endometrium. *Hum Reprod* 16(10):2103, 2001.

Mayani A, Barel S, et al. Dioxin concentrations. *Hum Reprod* 12(2):373, 1997.

McConnell HJ, O'Connor KA, et al. Validity of methods for analyzing urinary steroid data to detect ovulation in athletes. *Med Sci Sports Exerc* 34(11):1836, 2002.

McCord ML, Muram D, et al. Single serum progesterone as a screen for ectopic pregnancy: exchanging specificity and sensitivity to obtain optimal test performance. *Fertil Steril* 66(4):513, 1996.

McDonough PG. Puberty. In *Precis, Reproductive Endocrinology: an Update in Obstetrics and Gynecology.* Washington, DC: American College of Obstetricians and Gynecologists, 1998:32.

McElreavey K, Krausz C, et al. The human Y chromosome and male infertility. *Results Probl Cell Differ* 28:211, 2000.

McKenna TJ, Cunningham SK. Adrenal androgen production in polycystic ovary syndrome. *Eur J Endocrinol* 133:383, 1995.

McNatty KP, Makris A, et al. Metabolism of androstenedione by human ovarian tissues in vitro with particular reference to reductase and aromatase activity. *Steroids* 34(4):429, 1979.

Meade TW. Oral contraceptives, clotting factors, and thrombosis. *Am J Obstet Gynecol* 142(6 Pt 2):758, 1982.

Meunier PJ, Roux C, et al. The effects of strontium ranelate on the risk of vertebral fracture in women with postmenopausal osteoporosis. *N Engl J Med* 350(5):459, 2004.

Meyer WR, Castelbaum AJ, et al. Hydrosalpinges adversely affect markers of endometrial receptivity. *Hum Reprod* 12(7):1393, 1997.

Michaelsson K, Baron JA, et al. Oral-contraceptive use and risk of hip fracture: a case-control study. *Lancet* 353(9163):1481, 1999.

Migeon CJ, Wisniewski AB. Human sex differentiation and its abnormalities. *Best Pract Res Clin Obstet Gynaecol* 17(1):1, 2003.

Miller L, Hughes JP. Continuous combination oral contraceptive pills to eliminate withdrawal bleeding: a randomized trial. *Obstet Gynecol* 101(4):653, 2003.

REFERENCES

Miller JD, Shaw RW, et al. Historical prospective cohort study of the recurrence of pain after discontinuation of treatment with danazol or a gonadotropin-releasing hormone agonist. *Fertil Steril* 70(2):293, 1998.

Miller PB, Soules MR. The usefulness of a urinary LH kit for ovulation prediction during menstrual cycles of normal women. *Obstet Gynecol* 87(1):13, 1996.

Mishell DR, Jr. Noncontraceptive health benefits of oral steroidal contraceptives. *Am J Obstet Gynecol* 142(6 Pt 2):809, 1982.

Mishell DR, Darney PD, et al. Practice guidelines for OC selection: update. *Dialogues Contracept* 5(4):7, 1997.

Mitwally MF, Casper RF. Aromatase inhibition: a novel method of ovulation induction win women with polycystic ovarian syndrome. *Reprod Technol* 10:244, 2000.

Mitwally MF, Casper RF. Use of an aromatase inhibitor for induction of ovulation in patients with an inadequate response to clomiphene citrate. *Fertil Steril* 75(2):305, 2001.

Mittwally MF, Casper RF. P-486: Pregnancy outcome after the use of an aromatase inhibitor for ovarian stimulation. *Fertil Steril* 78(3, S1):S278, 2002.

Mitwally MF, Casper RF. Aromatase inhibition reduces gonadotrophin dose required for controlled ovarian stimulation in women with unexplained infertility. *Hum Reprod* 18(8):1588, 2003.

Mitwally MF, Casper RF. Single-dose administration of an aromatase inhibitor for ovarian stimulation. *Fertil Steril* 83(1):229, 2005.

Modan B, Hartge P, et al. Parity, oral contraceptives, and the risk of ovarian cancer among carriers and noncarriers of a BRCA1 or BRCA2 mutation. *N Engl J Med* 345(4):235, 2001.

Molitch ME. Pregnancy and the hyperprolactinemic woman. *N Engl J Med* 312(21):1364, 1985.

Molitch ME, Reichlin S. Hyperprolactinemic disorders. *Dis Mon* 28(9):1, 1982.

Morris JM, Mahesh BV. The syndrome of testicular feminization in male pseudohermaphrodites. *Am J Obstet Gynecol* 65:1192, 1953.

Morris RS, Paulson R. Ovarian hyperstimulation syndrome: classification and management. *Contemporary Ob/Gyn*, Sept:43, 1994.

Mortola JF, Girton L, et al. Diagnosis of premenstrual syndrome by a simple, prospective, and reliable instrument: the calendar of premenstrual experiences. *Obstet Gynecol* 76(2):302, 1990.

Muller P, Musset R, et al. [State of the upper urinary tract in patients with uterine malformations. Study of 133 cases]. *Presse Med* 75(26):1331, 1967.

Murphy AA, Green WR, et al. Unsuspected endometriosis documented by scanning electron microscopy in visually normal peritoneum. *Fertil Steril* 46(3):522, 1986.

Murray DL, Reich L, et al. Oral clomiphene citrate and vaginal progesterone sup-

REFERENCES

positories in the treatment of luteal phase dysfunction: a comparative study. *Fertil Steril* 51(1):35, 1989.

Murray MJ, Meyer WR, et al. A critical analysis of the accuracy, reproducibility, and clinical utility of histologic endometrial dating in fertile women. *Fertil Steril* 81(5):1333, 2004.

Muse KN, Cetel NS, et al. The premenstrual syndrome. Effects of "medical ovariectomy." *N Engl J Med* 311(21):1345, 1984.

Naftolin F, Taylor HS, et al. The Women's Health Initiative could not have detected cardioprotective effects of starting hormone therapy during the menopausal transition. *Fertil Steril* 81(6):1498, 2004.

Nagler et al. Varicocele: current concepts and treatment. In Lipschultz LI, Howards SS, eds. *Infertility in the Male* (3rd ed). St. Louis: Mosby, 1997.

Nakai Y, Plant TM, et al. On the sites of the negative and positive feedback actions of estradiol in the control of gonadotropin secretion in the rhesus monkey. *Endocrinology* 102(4):1008, 1978.

Nakajima ST, Brumsted JR, et al. Endometrial histology after first trimester spontaneous abortion. *Fertil Steril* 55(1):32, 1991.

Nakamura S, Douchi T, et al. Relationship between sonographic endometrial thickness and progestin-induced withdrawal bleeding. *Obstet Gynecol* 87(5 Pt 1):722, 1996.

Namnoum AB, Hickman TN, et al. Incidence of symptom recurrence after hysterectomy for endometriosis. *Fertil Steril* 64(5):898, 1995.

Narod SA, Risch H, et al. Oral contraceptives and the risk of hereditary ovarian cancer. Hereditary Ovarian Cancer Clinical Study Group. *N Engl J Med* 339(7):424, 1998.

Navot D, Rosenwaks Z, et al. Prognostic assessment of female fecundity. *Lancet* 2(8560):645, 1987.

Ness RB, Cramer DW, et al. Infertility, fertility drugs, and ovarian cancer: a pooled analysis of case-control studies. *Am J Epidemiol* 155(3):217, 2002.

Nestler JE. Metformin and the polycystic ovary syndrome. *J Clin Endocrinol Metab* 86(3):1430, 2001.

Nestler JE, Jakubowicz DJ, et al. Effects of metformin on spontaneous and clomiphene-induced ovulation in the polycystic ovary syndrome. *N Engl J Med* 338(26):1876, 1998.

Nestler JE, Powers LP, et al. A direct effect of hyperinsulinemia on serum sex hormone-binding globulin levels in obese women with the polycystic ovary syndrome. *J Clin Endocrinol Metab* 72(1):83, 1991.

Newfield L, Bradlow HL, et al. Estrogen metabolism and the malignant potential of human papillomavirus immortalized keratinocytes. *Proc Soc Exp Biol Med* 217(3):322, 1998.

REFERENCES

Nezhat CR, Nezhat FR, et al. *Operative Gynecologic Laparoscopy: Principles and Techniques.* New York: McGraw-Hill, 1995.

Ng EH, Ajonuma LC, et al. Adverse effects of hydrosalpinx fluid on sperm motility and survival. *Hum Reprod* 15(4):772, 2000.

Nielsen S, Hahlin M. Expectant management of first-trimester spontaneous abortion. *Lancet* 345(8942):84, 1995.

Nishida M, Nasu K, et al. Endometriotic cells are resistant to interferon-g-induced cell growth inhibition and apoptosis: a possible mechanism involved in the pathogenesis of endometriosis. *Mol Hum Reprod* 11(1):29, 2005.

Nisolle M, Donnez J. Endoscopic treatment of Mullerian anomalies. *Gynecol Endocrinol* 5:155, 1996.

Nisolle M, Donnez J. Peritoneal endometriosis, ovarian endometriosis, and adenomyotic nodules of the rectovaginal septum are three different entities. *Fertil Steril* 68(4):585, 1997.

Norman RJ. Metformin—comparison with other therapies in ovulation induction in polycystic ovary syndrome. *J Clin Endocrinol Metab* 89(10):4797, 2004.

North American Menopause Society. Treatment of menopause-associated vasomotor symptoms: position statement of the North American Menopause Society. *Menopause* 11(1):11, 2004.

Novak ER, Woodruff JD. *Gynecologic and Obstetric Pathology.* Philadelphia: WB Saunders, 1979.

Noyes RW, Hertig AT, et al. Dating the endometrial biopsy. *Fertil Steril* 1(1):3, 1950.

Nuojua-Huttunen S, Tomas C, et al. Intrauterine insemination treatment in subfertility: an analysis of factors affecting outcome. *Hum Reprod* 14(3):698, 1999.

Oates RD. The genetics of male reproductive failure: what every clinician needs to know. *Sex Reprod Menopause* 2(4):213, 2004.

Ober C, Karrison T, et al. Mononuclear-cell immunisation in prevention of recurrent miscarriages: a randomised trial. *Lancet* 354(9176):365, 1999.

Oei SG, Helmerhorst FM, et al. Effectiveness of the postcoital test: randomised controlled trial. *BMJ* 317(7157):502, 1998.

Ogasawara M, Aoki K, et al. Embryonic karyotype of abortuses in relation to the number of previous miscarriages. *Fertil Steril* 73(2):300, 2000.

Oktay K, Buyuk E, et al. Embryo development after heterotopic transplantation of cryopreserved ovarian tissue. *Lancet* 363(9412):837, 2004.

Oliveira FG, Abdelmassih VG, et al. Impact of subserosal and intramural uterine fibroids that do not distort the endometrial cavity on the outcome of in vitro fertilization-intracytoplasmic sperm injection. *Fertil Steril* 81(3):582, 2004.

Omland AK, Abyholm T, et al. Pregnancy outcome after IVF and ICSI in unexplained, endometriosis-associated and tubal factor infertility. *Hum Reprod* 20(3):722, 2005.

REFERENCES

Omland AK, Tanbo T, et al. Artificial insemination by husband in unexplained infertility compared with infertility associated with peritoneal endometriosis. *Hum Reprod* 13(9):2602, 1998.

Oral E, Arici A. Peritoneal growth factors and endometriosis. *Semin Reprod Endocrinol* 14:257, 1996.

Orio F, Jr., Palomba S, et al. The cardiovascular risk of young women with polycystic ovary syndrome: an observational, analytical, prospective case-control study. *J Clin Endocrinol Metab* 89(8):3696, 2004.

Osofsky JH, Blumenthal SJ, eds. *Premenstrual Syndrome: Current Findings and Future Directions*. Washington, DC: American Psychiatric Press, 1985.

Otis CL, Drinkwater B, et al. American College of Sports Medicine position stand. The Female Athlete Triad. *Med Sci Sports Exerc* 29(5):i, 1997.

Ottinger LW. *Fundamentals of Colon Surgery*. Boston: Little, Brown and Company, 1974.

Pache TD, de Jong FH, et al. Association between ovarian changes assessed by transvaginal sonography and clinical and endocrine signs of the polycystic ovary syndrome. *Fertil Steril* 59(3):544, 1993.

Page DC, de la Chapelle A, et al. Chromosome Y-specific DNA in related human XX males. *Nature* 315(6016):224, 1985.

Pagotto U, Marsicano G, et al. Normal human pituitary gland and pituitary adenomas express cannabinoid receptor type 1 and synthesize endogenous cannabinoids: first evidence for a direct role of cannabinoids on hormone modulation at the human pituitary level. *J Clin Endocrinol Metab* 86(6): 2687, 2001.

Pall M, Friden BE, et al. Induction of delayed follicular rupture in the human by the selective COX-2 inhibitor rofecoxib: a randomized double-blind study. *Hum Reprod* 16(7):1323, 2001.

Palmert MR, Boepple PA. Variation in the timing of puberty: clinical spectrum and genetic investigation. *J Clin Endocrinol Metab* 86(6):2364, 2001.

Palomba S, Orio F, Jr., et al. Raloxifene administration in women treated with gonadotropin-releasing hormone agonist for uterine leiomyomas: effects on bone metabolism. *J Clin Endocrinol Metab* 87(10):4476, 2002a.

Palomba S, Orio F, Jr., et al. Raloxifene administration in premenopausal women with uterine leiomyomas: a pilot study. *J Clin Endocrinol Metab* 87(8):3603, 2002b.

Palomba S, Orio F, Jr., et al. Metformin administration versus laparoscopic ovarian diathermy in clomiphene citrate-resistant women with polycystic ovary syndrome: a prospective parallel randomized double-blind placebo-controlled trial. *J Clin Endocrinol Metab* 89(10):4801, 2004.

Palomba S, Russo T, et al. Effectiveness of combined GnRH analogue plus raloxifene administration in the treatment of uterine leiomyomas: a prospective, randomized, single-blind, placebo-controlled clinical trial. *Hum Reprod* 17(12):3213, 2002c.

Panganiban W, Cornog JL. Endometriosis of the intestines and vermiform appendix. *Dis Colon Rectum* 15:253, 1972.

Papanikolaou EG, Tournaye H, et al. *Early Pregnancy Outcome Is Impaired in Early Ovarian Hyperstimulation Syndrome (OHSS) Comparing to Late OHSS.* St. Louis: American Society for Reproductive Immunology, 2004.

Parazzini F. Ablation of lesions or no treatment in minimal-mild endometriosis in infertile women: a randomized trial. Gruppo Italiano per lo Studio dell'Endometriosi. *Hum Reprod* 14(5):1332, 1999.

Parazzini F, Fedele L, et al. Postsurgical medical treatment of advanced endometriosis: results of a randomized clinical trial. *Am J Obstet Gynecol* 171(5):1205, 1994.

Parinaud J, Lesourd F. [Inhibin B is not a good marker of ovarian follicular reserve]. *Gynecol Obstet Fertil* 30(3):254, 2002.

Parsanezhad ME, Alborzi S, et al. Use of dexamethasone and clomiphene citrate in the treatment of clomiphene citrate-resistant patients with polycystic ovary syndrome and normal dehydroepiandrosterone sulfate levels: a prospective, double-blind, placebo-controlled trial. *Fertil Steril* 78(5):1001, 2002.

Pearlstein TB, Stone AB. Long-term fluoxetine treatment of late luteal phase dysphoric disorder. *J Clin Psychiatry* 55(8):332, 1994.

Pearlstone AC, Fournet N, et al. Ovulation induction in women age 40 and older: the importance of basal follicle-stimulating hormone level and chronological age. *Fertil Steril* 58(4):674, 1992.

Pellerito JS, McCarthy SM, et al. Diagnosis of uterine anomalies: relative accuracy of MR imaging, endovaginal sonography, and hysterosalpingography. *Radiology* 183(3):795, 1992.

Pellestor F, Andreo B, et al. Maternal aging and chromosomal abnormalities: new data drawn from in vitro unfertilized human oocytes. *Hum Genet* 112(2):195, 2003.

Phillips DR, Nathanson HG, et al. The effect of dilute vasopressin solution on blood loss during operative hysteroscopy: a randomized controlled trial. *Obstet Gynecol* 88(5):761, 1996.

Phipps WR. Polycystic ovary syndrome and ovulation induction. *Obstet Gynecol Clin North Am* 28(1):165, 2001.

Pierpoint T, McKeigue PM, et al. Mortality of women with polycystic ovary syndrome at long-term follow-up. *J Clin Epidemiol* 51(7):581, 1998.

Piippo S, Lenko H, et al. Use of percutaneous estrogen gel for induction of puberty in girls with Turner syndrome. *J Clin Endocrinol Metab* 89(7):3241, 2004.

Pisarska MD, Carson SA, et al. Ectopic pregnancy. *Lancet* 351(9109):1115, 1998.

REFERENCES

Polson DW, Adams J, et al. Polycystic ovaries—a common finding in normal women. *Lancet* 1(8590):870, 1988.

Pope CS, Cook EK, et al. Influence of embryo transfer depth on in vitro fertilization and embryo transfer outcomes. *Fertil Steril* 81(1):51, 2004.

Poppe K, Glinoer D, et al. Assisted reproduction and thyroid autoimmunity: an unfortunate combination? *J Clin Endocrinol Metab* 88(9):4149, 2003.

Poretsky L, Garber J, et al. Primary amenorrhea and pseudoprolactinoma in a patient with primary hypothyroidism. Reversal of clinical, biochemical, and radiologic abnormalities with levothyroxine. *Am J Med* 81(1):180, 1986.

Potlog-Nahari C, Catherino WH, et al. *Pregnancy Rates of Blastocyst-Staged Embryos Are Reduced If Transferred to an Endometrium Classified As Grade B by Transvaginal Ultrasound.* San Antonio, TX: American Society of Reproductive Medicine, 2003.

Potlog-Nahari C, Catherino WH, et al. A suboptimal endometrial pattern is associated with a reduced likelihood of pregnancy after a day 5 embryo transfer. *Fertil Steril* 83(1):235, 2005.

Prader A. Der genitalbefund beim ppseudohermaphroditismus femininus der kengenitalen adrenogenitalen syndroms. *Helv Paediatr Acta* 9:231, 1954.

Preston FE, Rosendaal FR, et al. Increased fetal loss in women with heritable thrombophilia. *Lancet* 348(9032):913, 1996.

Price TM, Allen S, et al. Lack of effect of topical finasteride suggests an endocrine role for dihydrotestosterone. *Fertil Steril* 74(2):414, 2000.

Pritts EA. Fibroids and infertility: a systematic review of the evidence. *Obstet Gynecol Surv* 56(8):483, 2001.

Pritts EA, Atwood AK. Luteal phase support in infertility treatment: a meta-analysis of the randomized trials. *Hum Reprod* 17(9):2287, 2002.

Proctor JA, Haney AF . Recurrent first trimester pregnancy loss is associated with uterine septum but not with bicornuate uterus. *Fertil Steril* 80(5):1212, 2003.

Propst AM, Storti K, et al. Lateral cervical displacement is associated with endometriosis. *Fertil Steril* 70(3):568, 1998.

Purvin VA. Visual disturbance secondary to clomiphene citrate. *Arch Ophthalmol* 113(4):482, 1995.

Quere I, Perneger TV, et al. Red blood cell methylfolate and plasma homocysteine as risk factors for venous thromboembolism: a matched case-control study. *Lancet* 359(9308):747, 2002.

Querleu D, Brasme TL, et al. Ultrasound-guided transcervical metroplasty. *Fertil Steril* 54(6):995, 1990.

Raga F, Bauset C, et al. Reproductive impact of congenital Mullerian anomalies. *Hum Reprod* 12(10):2277, 1997.

Rai R, Backos M, et al. Polycystic ovaries and recurrent miscarriage—a reappraisal. *Hum Reprod* 15(3):612, 2000.

REFERENCES

Rai R, Cohen H, et al. Randomised controlled trial of aspirin and aspirin plus heparin in pregnant women with recurrent miscarriage associated with phospholipid antibodies (or antiphospholipid antibodies). *BMJ* 314(7076):253, 1997.

Rai R, Shlebak A, et al. Factor V Leiden and acquired activated protein C resistance among 1000 women with recurrent miscarriage. *Hum Reprod* 16(5):961, 2001.

Raja SN, Feehan M, et al. Prevalence and correlates of the premenstrual syndrome in adolescence. *J Am Acad Child Adolesc Psychiatry* 31(5):783, 1992.

Ranke MB, Saenger P. Turner's syndrome. *Lancet* 358(9278):309, 2001.

Rarick LD, Shangold MM, et al. Cervical mucus and serum estradiol as predictors of response to progestin challenge. *Fertil Steril* 54(2):353, 1990.

Ray NF, Chan JK, et al. Medical expenditures for the treatment of osteoporotic fractures in the United States in 1995: report from the National Osteoporosis Foundation. *J Bone Miner Res* 12(1):24, 1997.

Rebar RW, Connolly HV. Clinical features of young women with hypergonadotropic amenorrhea. *Fertil Steril* 53(5):804, 1990.

Redmon JB, Carey P, et al. Varicocele—the most common cause of male factor infertility? *Hum Reprod Update* 8(1):53, 2002.

Regidor PA, Schindler AE, et al. Results of long-term follow-up in treatment of endometriosis with the GnRH agonist leuprorelin acetate depot (Enantone-Gyn monthly depot). *Zentralbl Gynakol* 118(5):283, 1996.

Reid IR, Brown JP, et al. Intravenous zoledronic acid in postmenopausal women with low bone mineral density. *N Engl J Med* 346(9):653, 2002.

Reid RL. Premenstrual syndrome. *Curr Probl Obstet Gynecol Fertil* 8:1, 1985.

Reindollar RH, Byrd JR, et al. Delayed sexual development: a study of 252 patients. *Am J Obstet Gynecol* 140(4):371, 1981.

Reindollar RH, Novak M, et al. Adult-onset amenorrhea: a study of 262 patients. *Am J Obstet Gynecol* 155(3):531, 1986.

Remohi J, Gallardo E, et al. Oocyte donation in women with recurrent pregnancy loss. *Hum Reprod* 11(9):2048, 1996.

Rey E, Kahn SR, et al. Thrombophilic disorders and fetal loss: a meta-analysis. *Lancet* 361(9361):901, 2003.

Rickenlund A, Carlstrom K, et al. Effects of oral contraceptives on body composition and physical performance in female athletes. *J Clin Endocrinol Metab* 89(9):4364, 2004.

Ridker PM, Miletich JP, et al. Factor V Leiden mutation as a risk factor for recurrent pregnancy loss. *Ann Intern Med* 128(12 Pt 1):1000, 1998.

Rivera JL, Lal S, et al. Effect of acute and chronic neuroleptic therapy on serum prolactin levels in men and women of different age groups. *Clin Endocrinol (Oxf)* 5(3):273, 1976.

Rivera-Tovar AD, Frank E. Late luteal phase dysphoric disorder in young women. *Am J Psychiatry* 147(12):1634, 1990.

411

REFERENCES

Roca CA, Schmidt PJ, et al. Effects of metergoline on symptoms in women with premenstrual dysphoric disorder. *Am J Psychiatry* 159(11):1876, 2002.

Rock JA, Jones HW. The clinical management of the double uterus. *Fertil Steril* 28(8):798, 1977.

Rock JA, Zacur HA. The clinical management of repeated early pregnancy wastage. *Fertil Steril* 39(2):123, 1983.

Rodrigues I, Grou F, et al. Effectiveness of emergency contraceptive pills between 72 and 120 hours after unprotected sexual intercourse. *Am J Obstet Gynecol* 184(4):531, 2001.

Romer T, Lober R. Hysteroscopic correction of a complete septate uterus using a balloon technique. *Hum Reprod* 12(3):478, 1997.

Ron-El R, Raziel A, et al. Birth of healthy male twins after intracytoplasmic sperm injection of frozen-thawed testicular spermatozoa from a patient with nonmosaic Klinefelter syndrome. *Fertil Steril* 74(4):832, 2000.

Rosen GF, Stone SC, et al. Ovulation induction in women with premature ovarian failure: a prospective, crossover study. *Fertil Steril* 57(2):448, 1992.

Rosenfeld CS, Wagner JS, et al. Intraovarian actions of oestrogen. *Reproduction* 122(2):215, 2001.

Rosenheim NB, Leichner PK, et al. Radiocolloids in the treatment of ovarian cancer. *Obstet Gynecol Surv* 34:708, 1979.

Rossato M, Popa FI, et al. Human sperm express cannabinoid receptor CB1 which activation inhibits motility, acrosome reaction and mitochondrial function. *J Clin Endocrinol Metab* 90:984, 2005

Rossouw JE, Anderson GL, et al. Risks and benefits of estrogen plus progestin in healthy postmenopausal women: principal results from the Women's Health Initiative randomized controlled trial. *JAMA* 288(3):321, 2002.

Rotterdam ESCHRE/ASRM-Sponsored PCOS Consensus Workshop Group, 2004.

Royar J, Becher H, et al. Low-dose oral contraceptives: protective effect on ovarian cancer risk. *Int J Cancer* 95(6):370, 2001.

Rubinek T, Hadani M, et al. Prolactin (PRL)-releasing peptide stimulates PRL secretion from human fetal pituitary cultures and growth hormone release from cultured pituitary adenomas. *J Clin Endocrinol Metab* 86(6):2826, 2001.

Sachdev R, Kemmann E, et al. Detrimental effect of hydrosalpinx fluid on the development and blastulation of mouse embryos in vitro. *Fertil Steril* 68(3):531, 1997.

Salat-Baroux J. [Recurrent spontaneous abortions]. *Reprod Nutr Dev* 28(6B):1555, 1988.

Saleh A, Morris D, et al. Effects of laparoscopic ovarian drilling on adrenal steroids in polycystic ovary syndrome patients with and without hyperinsulinemia. *Fertil Steril* 75(3):501, 2001.

Sammour A, Biljan MM, et al. Prospective randomized trial comparing the effects of letrozole (LE) and clomiphene citrate (CC) on follicular development, endome-

412

trial thickness and pregnancy rate in patients undergoing super-ovulation prior to intrauterine insemination (IUI). *Fertil Steril* 76[Suppl 1](3):S110, 2001.

Sampson JA. Peritoneal endometriosis due to menstrual dissemination of endometrial tissue into the peritoneal cavity. *Am J Obstet Gynecol* 14:422, 1927.

Sanborn CF, Jankowski CM. Physiologic considerations for women in sport. *Clin Sports Med* 13(2):315, 1994.

Sandlow JI, Zenni M, et al. Size of varicocele corresponds with pregnancy rates following surgical treatment: updated results. San Diego: American Society for Reproductive Medicine, *Fertil Steril*, 2000.

Sanson BJ, Friederich PW, et al. The risk of abortion and stillbirth in antithrombin, protein C-, and protein S-deficient women. *Thromb Haemost* 75(3):387, 1996.

Sargent IL, Wilkins T, et al. Maternal immune responses to the fetus in early pregnancy and recurrent miscarriage. *Lancet* 2(8620):1099, 1988.

Sarrel PM. Psychosexual effects of menopause: role of androgens. *Am J Obstet Gynecol* 180(3 Pt 2):S319, 1999.

Sawaya GF, Grady D, et al. Antibiotics at the time of induced abortion: the case for universal prophylaxis based on a meta-analysis. *Obstet Gynecol* 87(5 Pt 2):884, 1996.

Scheffer GJ, Broekmans FJ, et al. Antral follicle counts by transvaginal ultrasonography are related to age in women with proven natural fertility. *Fertil Steril* 72(5):845, 1999.

Schieve LA, Meikle SF, et al. Low and very low birth weight in infants conceived with use of assisted reproductive technology. *N Engl J Med* 346(10):731, 2002.

Schlaff WD, Hurst BS. Preoperative sonographic measurement of endometrial pattern predicts outcome of surgical repair in patients with severe Asherman's syndrome. *Fertil Steril* 63(2):410, 1995.

Schlaff WD, Zerhouni EA, et al. A placebo-controlled trial of a depot gonadotropin-releasing hormone analogue (leuprolide) in the treatment of uterine leiomyomata. *Obstet Gynecol* 74(6):856, 1989.

Schlechte J, Dolan K, et al. The natural history of untreated hyperprolactinemia: a prospective analysis. *J Clin Endocrinol Metab* 68(2):412, 1989.

Schlesselman JJ. Net effect of oral contraceptive use on the risk of cancer in women in the United States. *Obstet Gynecol* 85(5 Pt 1):793, 1995.

Schlesselman JJ, Collins JA. The influence of steroids on gynecologic cancers. In Fraser IS, Jansen RPS, et al., eds. *Estrogens and Progestogens in Clinical Practice*. London: Churchill Livingstone, 1999:831.

Schmidt PJ, Nieman LK, et al. Differential behavioral effects of gonadal steroids in women with and in those without premenstrual syndrome. *N Engl J Med* 338(4):209, 1998.

Schwartz D, Mayaux MJ. Female fecundity as a function of age: results of artificial

REFERENCES

insemination in 2193 nulliparous women with azoospermic husbands. Federation CECOS. *N Engl J Med* 306(7):404, 1982.

Schwimer SR, Lebovic J. Transvaginal pelvic ultrasonography. *J Ultrasound Med* 3(8):381, 1984.

Scott RT, Leonardi MR, et al. A prospective evaluation of clomiphene citrate challenge test screening of the general infertility population. *Obstet Gynecol* 82(4 Pt 1):539, 1993.

Scott RT, Opsahl MS, et al. Life table analysis of pregnancy rates in a general infertility population relative to ovarian reserve and patient age. *Hum Reprod* 10(7):1706, 1995.

Scott RT, Toner JP, et al. Follicle-stimulating hormone levels on cycle day 3 are predictive of in vitro fertilization outcome. *Fertil Steril* 51(4):651, 1989.

Scott RT, Jr., Hofmann GE, et al. Intercycle variability of day 3 follicle-stimulating hormone levels and its effect on stimulation quality in in vitro fertilization. *Fertil Steril* 54(2):297, 1990.

Seifer DB, Gutmann JN, et al. Comparison of persistent ectopic pregnancy after laparoscopic salpingostomy versus salpingostomy at laparotomy for ectopic pregnancy. *Obstet Gynecol* 81(3):378, 1993.

Seifer DB, Scott RT, Jr., et al. Women with declining ovarian reserve may demonstrate a decrease in day 3 serum inhibin B before a rise in day 3 follicle-stimulating hormone. *Fertil Steril* 72(1):63, 1999.

Seki K, Kato K, et al. Parallelism in the luteinizing hormone responses to opioid and dopamine antagonists in hyperprolactinemic women with pituitary microadenoma. *J Clin Endocrinol Metab* 63(5):1225, 1986.

Seligson U, Lebetsky A. Genetic susceptibility to venous thrombosis. *N Engl J Med* 16(344):1222, 2001.

Semino C, Semino A, et al. Role of major histocompatibility complex class I expression and natural killer-like T cells in the genetic control of endometriosis. *Fertil Steril* 64(5):909, 1995.

Shamma FN, Lee G, et al. The role of office hysteroscopy in in vitro fertilization. *Fertil Steril* 58(6):1237, 1992.

Sharara FI, Scott RT. Assessment of ovarian reserve. Is there still a role for ovarian biopsy? First do no harm! *Hum Reprod* 19(3):470, 2004.

Sharara FI, Scott RT, Jr., et al. The detection of diminished ovarian reserve in infertile women. *Am J Obstet Gynecol* 179(3 Pt 1):804, 1998.

Shelling AN, Burton KA, et al. Inhibin: a candidate gene for premature ovarian failure. *Hum Reprod* 15(12):2644, 2000.

Shifren JL, Braunstein GD, et al. Transdermal testosterone treatment in women with impaired sexual function after oophorectomy. *N Engl J Med* 343:682, 2000.

Shobokshi A, Shaarawy M. Correction of insulin resistance and hyperandrogenism

REFERENCES

in polycystic ovary syndrome by combined rosiglitazone and clomiphene citrate therapy. *J Soc Gynecol Investig* 10(2):99, 2003.

Shumaker SA, Legault C, et al. Conjugated equine estrogens and incidence of probable dementia and mild cognitive impairment in postmenopausal women: Women's Health Initiative Memory Study. *JAMA* 291(24):2947, 2004.

Siffroi JP, Le Bourhis C, et al. Sex chromosome mosaicism in males carrying Y chromosome long arm deletions. *Hum Reprod* 15(12):2559, 2000.

Silverberg KM. Ovulation induction in the ovulatory woman. *Semin Reprod Endocrinol* 14(4):339, 1996.

Silverberg SG, Haukkamaa M, et al. Endometrial morphology during long-term use of levonorgestrel-releasing intrauterine devices. *Int J Gynecol Pathol* 5(3):235, 1986.

Simpson J, Elias S, et al. Heritable aspects of endometriosis: genetic studies. *Am J Obstet Gynecol* 137:327, 1980.

Simpson JL, Carson SA, et al. Lack of association between antiphospholipid antibodies and first-trimester spontaneous abortion: prospective study of pregnancies detected within 21 days of conception. *Fertil Steril* 69(5):814, 1998.

Sinaii N, Cleary SD, et al. Autoimmune and related diseases among women with endometriosis: a survey analysis. *Fertil Steril* 77[Suppl 1]:S7, 2002.

Slater CA, Liang MH, et al. Preserving ovarian function in patients receiving cyclophosphamide. *Lupus* 8(1):3, 1999.

Slayden SM, Azziz R. The role of androgen excess in acne. In Azziz R, Nestler JE, Dewailly D. *Androgen Excess Disorders in Women.* Philadelphia: Lippincott–Raven Publishers: 131, 1997.

Sluijmer AV, Lappohn RE. Clinical history and outcome of 59 patients with idiopathic hyperprolactinemia. *Fertil Steril* 58(1):72, 1992.

Smith JS, Green J, et al. Cervical cancer and use of hormonal contraceptives: a systematic review. *Lancet* 361(9364):1159, 2003.

Smotrich DB, Widra EA, et al. Prognostic value of day 3 estradiol on in vitro fertilization outcome. *Fertil Steril* 64(6):1136, 1995.

Snyder PJ. The role of androgens in women. *J Clin Endocrinol Metab* 86(3):1006, 2001.

Soares SR, Barbosa dos Reis MM, et al. Diagnostic accuracy of sonohysterography, transvaginal sonography, and hysterosalpingography in patients with uterine cavity diseases. *Fertil Steril* 73(2):406, 2000.

Somigliana E, Ragni G, et al. Does laparoscopic excision of endometriotic ovarian cysts significantly affect ovarian reserve? Insights from IVF cycles. *Hum Reprod* 18(11):2450, 2003.

Somigliana E, Vigano P, et al. Human endometrial stromal cells as a source of soluble intercellular adhesion molecule (ICAM)-1 molecules. *Hum Reprod* 11(6):1190, 1996.

415

REFERENCES

Somigliana E, Vigano P, et al. Endometriosis and unexplained recurrent spontaneous abortion: pathological states resulting from aberrant modulation of natural killer cell function? *Hum Reprod Update* 5(1):40, 1999.

Soysal S, Soysal ME, et al. The effects of post-surgical administration of goserelin plus anastrozole compared to goserelin alone in patients with severe endometriosis: a prospective randomized trial. *Hum Reprod* 19(1): 160, 2004.

Spandorfer SD, Davis OK, et al. Relationship between maternal age and aneuploidy in in vitro fertilization pregnancy loss. *Fertil Steril* 81(5):1265, 2004.

Speiser PW. Congenital adrenal hyperplasia owing to 21-hydroxylase deficiency. *Endocrinol Metab Clin North Am* 30(1):31, vi, 2001.

Speiser PW, White PC. Congenital adrenal hyperplasia. *N Engl J Med* 349(8):776, 2003.

Speroff L, Fritz MA, eds. *Clinical Gynecologic Endocrinology and Infertility* (7th ed). Philadelphia: Lippincott Williams & Wilkins, 2005.

Stallings SP, Paling JE. New tool for presenting risk in obstetrics and gynecology. *Obstet Gynecol* 98:345, 2001.

Stampfer MJ, Colditz GA, et al. Postmenopausal estrogen therapy and cardiovascular disease. Ten-year follow-up from the nurses' health study. *N Engl J Med* 325(11):756, 1991.

Stearns V, Beebe KL, et al. Paroxetine controlled release in the treatment of menopausal hot flashes: a randomized controlled trial. *JAMA* 289(21):2827, 2003.

Steege JF, Stout AL, et al. Reduced platelet tritium-labeled imipramine binding sites in women with premenstrual syndrome. *Am J Obstet Gynecol* 167(1):168, 1992.

Stein ZA. A woman's age: childbearing and child rearing. *Am J Epidemiol* 121 (3):327, 1985.

Steinauer J, Pritts EA, et al. Systematic review of mifepristone for the treatment of uterine leiomyomata. *Obstet Gynecol* 103(6):1331, 2004.

Steinberger E, Smith KD, et al. Testosterone levels in female partners of infertile couples. Relationship between androgen levels in the woman, the male factor, and the incidence of pregnancy. *Am J Obstet Gynecol* 133(2):133, 1979.

Steiner AZ, Chang L, et al. 3alpha-hydroxysteroid dehydrogenase type III deficiency: a novel cause of hirsutism (O-307). *J Soc Gynecol Invest* 11(2S):307, 2004.

Steiner M, Romano SJ, et al. The efficacy of fluoxetine in improving physical symptoms associated with premenstrual dysphoric disorder. *BJOG* 108(5):462, 2001.

Steiner M, Steinberg S, et al. Fluoxetine in the treatment of premenstrual dysphoria. Canadian Fluoxetine/Premenstrual Dysphoria Collaborative Study Group. *N Engl J Med* 332(23):1529, 1995.

Stewart FH, Harper CC, et al. Clinical breast and pelvic examination requirements for hormonal contraception: current practice vs evidence. *JAMA* 285(17): 2232, 2001.

REFERENCES

Strandell A, Lindhard A. Why does hydrosalpinx reduce fertility? The importance of hydrosalpinx fluid. *Hum Reprod* 17(5):1141, 2002.

Strandell A, Lindhard A, et al. Hydrosalpinx and IVF outcome: a prospective, randomized multicentre trial in Scandinavia on salpingectomy prior to IVF. *Hum Reprod* 14(11):2762, 1999.

Strandell A, Lindhard A, et al. Hydrosalpinx and IVF outcome: cumulative results after salpingectomy in a randomized controlled trial. *Hum Reprod* 16(11):2403, 2001a.

Strandell A, Lindhard A, et al. Prophylactic salpingectomy does not impair the ovarian response in IVF treatment. *Hum Reprod* 16(6):1135, 2001b.

Strobelt N, Mariani E, et al. Fertility after ectopic pregnancy. Effects of surgery and expectant management. *J Reprod Med* 45(10):803, 2000.

Sung L, Mukherjee T, et al. Endometriosis is not detrimental to embryo implantation in oocyte recipients. *J Assist Reprod Genet* 14(3):152, 1997.

Surks MI. Commentary: Subclinical thyroid dysfunction: a joint statement on management from the American Association of Clinical Endocrinologists, the American Thyroid Association, and The Endocrine Society. *J Clin Endocrinol Metab* 90(1):586, 2005.

Surrey ES, Lietz AK, et al. Impact of intramural leiomyomata in patients with a normal endometrial cavity on in vitro fertilization-embryo transfer cycle outcome. *Fertil Steril* 75(2):405, 2001.

Surrey ES, Silverberg KM, et al. Effect of prolonged gonadotropin-releasing hormone agonist therapy on the outcome of in vitro fertilization-embryo transfer in patients with endometriosis. *Fertil Steril* 78(4):699, 2002.

Swerdloff RS, Wang C. Evaluation of male infertility. UpToDate Patient Information Web site: http://www.utdol.com. Accessed February, 2005.

Syrop CH, Dawson JD, et al. Ovarian volume may predict assisted reproductive outcomes better than follicle stimulating hormone concentration on day 3. *Hum Reprod* 14(7):1752, 1999.

Syrop CH, Hammond MG. Diurnal variations in midluteal serum progesterone measurements. *Fertil Steril* 47(1):67, 1987.

Syrop CH, Willhoite A, et al. Ovarian volume: a novel outcome predictor for assisted reproduction. *Fertil Steril* 64(6):1167, 1995.

Tanis BC, van den Bosch MA, et al. Oral contraceptives and the risk of myocardial infarction. *N Engl J Med* 345(25):1787, 2001.

Tarani L, Lampariello S, et al. Pregnancy in patients with Turner's syndrome: six new cases and review of literature. *Gynecol Endocrinol* 12(2):83, 1998.

Tartagni M, Schonauer MM, et al. Intermittent low-dose finasteride is as effective as daily administration for the treatment of hirsute women. *Fertil Steril* 82(3):752, 2004.

Taylor AE, Adams JM, et al. A randomized, controlled trial of estradiol replace-

REFERENCES

ment therapy in women with hypergonadotropic amenorrhea. *J Clin Endocrinol Metab* 81(10):3615, 1996.

Taylor DL, Mathew RJ, et al. Serotonin levels and platelet uptake during premenstrual tension. *Neuropsychobiology* 12(1):16, 1984.

Taylor JW. Plasma progesterone, oestradiol 17 beta and premenstrual symptoms. *Acta Psychiatr Scand* 60(1):76, 1979.

te Velde ER, Cohlen BJ. The management of infertility (editorial). *N Engl J Med* 340(3):224, 1999.

Teichmann AT, Brill K, et al. The influence of the dose of ethinylestradiol in oral contraceptives on follicle growth. *Gynecol Endocrincol* 9:229, 1995.

Telimaa S, Ronnberg L, et al. Placebo-controlled comparison of danazol and high-dose medroxyprogesterone acetate in the treatment of endometriosis after conservative surgery. *Gynecol Endocrinol* 1(4):363, 1987.

Thorneycroft IH, Stanczyk FZ, et al. Effect of low-dose oral contraceptives on androgenic markers and acne. *Contraception* 60(5):255, 1999.

Thys-Jacobs S, Ceccarelli S, et al. Calcium supplementation in premenstrual syndrome: a randomized crossover trial. *J Gen Intern Med* 4(3):183, 1989.

Tilford CA, Kuroda-Kawaguchi T, et al. A physical map of the human Y chromosome. *Nature* 409(6822):943, 2001.

Todd AS. Endothelium and fibrinolysis. *Bibl Anat* 12:98, 1973.

Toft A. Increased levothyroxine requirements in pregnancy—why, when, and how much? *N Engl J Med* 351(3):292, 2004.

Toma SK, Stovall DW, et al. The effect of laparoscopic ablation or danocrine on pregnancy rates in patients with stage I or II endometriosis undergoing donor insemination. *Obstet Gynecol* 80(2):253, 1992.

Toner JP. Age = egg quality, FSH level = egg quantity. *Fertil Steril* 79(3):491, 2003.

Toner JP, Philput CB, et al. Basal follicle-stimulating hormone level is a better predictor of in vitro fertilization performance than age. *Fertil Steril* 55(4):784, 1991.

Trio D, Strobelt N, et al. Prognostic factors for successful expectant management of ectopic pregnancy. *Fertil Steril* 63:469, 1995.

Trout SW, Seifer DB. Do women with unexplained recurrent pregnancy loss have higher day 3 serum FSH and estradiol values? *Fertil Steril* 74(2):335, 2000.

Trummer H, Tucker K, et al. Effect of storage temperature on sperm cryopreservation. *Fertil Steril* 70(6):1162, 1998.

Tulchinsky D, Hobel CJ. Plasma human chorionic gonadotropin, estrone, estradiol, estriol, progesterone, and 17 a-hydroxy-progesterone in human pregnancy. *Am J Obstet Gynecol* 117:884, 1973.

Tummon IS, Asher LJ, et al. Randomized controlled trial of superovulation and insemination for infertility associated with minimal or mild endometriosis. *Fertil Steril* 68(1):8, 1997.

418

Turek PJ. Male infertility. In Tanagho EA, McAninch JW, eds. *Smith's General Urology* (16th ed). Lange Medical Books. New York: McGraw-Hill, 2004.

Utian WH, Shoupe D, et al. Relief of vasomotor symptoms and vaginal atrophy with lower doses of conjugated equine estrogens and medroxyprogesterone acetate. *Fertil Steril* 75(6):1065, 2001.

Valbuena D, Simon C, et al. Factors responsible for multiple pregnancies after ovarian stimulation and intrauterine insemination with gonadotropins. *J Assist Reprod Genet* 13(8):663, 1996.

van Leeuwen I, Branch DW, et al. First-trimester ultrasonography findings in women with a history of recurrent pregnancy loss. *Am J Obstet Gynecol* 168(1 Pt 1):111, 1993.

van Montfrans JM, Dorland M, et al. Increased concentrations of follicle-stimulating hormone in mothers of children with Down's syndrome. *Lancet* 353(9167):1853, 1999.

van Montfrans JM, Hoek A, et al. Predictive value of basal follicle-stimulating hormone concentrations in a general subfertility population. *Fertil Steril* 74(1):97, 2000.

Van Voorhis BJ, Sparks AE. Semen analysis: what tests are clinically useful? *Clin Obstet Gynecol* 42(4):957, 1999.

Van Waart J, Kruger TF, et al. Predictive value of normal sperm morphology in intrauterine insemination (IUI): a structured literature review. *Hum Reprod Update* 7(5):495, 2001.

Vandenbroucke JP, Koster T, et al. Increased risk of venous thrombosis in oral-contraceptive users who are carriers of factor V Leiden mutation. *Lancet* 344(8935):1453, 1994.

Vandenbroucke JP, Rosing J, et al. Oral contraceptives and the risk of venous thrombosis. *N Engl J Med* 344(20):1527, 2001.

Vandermolen DT, Ratts VS, et al. Metformin increases the ovulatory rate and pregnancy rate from clomiphene citrate in patients with polycystic ovary syndrome who are resistant to clomiphene citrate alone. *Fertil Steril* 75(2):310, 2001.

Vanderpump MP, Tunbridge WM, et al. The incidence of thyroid disorders in the community: a twenty-year follow-up of the Whickham Survey. *Clin Endocrinol (Oxf)* 43(1):55, 1995.

Vanrell JA, Balasch J. Luteal phase defects in repeated abortion. *Int J Gynaecol Obstet* 24(2):111, 1986.

Vegetti W, Ragni G, et al. Laparoscopic ovarian drilling versus low-dose pure FSH in anovulatory clomiphene-resistant patients with polycystic ovarian syndrome: randomized prospective study. *Hum Reprod* 13(1):120 (abst), 1998.

Velazquez E, Acosta A, et al. Menstrual cyclicity after metformin therapy in polycystic ovary syndrome. *Obstet Gynecol* 90:392, 1997.

REFERENCES

Vercammen EE, D'Hooghe TM. Endometriosis and recurrent pregnancy loss. *Semin Reprod Med* 18(4):363, 2000.

Vercellini P, Aimi G, et al. Laparoscopic uterosacral ligament resection for dysmenorrhea associated with endometriosis: results of a randomized, controlled trial. *Fertil Steril* 80(2):310, 2003a.

Vercellini P, Chapron C, et al. Coagulation or excision of ovarian endometriomas? *Am J Obstet Gynecol* 188(3):606, 2003b.

Vercellini P, Cortesi I, et al. Progestins for symptomatic endometriosis: a critical analysis of the evidence. *Fertil Steril* 68(3):393, 1997a.

Vercellini P, De Giorgi O, et al. Menstrual characteristics in women with and without endometriosis. *Obstet Gynecol* 90:264, 1997b.

Vercellini P, Frontino G, et al. Continuous use of an oral contraceptive for endometriosis-associated recurrent dysmenorrhea that does not respond to a cyclic pill regimen. *Fertil Steril* 80(3):560, 2003c.

Vercellini P, Maddalena S, et al. Abdominal myomectomy for infertility: a comprehensive review. *Hum Reprod* 13:873, 1998.

Verhelst J, Abs R, et al. Cabergoline in the treatment of hyperprolactinemia: a study in 455 patients. *J Clin Endocrinol Metab* 84(7):2518, 1999.

Verp MS, Simpson JL. Abnormal sexual differentiation and neoplasia. *Cancer Genet Cytogenet* 25(2):191, 1987.

Volker P, Grundker C, et al. Expression of receptors for luteinizing hormone-releasing hormone in human ovarian and endometrial cancers: frequency, autoregulation, and correlation with direct antiproliferative activity of luteinizing hormone-releasing hormone analogues. *Am J Obstet Gynecol* 186(2):171, 2002.

Vollenhoven BJ, Lawrence AS, et al. Uterine fibroids: a clinical review. *Br J Obstet Gynecol* 97:285, 1990.

Waggoner W, Boots LR, et al. Total testosterone and DHEAS levels as predictors of androgen-secreting neoplasms: a populational study. *Gynecol Endocrinol* 13(6):394, 1999.

Waldenstrom U, Hellberg D, et al. Low-dose aspirin in a short regimen as standard treatment in in vitro fertilization: a randomized, prospective study. *Fertil Steril* 81(6):1560, 2004.

Walker AF, De Souza MC, et al. Magnesium supplementation alleviates premenstrual symptoms of fluid retention. *J Womens Health* 7(9):1157, 1998.

Walker-Bone K, Dennison E, et al. Epidemiology of osteoporosis. *Rheum Dis Clin North Am* 27(1):1, 2001.

Wallach EE, Vu KK. Myomata uteri and infertility. *Obstet Gynecol Clin N Am* 22:791, 1995.

Wamsteker K, Emanuel MH, et al. Transcervical hysteroscopic resection of submucous fibroids for abnormal uterine bleeding: results regarding the degree of intramural extension. *Obstet Gynecol* 82:736, 1993.

420

REFERENCES

Wang X, Chen C, et al. Conception, early pregnancy loss, and time to clinical pregnancy: a population-based prospective study. *Fertil Steril* 79(3):577, 2003.

Warburton D. De novo balanced chromosome rearrangements and extra marker chromosomes identified at prenatal diagnosis: clinical significance and distribution of breakpoints. *Am J Hum Genet* 49(5):995, 1991.

Warburton D, Fraser FC. Spontaneous abortion risks in man: data from reproductive histories collected in a medical genetics unit. *Am J Hum Genet* 16:1, 1964.

Warren MP, Vande Wiele RL. Clinical and metabolic features of anorexia nervosa. *Am J Obstet Gynecol* 117:435, 1973.

Weed JC, Ray JE. Endometriosis of the bowel. *Obstet Gynecol* 69:727, 1987.

Weiderpass E, Adami HO, et al. Use of oral contraceptives and endometrial cancer risk (Sweden). *Cancer Causes Control* 10(4):277, 1999.

Weiss MH, Teal J, et al. Natural history of microprolactinomas: six-year follow-up. *Neurosurg* 12:180, 1983.

White PC, Speiser PW. Congenital adrenal hyperplasia due to 21-hydroxylase deficiency. *Endocr Rev* 21(3):245, 2000.

Wilcox AJ, Baird DD, et al. On the frequency of intercourse around ovulation: evidence for biological influences. *Hum Reprod* 19(7):1539, 2004.

Wilcox AJ, Weinberg CR, et al. Timing of sexual intercourse in relation to ovulation. Effects on the probability of conception, survival of the pregnancy, and sex of the baby. *N Engl J Med* 333(23):1517, 1995.

Wild RA, Umstot ES, et al. Androgen parameters and their correlation with body weight in one hundred thirty-eight women thought to have hyperandrogenism. *Am J Obstet Gynecol* 146(6):602, 1983.

Wild S, Pierpoint T, et al. Cardiovascular disease in women with polycystic ovary syndrome at long-term follow-up: a retrospective cohort study. *Clin Endocrinol (Oxf)* 52(5):595, 2000.

Wilson WA, Gharavi AE, et al. International consensus statement on preliminary classification criteria for definite antiphospholipid syndrome: report of an international workshop. *Arthritis Rheum* 42(7):1309, 1999.

Wong IL, Morris RS, et al. A prospective randomized trial comparing finasteride to spironolactone in the treatment of hirsute women. *J Clin Endocrinol Metab* 80(1):233, 1995.

World Health Organization. *WHO Laboratory Manual for the Examination of Human Semen and Semen-Cervical Mucus Interaction.* New York: Cambridge University Press, 1999.

Yao M, Tulandi T. Current status of surgical and nonsurgical management of ectopic pregnancy. *Fertil Steril* 67:421, 1997.

Yates J, Barrett-Connor E, et al. Rapid loss of hip fracture protection after estrogen cessation: evidence from the National Osteoporosis Risk Assessment. *Obstet Gynecol* 103(3):440, 2004.

REFERENCES

Yokoyama Y, Shimizu T, et al. Prevalence of cerebral palsy in twins, triplets and quadruplets. *Int J Epidemiol* 24(5):943, 1995.

Yoshimura Y, Wallach EE. Studies of the mechanism(s) of mammalian ovulation. *Fertil Steril* 47(1):22, 1987.

Young RL, Goldzieher JW, et al. The endocrine effects of spironolactone used as an antiandrogen. *Fertil Steril* 48(2):223, 1987.

Yucelten D, Erenus M, et al. Recurrence rate of hirsutism after 3 different antiandrogen therapies. *J Am Acad Dermatol* 41(1):64, 1999.

Zhu BP, Rolfs RT, et al. Effect of the interval between pregnancies on perinatal outcomes. *N Engl J Med* 340(8):589, 1999.

Zreik TG, Garcia-Velasco JA, et al. Prospective, randomized, crossover study to evaluate the benefit of human chorionic gonadotropin-timed versus urinary luteinizing hormone-timed intrauterine inseminations in clomiphene citrate-stimulated treatment cycles. *Fertil Steril* 71(6):1070, 1999.

Zullo F, Pellicano M, et al. A prospective randomized study to evaluate leuprolide acetate treatment before laparoscopic myomectomy: efficacy and ultrasonographic predictors. *Am J Obstet Gynecol* 178(1 Pt 1):108, 1998.

Drug Index

DRUG INDEX

DRUG INDEX

DRUG INDEX

DRUG INDEX

DRUG INDEX

DRUG INDEX

Subject Index

SUBJECT INDEX

SUBJECT INDEX

Azoospermic factor region, Y
  chromosome
  microdeletions in, 312–313

B

Bardet-Biedl syndrome, and subfertility
  in males, 217
Behavioral differentiation in gender
  identity or sexuality, 3
Bicornuate uterus, 36
Biopsy
  endometrial
    in abnormal uterine bleeding,
      65–66, 69, 71
    in luteal phase deficiency, 263
  ovarian, in diminished ovarian
    reserve, 228
Birth defects
  after assisted reproductive
    techniques, 221
  risk related to maternal age, 310
Bleeding
  breakthrough, from oral
    contraceptives, 87
  in endometriosis, 154
  in fibroids, 160
  uterine, abnormal. See Abnormal
    uterine bleeding
  vaginal, in pediatric patients, 29–
    30
Body surface nomogram, 116
Bone mineral density
  measurements of, 337–338, 343–
    344
  in osteoporosis. See Osteoporosis
  in premature ovarian failure, 305
Bowel preparation in laparoscopy, 366
Breakthrough bleeding from oral
  contraceptives, 87
  in endometriosis, 154

Breast
  cancer of
    and endometriosis, 141
    estrogen therapy affecting, 324,
      326
    and hyperprolactinemia, 270
    and oral contraceptive use, 82
  chronic nerve stimulation causing
    hyperprolactinemia, 269
  development of, 18–20
    in amenorrhea, 101
Breast-feeding, oral contraceptives
  affecting, 84

C

Caffeine intake, and recurrent
  pregnancy loss, 292–293
Cancer. See Neoplasia
Candida infection, pediatric
  vulvovaginitis in, 28
Carbohydrate metabolism, oral
  contraceptives affecting,
    81
Cardiac disease
  myocardial infarction, and oral
    contraceptive use, 80
  in Turner syndrome, 45
Cardiolipin antibodies, and recurrent
  pregnancy loss, 288–290
Cardiovascular system, hormone
  therapy affecting, 324,
    326
Cauterization, ovarian, in polycystic
  ovary syndrome, 185–186,
    187
Central nervous system lesions. See
  Neurologic disorders
Cervical mucus
  changes in, 56, 60
  postcoital test, 200

438

SUBJECT INDEX

439

SUBJECT INDEX

SUBJECT INDEX

Fatigue, chronic, and endometriosis, 142
Females
  congenital adrenal hyperplasia, 6–8
  gonadal dysgenesis in, 8, 23
  masculinized, 6–8
  maternal androgen excess, 8
  sexual differentiation in, 1–5
    anomalies of, 6–8
  subfertility in, 193–209
  true hermaphroditism, 8
Femara
  in endometriosis, 155, 157
Ferning of cervical mucus, 56, 60
Ferriman-Gallway scores in
      polycystic ovary
      syndrome, 189–190
Fertility
  disorders of. *See* Subfertility in
      females; Subfertility in
      males
  in hypothyroidism, 277
  oral contraceptives affecting, 84
Fertilization
  dyssynchronous, spontaneous
      abortion in, 293
  in vitro (IVF), 229. *See also* Assisted
      reproductive technologies
    in endometriosis, 158
    luteal phase support in, 264
    in subfertility in males, 221
Fetus
  androgens affecting, 8
  chromosome abnormalities in
      abortuses, 285–286
  estrogens and progestins affecting,
      9
Fibroids, 160–166
  bleeding in, 160

infertility in, 161
intramural, 160
medical therapy in, 164–165
pain in, 161
and reproductive outcome, 162–164
submucosal, 160, 163
subserosal, 160
surgery in, 165–166
Fibromyalgia, and endometriosis, 142
Foley balloon in laparoscopy
      complications, 370
Follicle(s), ovarian
  antral follicle counts, 357
    and multiple pregnancy rate,
      358
  depletion of, 304
  dysfunction of, 305
Follicle-stimulating hormone, 50
  half-life of, 49
  screening in subfertility, 197–198
  serum levels
    in diminished ovarian reserve,
      226, 230
    in Down syndrome mothers, 198
    in menstrual cycle, 58
    in polycystic ovary syndrome,
      172, 174
    in puberty, 21
    in subfertility in males, 214,
      217
Follicular phase of menstrual cycle, 49,
      50
  endometrium in, 56
Foreign bodies, and vaginal bleeding in
      children, 30
Fractures in osteoporosis, 337, 339
Fragile X syndrome, 314–315
Frank's vaginal dilation technique, 35
  Ingram modification, 35
  Jaffe modification, 35

443

SUBJECT INDEX

G

Galactorrhea in hyperprolactinemia, 265–275. *See also* Hyperprolactinemia

Gallbladder disease, and oral contraceptive use, 81

Gamete intrafallopian transfer (GIFT), 229

Gamete preservation, 257–259
female, 257–258
indications for, 257
options for, 257–258
male, 259

Gamma knife in hyperprolactinemia, 273

Gastrointestinal disorders
in endometriosis, 146
pelvic pain in, 137

Genetic factors
in endometriosis, 143
in recurrent pregnancy loss, 279–285
in subfertility in males, 215–216

Genetic testing, 307–315
carrier testing in ethnic groups, 311
in cystic fibrosis, 307–309
male factors in, 312–313
risks for chromosomal abnormalities in, 310
and risks related maternal age, 310

Genital tract disorders, abnormal uterine bleeding in, 63

Genitalia
abnormalities of
in females, 12–13
in males, 9
ambiguous, 14
laboratory tests in, 14–15
management of, 16
embryology of, 1–3, 5

Gestrinone in endometriosis, 157

Glucocorticoids, excess levels of, and subfertility in males, 218

Glucose
intolerance in Turner syndrome, 46
tolerance test in polycystic ovary syndrome, 173

Gonad(s)
dysgenesis of
amenorrhea in, 102
in females, 8, 23
in males, 9, 23
embryology of, 1–2, 5

Gonadectomy in androgen insensitivity syndrome, 10

Gonadotropin
chorionic. *See* Chorionic gonadotropin
preparations, 231
releasing hormone secretion, pulsatile, 57
serum levels
in Sheehan syndrome, 125, 126
and subfertility in males, 217

Granulosa cells
luteinized, 53
in menstrual cycle, 50

Growth hormone
serum levels
in Sheehan syndrome, 125
and subfertility in males, 218
therapy in osteoporosis, 344

Growth hormone therapy in osteoporosis, 344

H

Hair removal systems in polycystic ovary syndrome, 180

Hams F-10 affecting sperm, 224

Harmonic scalpel, 372

Hearing loss in Turner syndrome, 45

SUBJECT INDEX

447

in ovulation, 51–52
serum levels
  in polycystic ovary syndrome, 167
  in puberty, 21
  in subfertility in males, 214
urine predictor kit
  in abnormal uterine bleeding, 65
  false positive with, 65
  before ovulation, 59, 196
Luteoplacental shift in progesterone in early pregnancy, 54, 55
Lymphedema in Turner syndrome, 46
Lymphoma, non-Hodgkin, and endometriosis, 141

M

Macroadenoma, pituitary, hyperprolactinemia in, 267
  management of, 270, 273
Magnetic resonance imaging
  in hyperprolactinemia, 269
  in premature ovarian failure, 306
  in uterine anomalies, 284
Males
  androgen insensitivity syndrome, 9–10
  factors in genetic testing, 312–313
  gonadal dysgenesis, 9, 23
  Leydig cell disorders
    function abnormalities, 10–11
    hypoplasia, 10
  Müllerian duct persistence, isolated, 11
  5α-reductase deficiency, 10
  sexual differentiation in, 1–5
    anomalies of, 9–11
  subfertility in, 208–224. See also Subfertility in males

true hermaphroditism, 11
undermasculinized, 9–11
Masculinized females, 6–8
Mayer-Rokitansky-Küster-Hauser syndrome, 22, 34
  amenorrhea in, 102–103
McCune-Albright syndrome, 25
Menarche, 18
  mean age of, 49
  precocious, 30
Menometrorrhagia, 61
Menopausal gonadotropin, human, in intrauterine insemination in endometriosis, 158
Menopause
  androgen production in, 318–320
  common complaints and symptoms in, 325
  hormone replacement therapy in, 324–334. See also Hormone replacement therapy, in the Drug Index
  mean age of, 49
  surgical, 318, 324
  vaginal bleeding in, transvaginal ultrasound in, 362
Menorrhagia, 61
  in adolescence, 31–32
  treatment of, 67
Menstrual cycle, 49–59
  follicular phase in, 49, 50
  and halting of vaginal bleeding in hematology/oncology patients, 57
  luteal phase in, 49, 53–55
    deficiency of, 260–267
  migraines in, 57
  normal characteristics of, 49
  ovulation in, 51–52
    control of, 57

SUBJECT INDEX

SUBJECT INDEX

SUBJECT INDEX

SUBJECT INDEX

SUBJECT INDEX

Uterus—*continued*
    causing abnormal bleeding,
        63
    pelvic pain in, 137
    embryology of, 1–2
    evaluation before assisted
        reproductive technologies,
        230
    fibroids, 160–166
    hypoplasia or agenesis of,
        42
    hysteroscopy, 363–365
    malformations of, 42–43
        from diethylstilbestrol, 43
    septate, 36–43
        adverse outcomes with, 38
        diagnosis of, 37–38
        embryology of, 36
        surgery in, 38–40, 41
    synechiae in, and amenorrhea,
        104–105
    unicornuate, 42

V

Vacuum aspiration, manual, in early
        pregnancy failure, 299,
        301–302
Vagina
    agenesis of, 34–35
    atresia of, 13
    bleeding in pediatric patients, 29–
        30
    changes in menstrual cycle, 56
    dilators in müllerian agenesis, 35
    embryology of, 1–2
    longitudinal septa in, 13
    lubricants affecting sperm,
        224
    in pediatric patients, 27
    transverse septa in, 13

Vaginitis in children, 29
Vaginosis, bacterial, in pediatric
        patients, 28
Vanishing testis syndrome, 218
Varicocele, and subfertility in males,
        213–214, 219
Vas deferens examination in
        subfertility, 213
Vasectomy reversal, and pregnancy
        rate, 220
Vecchietti procedure in müllerian
        agenesis, 35
Veress needle in laparoscopy, 368
Virilization of females, 6–8
Virilizing tumors, ovarian or adrenal,
        175
Vision disorders in Turner syndrome,
        46
Vomiting, and hyperemesis in
        pregnancy, 254–256
Vulva disorders causing abnormal
        uterine bleeding, 63
Vulvodynia, 139
Vulvovaginitis in pediatric patients,
        treatment of, 28

W

Waist-hip ratio, and insulin sensitivity,
        168
Weight gain
    and oral contraceptive use,
        88
    in ovarian hyperstimulation
        syndrome, 247
Weight loss
    and amenorrhea, 105
    in treatment of polycystic ovary
        syndrome, 183
Wilms tumor suppressor gene in males,
        4, 23

NOTES

NOTES